Febrile Seizures

Febrile Seizures

Edited by

Tallie Z. Baram, M.D., Ph.D.

Professor, Departments of Pediatrics,
Anatomy/Neurobiology, and Neurology
Danette D. Shepard Professor of Neurological Sciences
University of California at Irvine
Irvine, California

Shlomo Shinnar, M.D., Ph.D.

Professor, Departments of Neurology and Pediatrics
Director, Comprehensive Epilepsy Management Center
Martin A. and Emily L. Fisher Fellow in Neurology and Pediatrics
Montefiore Medical Center
Albert Einstein College of Medicine
Bronx, New York

ACADEMIC PRESS

A Harcourt Science and Technology Company

San Diego   San Francisco   New York   Boston   London   Sydney   Tokyo

2002

Academic Press
A division of Harcourt, Inc.
525 B Street, Suite 1900, San Diego, California 92101-4495, USA
http://www.academicpress.com

Academic Press
Harcourt Place, 32 Jamestown Road, London NW1 7BY, UK
http://www.academicpress.com

Library of Congress Catalog Card Number: 2001094374

International Standard Book Number: 0-12-078141-7

PRINTED IN THE UNITED STATES OF AMERICA
01   02   03   04   05   06   EB   9   8   7   6   5   4   3   2   1

CONTENTS

PART I

Epidemiology of Febrile Seizures

PART **II**

*Population Studies on the Outcome
of Febrile Seizures*

5 Febrile Seizures and the Risk for Epilepsy

Dale C. Hesdorffer and W. Allen Hauser

6 Do Febrile Seizures Promote Temporal Lobe Epilepsy? Retrospective Studies

Fernando Cendes and Frederick Andermann

7 Do Febrile Seizures Lead to Temporal Lobe Epilepsy? Prospective and Epidemiological Studies

Shlomo Shinnar

PART **III**

Do Prolonged Febrile Seizures Cause
Acute Neuronal Injury?

8 Do Prolonged Febrile Seizures Injure the Hippocampus? Human MRI Studies

Teresa V. Mitchell and Darrell V. Lewis

9 Do Prolonged Febrile Seizures Injure Hippocampal Neurons? Insights from Animal Models

Roland A. Bender and Tallie Z. Baram

10 Do Effects of Febrile Seizures Differ in Normal and Abnormal Brain?

Ellen F. Sperber, Solomon L. Moshé, and Isabelle M. Germano

PART **IV**

The Neurobiology of Febrile Seizures and of Their Consequences: Experimental Approaches

11 Why Does the Developing Brain Demonstrate Heightened Susceptibility to Febrile and Other Provoked Seizures?

Frances E. Jensen and Russell M. Sanchez

12 Mechanisms of Fever and Febrile Seizures: Putative Role of the Interleukin-1 System

S. Gatti, A. Vezzani, and T. Bartfai

13 Animal Models for Febrile Seizures

Tallie Z. Baram

14 Physiology of Limbic Hyperexcitability after Experimental Complex Febrile Seizures: Interactions of Seizure-Induced Alterations at Multiple Levels of Neuronal Organization

Niklas Thon, Kang Chen, Ildiko Aradi, and Ivan Soltesz

15 Do Prolonged Febrile Seizures in an Immature Rat Model Cause Epilepsy?

Celine Dube

16 Basic Electrophysiology of Febrile Seizures

Robert S. Fisher and Jie Wu

PART **V**

Genetics of Febrile Seizures

17 The Genetics of Febrile Seizures

David A. Greenberg and Gregory L. Holmes

PART **VI**

Current Management of Febrile Seizures

18 Evaluation of the Child with Febrile Seizures

N. Paul Rosman

19 Practical Management Approaches to Simple and Complex Febrile Seizures

Finn Ursin Knudsen

20 What Do We Tell Parents of a Child with Simple or Complex Febrile Seizures?

Christine O'Dell

PART **VII**

Current State of the Art: Implications for Future Study and Treatment

21 Human Data: What Do We Know about Febrile Seizures and What Further Information Is Needed

Shlomo Shinnar

22 Mechanisms and Outcome of Febrile Seizures: What Have We Learned from Basic Science Approaches, and What Needs Studying?

Tallie Z. Baram

CONTRIBUTORS

FREDERICK ANDERMANN, M.D., FRCP(C), Professor, Department of Neurology and Neurosurgery, Montreal Neurological Institute and Hospital, McGill University, Montreal, Quebec, Canada H3A 2B4

ILDIKO ARADI, Ph.D., Postdoctoral Researcher, Department of Anatomy/Neurobiology, University of California at Irvine, Irvine, California 92697

TALLIE Z. BARAM, M.D., Ph.D., Professor, Departments of Pediatrics, Anatomy/Neurobiology, and Neurology, Danette D. Shepard Professor of Neurological Sciences, University of California at Irvine, Irvine, California 92697

T. BARTFAI, Ph.D., Professor, The Harold L. Dorris Neurological Research Center, Department of Neuropharmacology, The Scripps Research Institute, La Jolla, California 92037

ROLAND A. BENDER, Ph.D., Postdoctoral Researcher, Departments of Pediatrics and Anatomy/Neurobiology, University of California at Irvine, Irvine, California 92697

ANNE T. BERG, Ph.D., Associate Professor, Department of Biological Sciences, Northern Illinois University, DeKalb, Illinois 60115

CAROL CAMFIELD, M.D., FRCP(C), Professor, Department of Pediatrics, Dalhousie University and IWK Health Centre, Halifax, Nova Scotia, Canada B3J 3G9

PETER CAMFIELD, M.D., FRCP(C), Department of Pediatrics, Dalhousie University and IWK Health Centre, Halifax, Nova Scotia, Canada B3J 3G9

FERNANDO CENDES, M.D., Ph.D., Department of Neurology and Neurosurgery, Montreal Neurological Institute and Hospital, McGill University, Montreal, Quebec, Canada H3A 2B4

KANG CHEN, M.D., Postdoctoral Researcher, Department of Anatomy/Neurobiology, University of California at Irvine, Irvine, California 92697

CELINE DUBE, Ph.D., Postdoctoral Researcher, Departments of Pediatrics and Anatomy/Neurobiology, University of California at Irvine, Irvine, California 92697

ROBERT S. FISHER, M.D., Ph.D., Maslah Saul M.D. Professor of Neurology, Neurological Sciences, and Neurosurgery, Stanford University School of Medicine, Stanford, California 94305

S. GATTI, Ph.D., Researcher, CNS Preclinical Research, Pharmaceutical Division Hoffmann-LaRoche, 4070 Basel, Switzerland

ISABELLE M. GERMANO, M.D., Assistant Professor, Department of Neurosurgery, Mt. Sinai School of Medicine, New York, New York 10024

KEVIN GORDON, M.D., FRCP(C), Associate Professor, Department of Pediatrics, Dalhousie University and IWK Health Centre, Halifax, Nova Scotia, Canada B3J 3G9

DAVID A. GREENBERG, Ph.D., Professor of Biostatistics and Psychiatry, Co-Director, Mathematical Genetics Unit, Division of Clinical-Genetic Epidemiology, New York State Psychiatric Institute, New York, New York 10032; and Director, Division of Statistical Genetics, Department of Biostatistics, Mailman School of Public Health, Columbia University, New York, New York 10029

W. ALLEN HAUSER, M.D., Gertrude H. Sergievsky Center, Professor, Departments of Neurology and Epidemiology, Columbia University, New York, New York 10032; and Department of Neurology, New York Presbyterian Hospital, New York, New York 10032

DALE C. HESDORFFER, Ph.D., Gertrude H. Sergievsky Center, Assistant Professor, Department of Epidemiology, Columbia University, New York, New York 10032

DEBORAH HIRTZ, M.D., Program Director, Clinical Trials, National Institute of Neurological Disorders and Stroke, Neuroscience Center, National Institutes of Health, Rockville, Maryland 20892

GREGORY L. HOLMES, M.D., Departments of Psychiatry and Biomathematics, Mt. Sinai School of Medicine and the Columbia University Genome Center, New York, New York 10029; and Director, Clinical Neurophysiology Laboratory, Department of Neurology, Harvard Medical School, Children's Hospital, Boston, Massachusetts 02115

FRANCES E. JENSEN, M.D., Associate Professor, Department of Neurology,

Children's Hospital and Program in Neuroscience, Harvard Medical School, Boston, Massachusetts 02115

FINN URSIN KNUDSEN, Ph.D., Senior Neuropediatric Consultant, Lecturer, Department of Pediatrics, Glostrup University Hospital, DK-2600 Glostrup, Denmark

DARRELL V. LEWIS, M.D., Professor, Departments of Pediatrics (Neurology) and Neurobiology, Duke University Medical Center, Durham, North Carolina 27710

TERESA V. MITCHELL, Ph.D., Research Associate, Brain Imaging and Analysis Center, Department of Radiology, Duke University Medical Center, Durham, North Carolina 27710

SOLOMON L. MOSHÉ, M.D., Professor, Departments of Neurology, Neuroscience, and Pediatrics, Director of Pediatric Neurology and Clinical Neurophysiology, Martin A. and Emily L. Fisher Fellow, Albert Einstein College of Medicine, Bronx, New York 10461

CHRISTINE O'DELL, RN, MSN, Clinical Nurse Specialist, Comprehensive Epilepsy Management Center, Montefiore Medical Center, Bronx, New York 10467

N. PAUL ROSMAN, M.D., Professor of Pediatrics and Neurology, Tufts University School of Medicine; Chief, Division of Pediatric Neurology, Floating Hospital for Children; Director, Center for Children with Special Needs, New England Medical Center, Boston, Massachusetts 02111

RUSSELL M. SANCHEZ, M.D., Postdoctoral Researcher, Department of Neurology, Children's Hospital and Program in Neuroscience, Harvard Medical School, Boston, Massachusetts 02115

SHLOMO SHINNAR, M.D., Ph.D., Professor, Departments of Neurology and Pediatrics, and Director, Comprehensive Epilepsy Management Center, Martin A. and Emily L. Fisher Fellow in Neurology and Pediatrics, Montefiore Medical Center, Albert Einstein College of Medicine, Bronx, New York 10467

IVAN SOLTESZ, Ph.D., Associate Professor, Department of Anatomy/Neurobiology, University of California at Irvine, Irvine, California 92697

ELLEN F. SPERBER, Ph.D., Associate Professor, Departments of Neurology and Neuroscience, Albert Einstein College of Medicine, Bronx, New York 10461; and Department of Psychology, Mercy College, Dobbs Ferry, New York 10522

CARL E. STAFSTROM, M.D., Ph.D., Associate Professor, Departments of Neurology and Pediatrics, University of Wisconsin, Madison, Wisconsin 53792

NIKLAS THON, Department of Anatomy/Neurobiology, University of California at Irvine, Irvine, California 92697

A. VEZZANI, Ph.D., Chief, Laboratory of Experimental Neurology, Department of Neuroscience, Mario Negri Institute for Pharmacological Research, 20157 Milan, Italy

JIE WU, M.D., Ph.D., Senior Staff Scientist, Department of Neurology, Barrow Neurological Institute/St. Joseph's Hospital and Medical Center, Phoenix, Arizona 85013

PREFACE

With all the new books on epilepsy, why do we need a book on febrile seizures? There are several reasons. Febrile seizures are the most common form of childhood seizures, occurring in 2 to 5% of children in Western Europe and North America. As such, these seizures are of great interest to those specializing in clinical and basic research on seizures, especially developmental seizures, as well as to all involved in the care of children. Febrile seizures have specific features that make them distinct from all other forms of seizures and epilepsy, and a controversy about their relationship to subsequent epilepsy has been ongoing for many years. The last book devoted to febrile seizures appeared 20 years ago and much has been learned since. In the clinical arena, epidemiological studies have provided a better understanding of the incidence of febrile seizures, risk factors for their occurrence, and their short- and long-term outcomes. Imaging techniques now allow us to study the possible effects of seizures in children. Advances in genetics should allow us to define the role of genetic factors in this common disorder. In the basic sciences, the availability of animal models, combined with a better understanding of mechanisms of excitation and injury that are unique to the developing brain, has resulted in major advances in our understanding of the pathophysiology of febrile seizures and their possible consequences. The bottom line in terms of treatment has also changed in the past 20 years. For all these reasons, a new book is both timely and necessary.

Fortunately, we, the editors, are not the only people who feel this way. We received a tremendous and enthusiastic response and commitment, with outstanding chapters, from a stellar group of scientists and clinicians who are leaders in their field. We were thus able to assemble a book that truly reflects the state of the art. It includes the latest clinical research findings on incidence and outcome and the most recent and exciting basic science work on mechanisms and consequences, including work published in 2001. The latest treatment recommendations, such as the recent practice parameters of the American Academy of Pediatrics, are also included.

As clinician scientists, the editors firmly believe that, whether you are a clinician taking care of patients or a basic scientist working in the laboratory, it is important to have an understanding of both the clinical problem and what is known about the basic mechanisms of the disorder. The book is therefore intended to be a comprehensive overview of the state of the art that is detailed enough for the specialist while at the same time presents the data in a manner that is accessible to the nonspecialist. For this reason we have avoided the use of most abbreviations and have included brief explanations of technical terms. In the basic science sections, clinicians will find data that are both useful and informative, while in the clinical sections, basic scientists will find the information they need to understand the phenomenon they are attempting to model. This approach should also make the book accessible to the educated layman interested in febrile seizures.

As editors, it is our hope that this book will serve at least two purposes. The first is to provide a comprehensive review of the current state of the art. We have come a long way in our understanding of the clinical phenomenon and the basic mechanisms underlying it. This book both documents and celebrates these accomplishments. The second goal is to provide a road map of where we are headed. While much has been accomplished, much work remains to be done in both the clinical and the basic science arenas. The various sections of this book address the problems that remain and suggest ways to approach them. The editors' individual perspectives on where we are and where we are headed are presented at the end of the book. We hope that this book will not only inform the reader about the current state of the art but also help the next generation of researchers get started.

One of the real pleasures of editing this book was that we the editors, even though we have both worked in this field for many years, learned new data and novel approaches and perspectives. This is almost inevitable in a productive collaboration, especially when so many of the leaders in the field agree to contribute and two editors with different perspectives but a shared passion for finding solutions to the problem are involved. We hope that you the reader share our excitement and pleasure.

Tallie Z. Baram
Shlomo Shinnar

ACKNOWLEDGMENTS

A book such as this is a quilt, involving unique, individual contributions as well as a cohesive, unifying theme. The editors thank the contributors for their excellent and creative contributions as well as for their forbearance with the editors' prompts and nagging. Also appreciated are the excellent support and contributions of Michele Hinojosa and the Academic Press staff, specifically Hilary Rowe and Kathy Nida. We thank all our colleagues and friends for their input and advice.

Each of us also thanks those who have assisted us with our work over the years. In addition, each of us acknowledges the input of special people in our lives. Tallie Z. Baram: I thank my parents, who have nurtured (and put up with) my determined individualism and unyielding intellectual curiosity. I especially thank Craig LaFrance for his unwavering love, support, and understanding. Shlomo Shinnar: I thank my family, several generations of whom have provided love, support, and advice. I also acknowledge two of my mentors: my father, Professor Reuel Shinnar, who introduced me to science and the joys of scientific injury; and my clinical mentor, Professor John Freeman, who showed me that clinical work could be both rewarding and intellectually stimulating.

Finally, we are indebted to all our patients and their families. It is from you we learn.

CHAPTER 1

The Incidence and Prevalence of Febrile Seizures

CARL E. STAFSTROM

Departments of Neurology and Pediatrics, University of Wisconsin, Madison, Wisconsin 53792

Epidemiological studies have made substantial contributions to our understanding of the frequency, natural history, and prognosis of febrile seizures. Using a wide variety of methodologies, epidemiological studies have consistently estimated that febrile seizures occur in 2–5% of children under 5 years of age. In certain populations (e.g., Japan, Guam), febrile seizures may be even more common (8–14%). The reason for this geographical discrepancy remains unexplained, but may be related to genetic predisposition, environmental factors, or both. This chapter critically reviews the studies that have led to the widely accepted febrile seizure occurrence rates (incidence, prevalence) and examines the assumptions and methods underlying those studies. © 2002 Academic Press.

I. INTRODUCTION

Nearly every article or text written about febrile seizures contains a statement relating that "febrile seizures are the most common type of seizure in childhood, occurring in 2–5% of children." How is this percentage derived, and from what population(s)? Is there geographical, seasonal, or sexual variation in febrile seizure rates? Has the occurrence of febrile seizures changed over time, as different management approaches have evolved? Does the incidence differ according to febrile seizure type (e.g., simple vs. complex)? How can such data help us understand the pathogenesis of febrile seizures and arrive at a consensus for managing them? These are some of the questions considered in this chapter, as a prelude to more detailed discussions of febrile seizure natural history, prognosis, and pathophysiology in subsequent chapters. First, febrile seizure definitions, past and present, are discussed. Next, epidemiological concepts and methods for measuring febrile seizure incidence and prevalence are reviewed. Finally, some pivotal epidemiological studies that have contributed to our current understanding of febrile seizure frequency are considered.

II. WHAT IS A FEBRILE SEIZURE?

A. HISTORICAL PERSPECTIVE

Before embarking on an analysis of epidemiological studies of febrile seizures, the fundamental question must be considered: What is a febrile seizure? Over the past several decades there has been an evolution in what the term "febrile seizure" connotes. Some series, especially prior to about 1980, did not exclude seizures precipitated by fever that may have been accompanied by an underlying neurologic disturbance such as meningitis, encephalitis, or toxic encephalopathy (van den Berg and Yerushalmy, 1969; Millichap, 1981). The prognosis of febrile seizures in the early literature was fairly pessimistic, due to the inclusion of symptomatic causes of seizure other than fever and to patient selection bias (Wallace, 1980). In addition, early studies were predominantly performed at tertiary care facilities and selected the more severe cases (Ellenberg and Nelson, 1980). The modern viewpoint is that the vast majority of febrile seizures have a benign outcome, with no lasting neurologic sequelae.

The consensus that febrile seizures do not constitute a form of epilepsy is an important conceptual advance with relevance to the consideration of febrile seizure incidence and prevalence. The distinction between febrile seizures and epilepsy has been fairly recent; it was formerly thought that febrile seizures represented "epilepsy unmasked by fever" and that they were a frequent harbinger of afebrile seizures (epilepsy) (Lennox, 1953, 1960; Livingston, 1958). Peterman stated emphatically that a febrile convulsion "does not occur in a normal child" (Peterman, 1952). E. M. Bridge (quoted in Millichap, 1968, p. 3) stated, in 1949, "There is no good reason for considering febrile convulsions as a clinical entity distinct from epilepsy. In reality, both belong in a single group, best described with the name of convulsive disorders. The differences are not of a fundamental nature but only of type and degree" (Bridge, 1949). The current definition of epilepsy as unprovoked, recurrent seizures excludes febrile seizures, which are always provoked by fever. Of course, some children experience a febrile seizure as the first manifestation of what will subsequently emerge as epilepsy, but it is not possible to predict with certainty which child will develop afebrile seizures (Berg and Shinnar, 1994).

Large epidemiological studies in the 1970s were pivotal in differentiating febrile seizures from epilepsy (van den Berg and Yerushalmy, 1969; Nelson and Ellenberg, 1976, 1978; Annegers *et al.*, 1979). The natural history of febrile seizures is quite different from that of epilepsy, as supported by several observations (Berg, 1992): (1) The risk of developing epilepsy after febrile seizures is small, on the order of 2–4%. (2) There are different risk factors for developing febrile seizures vs. epilepsy. About one-third of children with febrile seizures will experience another febrile seizure in a subsequent febrile illness, whereas 2–4% will later develop afebrile seizures (epilepsy) (van den Berg and Yerushalmy, 1969; Hauser and Kurland, 1975; Nelson and Ellenberg, 1978; Verity *et al.*, 1985; Annegers *et al.*, 1987; Berg *et al.*, 1990; Hackett *et al.*, 1997). The major predictors of recurrent febrile seizures are (1) occurrence before 1 year of age, (2) a positive family history of febrile seizures (not a family history of epilepsy), and (3) a low degree of fever (Berg *et al.*, 1997). These risk factors are *not* predictive of later epilepsy. Rather, the risk factors for epilepsy in children with febrile seizures are (1) complex febrile seizures, (2) a family history of epilepsy, and (3) neurologic impairment prior to the febrile seizure (Berg *et al.*, 1990). [One study did find that a complex initial febrile seizure increased the risk for febrile seizure recurrence (Al-Eissa, 1995).] Notably, prevention of recurrent febrile seizures does not appear to alter the risk of developing afebrile seizures (see Chapters 3, 7, and 19, this volume). Several randomized studies of febrile seizure prevention showed that although febrile seizure recurrence could be reduced, the development of later afebrile seizures was not altered by treatment (Knudsen, 1985; Wolf and Forsythe, 1989; Rosman *et al.*, 1993; Berg and Shinnar, 1994).

The controversy as to whether febrile seizures initiate a pathophysiological cascade that ultimately results in mesial temporal sclerosis and hence temporal lobe epilepsy (TLE) has been unresolved for decades (Liu *et al.*, 1995). A disproportionate number of patients (up to 20%) with TLE had febrile seizures (especially prolonged ones) as young children (Falconer *et al.*, 1964; Cendes *et al.*, 1993). However, prospective series cite only a minority of children with febrile seizures going on to develop epilepsy (2–4%) (Nelson and Ellenberg, 1976, 1978; Camfield *et al.*, 1994; Hamati-Haddad and Abou-Khalil, 1998). This controversy is discussed in detail elsewhere in this volume (Chapters 5–8, 21, 22).

B. MODERN DEFINITIONS

1. National Institutes of Health and International League Against Epilepsy Definitions

According to the International League Against Epilepsy classification of the epilepsies, febrile seizures are an acute, symptomatic type, i.e., a "special," situation-related seizure (Commission, 1989). Because they are always evoked by a specific precipitant (fever), febrile seizures cannot be considered a true form of epilepsy. Nevertheless, febrile seizures do constitute a "syndrome" because they fulfill several characteristics that are similar among affected children:

1. Febrile seizures generally occur within a restricted age range.
2. The majority of febrile seizures occur in children who are neurologically normal and continue to develop normally after the febrile seizures.
3. Febrile seizures are not associated with a structural or maldevelopmental anomaly of brain, though the existence of such pathology may enhance the susceptibility to febrile seizures (Germano et al., 1996).

Two operational definitions of febrile seizures have been published, one from a National Institutes of Health (NIH) Consensus Conference (National Institutes of Health, 1980; Nelson and Ellenberg, 1981), and the other from the International League Against Epilepsy (ILAE) (Commission, 1993). These definitions are compared in Table 1. In light of the huge disparities in epidemiological studies of febrile seizures, especially prior to 1980, the NIH conference represented a major advance, forming a coherent definition that has been used subsequently in many epidemiological and therapeutic investigations (e.g., Verity et al., 1985; Offringa et al., 1991; Okan et al., 1995). The ILAE proposed guidelines for epidemiological studies of epilepsy in general, as an attempt to standardize methods of case ascertainment, diagnostic accuracy, and seizure classification, and these recommendations are relevant to studies of febrile seizures as well.

Although the NIH and ILAE definitions are similar, their differences are worth noting. The lower age limit for febrile seizures is 1 month in the ILAE definition and 3 months in the NIH definition, although the NIH guideline is made purposefully flexible by use of the phrase "usually occurs." Each of these lower age limits have been employed in epidemiological studies of febrile

TABLE 1   Definitions of Febrile Seizures

National Institutes of Health Consensus Conference (1980)	International League Against Epilepsy Commission on Epidemiology and Prognosis (1993)
Febrile seizure: A febrile seizure is an event in infancy or childhood, usually occurring between 3 months and 5 years of age, associated with fever but without evidence of intracranial infection or defined cause. Seizures with fever in children who have suffered a previous nonfebrile seizure are excluded	**Febrile seizure**: A seizure occurring in childhood after age 1 month, associated with a febrile illness not caused by an infection of the CNS, without previous neonatal seizures or a previous unprovoked seizure, and not meeting criteria for other acute symptomatic seizures **Febrile seizure with neonatal seizure**: One or more neonatal seizures in a child who has also experienced one or more febrile seizures as herein defined

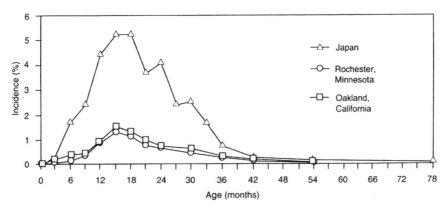

FIGURE 1   Age-specific incidence of febrile seizures among children in Japan; Rochester, Minnesota; and Oakland, California. From Hauser (1994). The prevalence and incidence of convulsive disorders in children. *Epilepsia* **35** (Suppl. 2), S1–S6. Reprinted by permission of Blackwell Science, Inc.

seizures [1 month (Nelson and Ellenberg, 1976, 1978; Berg *et al.*, 1997); 3 months (Verity *et al.*, 1985; Al-Eissa, 1995)]. Other studies do not state a lower age limit (Hauser and Kurland, 1975) or use another definition [e.g., 6 months (Hackett *et al.*, 1997)]. Both of the NIH and ILAE definitions exclude children with prior afebrile seizures and those with seizures due to an intracranial infection or other specific cause, but neither definition excludes children with prior neurologic impairment. However, the ILAE definition subdivides febrile seizures into those with and without prior neonatal seizures. Seizures with fever occurring during the second and third months of life, included in the ILAE definition, might not be included under the NIH definition. Practically speaking, children in this young age range probably account for a very small proportion of cases (Figure 1) (Hauser, 1994). The specific age during the first few months of life when the maturing brain first expresses an increased susceptibility to fever-induced seizures is not known precisely and may vary somewhat between children; this variability theoretically could impact epidemiological data.

Another notable difference is the lack of an upper age limit in the ILAE definition. The majority of febrile seizures occur between 6 months and 3 years of age, with the peak incidence at about 18 months (Figure 1) (Friderichsen and Melchior, 1954; van den Berg and Yerushalmy, 1969; Hauser and Kurland, 1975; Nelson and Ellenberg, 1976; Tsuboi, 1986; Annegers *et al.*, 1987; Offringa *et al.*, 1991). The observation that these data comprise a bell-shaped curve, regardless of the population studied, attests to the unique age specificity of the brain's sensitivity to fever. Only about 6–15% of first febrile seizures occur after 4 years of age (Hauser and Kurland, 1975; Aicardi, 1994) and onset after 6 or 7 years of age is unusual.

Neither definition includes a specific criterion as to what temperature defines "fever." A temperature of at least 38.4°C (101°F) would probably be accepted by most authorities and has been utilized in many epidemiological studies. Some researchers have accepted lower values (38°C) (Tsuboi, 1984; Al-Eissa, 1995). The route of temperature determination is not always mentioned (Tsuboi, 1984). Other rigorous studies have differentiated axillary (37.8°C) from rectal (38.3°C) temperatures, and have required that these be documented by emergency room personnel (Berg et al., 1997). Despite the common belief that the rate of temperature rise is more important than the ultimate temperature achieved, there are no data supporting that view (Michon and Wallace, 1984; Berg, 1993). Many febrile seizures (at least half) occur early in the course of a febrile illness, especially within the first 24 hours, and can even be the presenting sign of the febrile illness (Wolf et al., 1977; Berg et al., 1992, 1997). In clinical practice, it is difficult to establish the exact temperature just prior to or at the onset of a febrile seizure. Such a determination would ordinarily be in the hands of the parent or other caretaker. In most cases, a temperature is not recorded by the parent at the time of the seizure, and by the time the child's temperature is recorded at the physician's office or emergency room, the seizure is likely to be over and the information may be of limited relevance. Despite the lack of a uniform temperature criterion, several studies have shown that the height of the fever is related to febrile seizure recurrence (El-Radhi et al., 1986; Berg, 1993; Berg et al., 1997).

The definition of "seizure" is not specified in either the NIH or the ILAE definition. Some authorities emphasize the presence of convulsive activity (Millichap, 1981; Camfield and Camfield, 1995); indeed, febrile seizures are also known as "febrile convulsions." But is convulsive activity necessary? The lack of tonic–clonic rhythmic motor activity certainly makes the diagnosis of febrile seizure less secure, but clinicians routinely diagnose febrile seizures in children who present with limpness, altered consciousness, apnea, or nonconvulsive activity suggestive of partial complex symptomatology. In fact, the NIH definition uses the vague term "event" rather than seizure, perhaps to emphasize that some febrile seizures may not involve convulsive activity. Other clinical phenomena in the differential diagnosis of febrile seizures are mentioned in Section III,C. Inclusion of nonconvulsive activity under the febrile seizure umbrella could alter epidemiological results.

2. Simple and Complex Febrile Seizures

Febrile seizures are typically divided into two types, simple and complex. A *complex febrile seizure* has one or more of the following features (Commission 1993): (1) partial onset or focal features during the seizure, (2) prolonged duration [>10 minutes (Annegers et al., 1987; Berg et al., 1997) or >15 minutes

(Berg and Shinnar, 1996; Nelson and Ellenberg, 1978)], or (3) recurrent febrile seizures within 24 hours of the first episode (Nelson and Ellenberg, 1976; Annegers *et al.*, 1987). Some authors use a phrase such as "within the same febrile illness" instead of "within 24 hours" (Camfield and Camfield, 1995; Shinnar, 1999). A *simple febrile seizure* consists of less than 10 or 15 minutes of generalized tonic–clonic activity, resolving spontaneously, in the context of a febrile illness, without focal features or recurrence during the subsequent 24 hours. Approximately 20–30% of febrile seizures are complex (Nelson and Ellenberg, 1976; Verity *et al.*, 1985; Annegers *et al.*, 1990; Berg and Shinnar, 1996; Offringa *et al.*, 1991; Al-Eissa, 1995). Early studies that showed a much higher percentage of complex febrile seizures [e.g., 62% in Wallace (1974)], but these series comprised hospitalized patients, representing the more severe end of the spectrum. In the large National Collaborative Perinatal Project (NCPP), a cohort of 54,000 children was followed from before birth until 7 years of age. In this study, 1706 children with febrile seizures were identified. Focal features were present in 4%, prolonged durations (>15 minutes) in 8%, and recurrent febrile seizures within 24 hours of the first one in 15–20% (Nelson and Ellenberg, 1976). Complex febrile seizures are associated with a higher risk of afebrile seizures but not of febrile seizure recurrence (Verity *et al.*, 1985; Berg, 1992). Because complex febrile seizures are associated with a higher risk of subsequent epilepsy, it is important to establish whether complex features are present when evaluating a child with a febrile seizure. Of the complex features, recurrence within 24 hours is perhaps the easiest to document. The presence of focal features can often be overlooked by the observer. Finally, as discussed in Section III,C, seizure duration is likely to be quite inaccurate. As discussed in depth in other chapters, the two subtypes of febrile seizures may form biologically distinct conditions with different risks for future seizures and neurologic deficits.

In summary, epidemiological studies vary in their operational definitions of febrile seizures, age limits employed, methods for determining whether they are simple vs. complex, seizure duration, and other factors. Such variations should be considered when comparing studies.

III. DETERMINING FEBRILE SEIZURE INCIDENCE AND PREVALENCE

A. DEFINITIONS OF EPIDEMIOLOGICAL TERMS

Much of our understanding of the risk factors, natural history, and prognosis of febrile seizures comes from epidemiological studies. However, epidemiological conclusions are only as reliable as the initial data obtained. To analyze the literature on febrile seizure frequency, certain epidemiological terms must be de-

TABLE 2   Epidemiological Terminology

Term	Definition
Incidence (or incidence rate)	The number of new cases in a defined population over a specified time period; expressed as individuals at risk per standard population per unit time
Age-specific incidence	Incidence adjusted for age
Cumulative incidence	The expected risk of developing the disorder by a specific age, i.e., the summation of age-specific incidence
Prevalence	The proportion of individuals in a population with the disorder at a specific time point; a function of incidence and average duration of illness
Lifetime prevalence	The proportion of the population with a history of the disorder, active or not

fined (Table 2) (Sander and Shorvon, 1987; Hauser and Hersdorffer, 1990; Berg, 1995). Unfortunately, incidence and prevalence are not always used correctly in the literature, and the terms are sometimes used interchangeably.

Incidence (or incidence rate) is the number of new cases occurring in a defined population over a specified period of time. For example, febrile seizure incidence is often denoted as the number of new cases per 1000 persons in a population, per year. Incidence can only be determined from longitudinal studies. *Prevalence* is the proportion of individuals in a population that has ever had the disorder, determined at a specific time point. Prevalence can be obtained from cross-sectional surveys. For example, prevalence is often specified as the number of children with a history of febrile seizures on a given date that a population survey is performed. Prevalence is dependent on both the incidence of the disorder and its average duration. Because the number of cases accumulate over time, prevalence can be high even if incidence is low, and knowledge of prevalence does not always lead to accurate incidence statistics. Although both incidence and prevalence can be adjusted for age, prevalence is not as useful in an age-specific syndrome such as febrile seizures. Febrile seizure incidence should decrease with age and become zero after about 7 years of age (Figure 1).

Cumulative incidence is the summation of age-specific incidence rates, i.e., expected risk of developing febrile seizures by a specific age. Therefore, this term is probably the most appropriate one to compare febrile seizure occurrence between populations, because all cases are expected to occur by about 5 years of age. Cumulative incidence should approach the *lifetime prevalence,* that is, the proportion of the population that has ever had a febrile seizure. This point is illustrated well in van den Berg and Yerushalmy (1969), which showed that cumulative incidence reaches a plateau by about 4 years of age. *Annual incidence* refers to the incidence only within the year studied; this value should be summated over the years of febrile seizure susceptibility to arrive at a rate approximating the cumulative incidence. Finally, the *first attendance rate* (Forsgren *et al.*, 1990) is defined as the number of new cases in the population at risk per year, including both new cases during the study period and those who had their first febrile seizure prior to the study period but were diagnosed during the study period.

B.   STUDY DESIGNS TO DETERMINE INCIDENCE AND PREVALENCE

The wide variety of study designs may strongly impact incidence and prevalence figures. To determine those rates, a number of techniques have been used. The goal of any method is to determine the number of cases (numerator) and the total population from which the cases are drawn (denominator). The two main types of study designs are clinic based and population based. Clinic-based studies are often performed in a specialized clinic, hospital setting, or other tertiary care facility. They have the advantage of providing a ready-made set of patients with detailed clinical information available. However, the type of patient that seeks care or has access to such a facility may skew the results. In general, these would be the most severely affected patients, with poorest outcomes (Ellenberg and Nelson, 1980). Clinic-based studies of febrile seizure occurrence are rarely performed anymore; older studies are reviewed by Rose *et al.* (1973).

Many studies have used larger populations to investigate febrile seizure incidence and prevalence, using case-finding methods such as medical record reviews, mailed questionnaires, telephone interviews, and door-to-door surveys (Table 3). Although these techniques are useful to investigate a much larger population base and thus better reflect the spectrum of disease severity and frequency, they are also subject to methodological biases. Such large-scale surveys are ordinarily carried out by personnel with limited medical training. Home visits are expensive and time consuming. Medical records are subject to some of the same biases discussed above, with documentation dependent on the training, time, and interest of the personnel collecting the data.

Population-based data are more difficult to obtain but have the advantage of surveying a large number of people. Population-based studies are of two basic types: cohort/cumulative incidence studies (Nelson and Ellenberg, 1976; Verity *et al.*, 1985) and prevalence surveys (Tsuboi, 1984; Forsgren *et al.*, 1990; Offringa *et al.*, 1991). A cohort may be followed from birth, allowing a prospec-

TABLE 3 Selected Studies of Febrile Seizure Incidence and Prevalence

Author	Location	Study type	Case ascertainment	Population size	Febrile seizures
Lessell et al. (1962)	Guam	Population based	First phase, survey of all 5- to 13-year old school registrants, followed by home visits; second phase, total community survey	1350	14% (age-specific prevalence in children 0–14 years old)
Schuman and Miller (1966)	Tecumseh, Michigan	Population based	Retrospective survey	3953	3.6% (prevalence)
Mathai et al. (1968)	Guam	Population based	Door-to-door total community survey, followed by screening examination by physician	6967	8.9% (age-specific incidence in children 0–4 years old)
van den Berg and Yerushalmy (1969)	Oakland, California	Cohort	Hospital and clinical records of children born 1960-1967 (Kaiser Foundation)	18,500	2% (cumulative incidence by 5 years old)
Stanhope et al. (1972)	Guam	Cohort and Population based	Retrospective; follow up of two birth cohorts in four villages—mailed questionnaires, interviews, and medical record review	419	11% (prevalence by 5 years old)
Rose et al. (1973)	Washington County, Maryland	Population based	Mailed questionnaire to families of all third graders; follow-up examinations in random subset	1866	4.8% (prevalence at 8–9 years old)
Hauser and Kurland (1975)	Rochester, Minnesota	Population based	Retrospective review of records (patient registry); children born 1935–1967	472 (city population, ~55,000)	0.4% (mean annual incidence in children <5 years old)
Rossiter et al. (1977)	Geelong, Australia	Cohort	Prospective study of consecutive births	580	34.0% (cumulative incidence, 0–3 years old)

Reference	Location	Study type	Method	Sample size	Prevalence/incidence
Nelson and Ellenberg (1976, 1978)	United States	Cohort	Prospective study of children born 1959–1966 at 12 urban teaching hospitals (National Collaborative Perinatal Project)	~54,000	3.5% (prevalence by age 7 years)
Bauman et al. (1978)	Rural Kentucky	Population based	Questionnaire, interview with neurologist	4023	1.7% (prevalence in children 6–16 years old)
Chiofalo et al. (1979)	Chile	Population based	Interview, examination by neurologist in positive cases; children born in 1966	2085	5.2% (prevalence at age 9 years)
Ross et al. (1980)	United Kingdom	Cohort	Questionnaire to all children born during one week of March 1958 (National Child Development Study)	15,496	2.4% (prevalence at age 11 years)
Heijbel et al. (1980)	Northern Sweden	Population based	Prospective	15,284	0.7% (annual incidence in children 0–5 years old)
Tsuboi (1984)	Fuchu, Tokyo Miyake, Tokyo	Population based	Retrospective. All 3-year-old children presenting to physicians for regular health examinations; urban and rural populations	17,587	8.3% (prevalence)
Verity et al. (1985)	United Kingdom	Cohort	Prospective study of children born during one week in April 1970; interviews by local health visitors at age 5 years	13,135	2.3% (cumulative incidence by age 5 years)
Zhao et al. (1987, 1991)	China—six cities	Population based	Door-to-door survey by neurologist; case-control study	63,195 (9198 under age 12; calculated from data in paper)	1.7% (prevalence in children <4 years old); 2.1% (prevalence through age 12 years); 0.6% (incidence in children <4 years old)

(continues)

TABLE 3 (continued)

Author	Location	Study type	Case ascertainment	Population size	Febrile seizures
Forsgren et al. (1990)	Northern Sweden	Population based	Prospective	15,420	4.1% (cumulative incidence by age 5 years); 0.46% (annual first attendance rate)
Offringa et al. (1991)	Rotterdam suburbs	Population based	Cross sectional prevalence survey	3570	3.9% (cumulative incidence by age 6 years)
Monetti et al. (1995)	Northeastern Italy	Population based	Questionnaire, interview by M.D.; compare with clinic files	165 controls without epilepsy	1.8% (cumulative incidence)
Okan et al. (1995)	Turkey	Population based	Retrospective survey; interviews by medical students, examinations by pediatricians	5002	4.5% (prevalence, 0–5 years)
Hackett et al. (1997)	Southern India	Population based	Home interview of 8- to 12-year-olds in a defined district, by psychologist or psychiatrist	4340	10.1% (lifetime incidence)
Pal (1999)	West Bengal, India	Population based	Structured questionnaire, home visit; unmatched case-control study	59 controls	5.1% (prevalence among controls)
Huang et al. (1999) Chang et al. (2000)	Taiwan	Population based	Prospective survey, case-control study: telephone interview, home visit	10,460	2.4% (prevalence among children 3 years old)

tive evaluation of febrile seizure occurrence. A potential disadvantage is that a cohort born on the same day may reach the age of peak incidence for febrile seizures during a month or season that is not the peak for the disorder (see Section IV,C).

The major differences between outcomes of clinic-based and population-based studies of febrile seizures are illustrated in a metaanalysis of twenty-six studies (Ellenberg and Nelson, 1980). Clinic-based studies reported the development of epilepsy in a much higher proportion of children with febrile seizures (median 17%) than was found in population-based studies (median 3%). These results support the notion that clinic-based studies are skewed toward disproportionately severe cases (Berg and Shinnar, 1994).

C. CASE ASCERTAINMENT: WAS IT A FEBRILE SEIZURE?

In studying the frequency of febrile seizures, the initial and most obvious task is to figure out if a clinical event was actually a febrile seizure. This determination can be challenging, as most pediatricians and pediatric neurologists will attest. To determine whether an event was a seizure, we must usually rely on the history given by a witness, usually a parent. The historical details are often colored by vague recollections of the child's abnormal behavior at a time of extreme stress. Important variables such as height (or even presence) of the preceding fever, seizure onset characteristics (focal versus generalized), and duration of the event are rarely recalled clearly. It is unlikely that the seizure duration will be accurately estimated by the caretaker, especially for shorter events, which are often overestimated. For longer febrile seizures, i.e., those still ongoing on arrival of emergency medical personnel or at the emergency room, durations may be easier to estimate. In addition, there is uncertainty inherent in parental reporting of febrile seizures. Based on their personal perceptions, cultural background, and medical sophistication, parents may underplay the episode (e.g., if they fear the stigma of an epilepsy diagnosis) or exaggerate its severity or duration [many parents feel their child is dying during a febrile seizures (Baumer et al., 1981)]. In an interesting study, approximately 25% of patients with known epilepsy (from medical records) denied having epilepsy on a questionnaire (Beran et al., 1985).

Even physicians have a variable degree of comfort evaluating spells such as febrile seizures. Other episodic conditions that may occur during a febrile illness must be differentiated from a bona fide febrile seizure (Baumann, 1981). The most frequent mimic of febrile seizures is a shaking rigor (shiver) (Rosman, 2000). Other conditions include febrile syncope (Stephenson, 1990), breath-holding spells, febrile "toxic delirium," and even temper tantrums. Like a seizure, many of these behaviors are exhausting and are followed by sleep, so postictal fatigue cannot be used as a differentiating factor. All these issues may affect case ascertainment and hence febrile seizure incidence, and these problems can be even more pronounced when data are collected by persons with limited experience dealing with the clinical vagaries of such episodes.

Methods of case ascertainment differ widely, and include medical record reviews, patient registries (Hauser and Kurland, 1975), reports from general practitioners, routine pediatric examinations, and questionnaires. Sampling methods include total population surveys (e.g., all residents of a geographical area) and selected population surveys (e.g., birth cohorts, schoolchildren, and children admitted to hospitals). In community studies, case ascertainment is independent of the medical record, reducing the chance that investigators are influenced by a preexisting diagnosis (Sander and Shorvon, 1987). Highly sensitive questionnaires must be designed. To reduce the number of false positive and false negative cases, some studies have used a combination of approaches [e.g., clinical sources vs. field techniques; medically trained vs. untrained personnel (Stanhope *et al.*, 1972)], allowing comparison of ascertainment methods. In that study, which took place on Guam, febrile seizure incidence rates from 17 to 35 per 100,000 persons were found; field studies found incidences twice as high as those found using the medical record alone. Medical record reviews may miss cases if there is insufficient documentation in the initial report. Children with febrile seizures, especially simple ones, may not even come to medical attention.

Surveys may cover the entire community or a smaller sample/subset. Door-to-door surveys have been quite popular and useful in epidemiological studies of febrile seizures. Again, proper training of paramedical personnel and a highly sensitive questionnaire are critical. Sensitivity can be checked by comparison with existing medical records, and specificity can be assessed by a medical examination of positive cases (Sander and Shorvon, 1987). One study found that adding door-to-door surveys to medical record review doubled the prevalence of partial seizures (Zielinski, 1974). Questionnaires are frequently used for large-scale surveys of populations. Although this method allows assessment of large numbers of persons, results may be complicated by several factors, including the response rate and poor memory for an event that occurred years earlier. By adding an examination by a neurologist to the questionnaire, incidence rate of febrile seizures tripled in one study (Rose *et al.*, 1973).

Although case ascertainment (numerator) remains a challenging problem in any epidemiological study, the population base (denominator) is equally important (Ellenberg and Nelson, 1980). The investigator must ensure that the population from which the cases are drawn reflects the entire group susceptible to the disorder, in this case all children within the vulnerable age range.

Unfortunately, all types of epidemiological studies are subject to a number of inherent or methodological biases, which must be considered when interpreting findings. As mentioned above, the imprecise use of definitions makes comparisons between many studies difficult, though this problem has improved since the adoption of the NIH and ILAE guidelines. Patient selection bias, duration and reliability of follow-up, intensity of observation, types of adverse outcomes, and training of personnel obtaining data are all important considerations (Baumann, 1981). Investigators must consider and attempt to control for all sources of bias when designing and performing an epidemiological study.

IV. HOW COMMON ARE FEBRILE SEIZURES?

A. KEY STUDIES

Despite the caveats and methodological difficulties described above, the various population-based studies show a remarkable similarity of febrile seizure incidence and prevalence across time periods and geographical regions. As can be seen in Table 3 and Figure 2, most studies carried out in the United States or western Europe found the cumulative incidence or prevalence of febrile seizures to be within the 2–5% range, despite the wide variety of study designs and case ascertainment methods. A few of the key studies deserve more in-depth discussion.

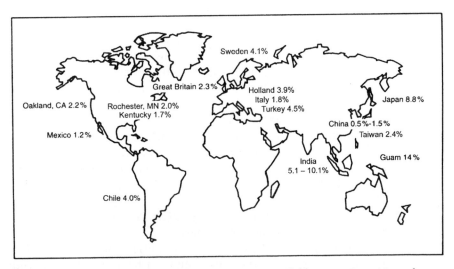

FIGURE 2 Cumulative incidence of febrile seizures among children in various cities and countries of the world. Revised and updated from Hauser (1994). The prevalence and incidence of convulsive disorders in children. *Epilepsia* 35 (Suppl. 2), S1–S6. Reprinted by permission of Blackwell Science, Inc.

Using a cohort of 18,500 babies born at the Kaiser Foundation Hospital in Oakland, California between 1960 and 1967, van den Berg and Yerushalmy (1969) assessed seizure incidence, including febrile seizures, retrospectively using outpatient and inpatient records. This study consisted of members of a pre-paid healthcare plan comprising a largely middle class, employed populace. By 5 years of age, 2% of the children experienced a febrile convulsion, with the peak incidence in the second year of life. One-third of the children had recurrent febrile seizures and about 3% later developed afebrile seizures. Strengths of this study were the large cohort size, relatively long follow-up period, and ability to compare records of children with febrile seizures and those affected by afebrile seizures or no seizures. A weakness of the study was the inclusion of children with intracranial infections, which accounted for 4% of those with febrile convulsions.

In perhaps the most comprehensive of all published epilepsy epidemiology studies, the entire population of Rochester, Minnesota (approximately 55,000) was assessed over 33 years (Hauser and Kurland, 1975; Hauser and Hersdorffer, 1990; Hauser et al., 1993). Meticulous attention was paid to methodology, including seizure definitions and classification, case ascertainment, and epidemiological techniques. Patients were identified from the Mayo Clinic registry, with telephone follow-up of positive cases. Febrile seizures were considered separately from epilepsy. Febrile seizures were defined as any seizure occurring during a febrile illness, excluding cases of a prior afebrile seizures and central nervous system (CNS) infection. No age limits were set. Over the 33 years, 472 children had a seizure with fever in the absence of CNS infection. The mean annual incidence rate was 3.9 cases per 1000 children under 5 years old. When incident cases were considered as a function of time, the incidence was similar throughout the 33-year study period, except that the earliest decade of the study had a slightly lower rate (probably due to lower case ascertainment after such a long delay). The stability of these data is especially impressive considering the evolving definitions and management of febrile seizures over the 33-year study period. The authors concluded that about 2% of children under 5 years old experienced at least one febrile seizure, a figure they considered to be an underestimate. Thirty-five percent of children had a recurrent febrile seizure during a subsequent febrile illness; this recurrence rate did not vary over the 33-year study period.

The National Collaborative Perinatal Project (NCPP) followed a cohort of about 54,000 pregnancies from birth to 7 years of age. Data were collected from 12 urban teaching hospitals in the United States (Nelson and Ellenberg 1976, 1978). This study differed from the Kaiser study in being prospective, with children receiving periodic examinations and interval histories by a variety of ancillary medically trained personnel. Febrile seizures were experienced by

1706 children (about 3.5%), and risk factors for the development of recurrent febrile seizures and epilepsy were determined, as discussed in Section II,A. The main advantages of this study are its prospective nature, large cohort size (essentially equivalent to a population-based study), and accurate, long-term follow-up. A possible complicating factor is that urban teaching hospitals were used as the study population, and these tend to entail a large proportion of high-risk pregnancies. Nevertheless, the study is monumental in its size and importance for our understanding of febrile seizures and many other neurologic disorders.

Several studies from a well-defined population in the county of Västerbotten in northern Sweden illustrate other aspects of febrile seizure epidemiology. In a prospective incidence study of over 15,000 children under age 5 years, 107 children developed a first febrile seizure during the study (essentially covering the year 1973), for an annual incidence of 700 affected out of 100,000 children at risk (0.7%) (Heijbel et al., 1980). A later study of the same population base, covering a 20-month period beginning in November 1985, found a lower annual incidence rate of 0.46% and a cumulative incidence of 4.1% among children under 5 years of age (Forsgren et al., 1990). During the study period, one recurrence was documented in 18% and two recurrences in 10%. Therefore, even in the same population and geographical region, there may be variation in febrile seizure incidence over time. It is unlikely that different medical conditions or treatments account for this discrepancy, although the authors speculate that a difference in vaccination rates in the two time periods may have played a role.

A large British study followed a cohort of over 13,000 children born during one week in April 1970. Detailed prenatal and postnatal data were documented on these children. When the children turned 5 years old, they were contacted by local health visitors, who administered detailed questionnaires; data on 80% of the original cohort were available. If a seizure was suspected, further information was obtained by a physician. Three-hundred and three children (2.3%) had a febrile seizure by age 5 years, and 35% of these had at least one recurrence. These rates were similar to another British cohort study performed a decade earlier (Ross et al., 1980).

Finally, a Dutch study evaluated 3570 children at the age of 6 years in the suburbs of Rotterdam (Offringa et al., 1991). Each child was seen by a school physician. Prior to that examination, parents filled out a questionnaire that inquired about possible seizures. The cumulative incidence of febrile seizures by age 6 years was 3.9%, with 26% having recurrences. This and other studies (Annegers et al., 1979; Tsuboi and Endo, 1991) found a strikingly increased risk of febrile seizures among family members, attesting to the strong genetic predisposition to febrile seizures.

B. Geographical Variation
in Febrile Seizures

Although incidence figures of 2–5% are documented consistently in population studies from the United States and western Europe (Hauser and Kurland, 1975; Nelson and Ellenberg, 1978; Hauser, 1981; Verity *et al.*, 1985), febrile seizures are reported to be much more common in certain geographical regions (Figure 2). In Japan, 8.3% of children were found to have febrile seizures in a carefully designed study involving total population surveys of two populations: an urban Tokyo community (Fuchu) and five villages on the Miyake Island 200 km south of Tokyo (Tsuboi, 1984). At the age of 3 years, all children in each community underwent health examinations; children identified with any type of seizure were followed up with neurologic examinations and electroencephalograms (EEGs). In the Fuchu group (17,044 children), febrile seizure prevalence was 8.7% over a 5-year period. On Miyake Island, five villages were assayed separately over 10 years, and the prevalence rates varied from 0.9 to 20.6% (mean 10.7%). The most dramatic finding was the consistently high prevalence of febrile seizure in both areas of Japan, much higher rates than in any other area of the world except Guam.

In the Mariana Islands (Guam), an even higher incidence of febrile seizures was reported (14%) in a series of detailed population-based studies (Mathai *et al.*, 1968; Stanhope *et al.*, 1972). Studies from India found prevalence rates of 5–10% (Hackett *et al.*, 1997; Pal, 1999). In the unmatched case-control study of 2- to 18-year-old children, a door-to-door survey with a structured questionnaire was supplemented by examination by a pediatric neurologist (Pal, 1999). Of the controls, 5% had febrile seizures, compared with 18% of children with epilepsy. There are several possible explanations for these geographical discrepancies: the data may be tainted by some form of bias in case ascertainment or study design, there may be an underlying genetic predilection for febrile seizures in that population, or a specific environmental factor may predispose to febrile seizures. Of course, these are not mutually exclusive.

Tsuboi attempted to explain the high rate of febrile seizures in Japan on the basis of extensive cosleeping that exists in that country. Because parents and children sleep in close proximity, fevers and febrile seizures are more likely to be detected. However, the data cannot be fully explained on that basis, because other countries in which cosleeping is common do not have inordinately high rates of febrile seizures [e.g., China, 1.7% (Zhao *et al.*, 1987)]. The even greater incidence on the Mariana Islands also defies explanation. Cosleeping occurs in that culture as well. However, unlike most of the western world, seizures are not stigmatized on Guam (Lessell *et al.*, 1962; Mathai *et al.*, 1968); the willingness of parents to openly discuss seizures in their children could lead to an enhanced ability to identify cases. This observation emphasizes the importance of cultural factors in case ascertainment, which is not often acknowledged.

In tropical regions, there could be a higher frequency of infectious illnesses and thus febrile seizures. The high rate of reported febrile seizures could relate to local infection profiles (Senanayake and Roman, 1993). In western countries, most cases of febrile seizures are due to illnesses such as upper respiratory infections, otitis media, *Shigella* gastroenteritis, human herpes virus-6 infections (roseola), or undefined viral illnesses (Barone *et al.*, 1995; Hirtz *et al.*, 1997). However, in Africa, endemic malaria accounts for at least one-third of fever-related seizures (Obi *et al.*, 1994; Birbeck, 2000), and inclusion of these cases could lead to a high false positive rate, because seizures in the context of active malaria should not be considered a febrile seizure (Akpede *et al.*, 1993). Other developing nations report febrile seizures rates approaching those of western Europe and the United States (Figure 2), so much of the geographical disparity remains unexplained.

In terms of racial predilection, results have been inconsistent. The NCPP data reported febrile seizures in 3.5% of Caucasian children and 4.2% of black children, a difference that, although small, was found to be statistically significant (Nelson and Ellenberg, 1978). As indicated in the Kaiser Foundation study, socioeconomic and other factors rather than purely racial ones could account for the difference in racial incidence (van den Berg and Yerushalmy, 1969). There was no racial propensity in the large British (Verity *et al.*, 1985) or Dutch (Offringa *et al.*, 1991) studies, although only a few percent of noncaucasians were present in these studies of relatively homogeneous populations.

C. Seasonal Variation in Febrile Seizures

Intuitively, one would expect febrile seizure incidence to vary according to fever incidence. Because children incur a greater number of fevers during the winter months, febrile seizures would be predicted to occur more frequently then. Indeed, analysis of the cohort data of Tsuboi showed that there were two peaks in febrile seizure incidence, November–January (corresponding to the peak of viral infections involving the upper respiratory tract) and June–August (when gastrointestinal viral illnesses are common) (Tsuboi and Okada, 1984). However, Berg and colleagues (1995) have reported that febrile seizures are less likely to accompany a gastrointestinal illness than an upper respiratory illness. The Swedish prospective study also found a higher rate of febrile seizures during fall months, when it was speculated that viral illnesses increased as children returned to daycare after their summer vacation (Forsgren *et al.*, 1990). Other researchers failed to find that febrile seizure incidence correlated with specific months, but did note a seasonal variation based on the month of birth of affected children (Sunderland *et al.*, 1982). These workers suggested caution when analyzing data from cohort studies that utilize a single week or month of birth and extrapolate that data to the entire year (Ross *et al.*, 1980; Verity *et al.*, 1985). Of note, the patients in the study of Sunderland *et al.* (1982) were all hospitalized for their febrile seizures, so probably represented sicker children.

D. FEBRILE SEIZURES ARE SLIGHTLY MORE COMMON IN BOYS

Regardless of the era of the study or particulars of the experimental design, boys have consistently emerged with a higher frequency of febrile seizures. Incidence ratios of boys:girls have ranged from 1.1:1 to 2:1 (Lennox-Buchtal, 1973; Nelson and Ellenberg, 1978; Hauser, 1981; Tsuboi, 1984; Forsgren *et al.*, 1990). However, some large studies showed no significant difference on the basis of gender (Vandenberg and Yerushalmy, 1969; Verity *et al.*, 1985; Offringa *et al.*, 1991), and the NCPP study showed more frequent febrile seizures in boys only among blacks (Nelson and Ellenberg, 1978). Complex febrile seizure incidence is not gender-related (Nelson and Ellenberg, 1978; Verity *et al.*, 1985). Whether there is a biological basis for the gender-specific differences in febrile seizure susceptibility, or whether boys simply contract more fevers and therefore are at greater risk, is currently unknown.

V. WHY DO WE NEED EPIDEMIOLOGICAL DATA?

Our current understanding of the nature and natural history of febrile seizures owes much to the evidence collected in epidemiological studies (Berg, 1992). Data obtained from epidemiological studies can help us understand the genetics and prognosis of febrile seizures, and perhaps even give insights into their mechanism. Knowledge gained from epidemiological studies has allowed us to counsel families that the vast majority of febrile seizures are benign, that the chance of febrile seizures progressing to epilepsy is small, and that in most cases, prophylactic treatment is unnecessary or even detrimental. In terms of diagnostic evaluation, epidemiological findings have contributed to our clinical approach, obviating unnecessary blood draws, lumbar punctures, neuroimaging, and electroencephalograms. Population data first suggested a heritable component in febrile seizures and set the stage for modern molecular genetic investigations (Annegers *et al.*, 1979; Berkovic and Scheffer, 1998; Kugler and Johnson, 1998; Racacho *et al.*, 2000). Thus, epidemiological data are the cornerstone of our information about febrile seizures. Because there is no laboratory test or other method to verify febrile seizures, epidemiological studies are likely to retain their paramount importance. Appropriate methodological caveats should be kept in mind when reviewing these data.

ACKNOWLEDGMENT

The author is grateful to Dr. Anne T. Berg for insightful comments and suggestions.

REFERENCES

Aicardi, J. (1994). Febrile convulsions. *In* "Epilepsy in Children," pp. 253–275. Raven Press, New York.

Akpede, G. O., Sykes, R. M., and Abiodun, P. O. (1993). Convulsions with malaria: Febrile or indicative of cerebral involvement? *J. Trop. Pediatr.* **39**, 350–355.

Al-Eissa, Y. A. (1995). Febrile seizures: Rate and risk factors of recurrence. *J. Child Neurol.* **10**, 315–319.

Annegers, J. F., Hauser, W. A., Elveback, L. R., and Kurland, L. T. (1979). The risk of epilepsy following febrile convulsions. *Neurology* **29**, 297–303.

Annegers, J. F., Hauser, W. A., Shirts, S. B., and Kurland, L. T. (1987). Factors prognostic of unprovoked seizures after febrile convulsions. *N. Engl. J. Med.* **316**, 493–498.

Annegers, J. F., Blakely, S. A., Hauser, W. A., and Kurland, L.T. (1990). Recurrence risk of febrile convulsions in a population-based cohort. *Epilepsy Res.* **5**, 209–216.

Barone, S. R., Kaplan, M. H., and Krilov, L. R. (1995). Human herpesvirus-6 infection in children with first febrile seizures. *J. Pediatr.* **127**, 95–97.

Baumann, R. J. (1981). Problems in epidemiologic studies of the consequences of febrile seizures in children. *In* "Febrile Seizures" (K. B. Nelson and J. H. Ellenberg, eds.), pp. 27–33. Raven Press, New York.

Baumann, R. J., Marx, M. B., and Leonidakis, M. G. (1978). Epilepsy in rural Kentucky: Prevalence in a population of school age children. *Epilepsia* **19**, 75–80.

Baumer, J. H., David, T. J., Valentine, S. J., Roberts, J. E., and Hughes, B. R. (1981). Many parents think their child is dying when having a first febrile convulsion. *Dev. Med. Child Neurol.* **23**, 462–464.

Beran, R. G., Michelazzi, J., Hall, L., Tsimnadis, P., and Loh, S. (1985). False-negative response rate in epidemiologic studies to define prevalence ratios of epilepsy. *Neuroepidemiology* **4**, 82–85.

Berg, A. T. (1992). Febrile seizures and epilepsy: The contribution of epidemiology. *Paediatr. Perinat. Epidemiol.* **6**, 145–152.

Berg, A. T. (1993). Are febrile seizures provoked by a rapid rise in temperature? *Am. J. Dis. Child.* **147**, 1101–1103.

Berg, A. T. (1995). The epidemiology of seizures and epilepsy in children. *In* "Childhood Seizures" (S. Shinnar, N. Amir, and D. Branski, eds.),Vol. 6, pp. 1–10. Karger, Basel.

Berg, A. T., and Shinnar, S. (1994). The contributions of epidemiology to the understanding of childhood seizures and epilepsy. *J. Child Neurol.* **9**, 2S19–2S26.

Berg, A. T., and Shinnar, S. (1996). Complex febrile seizures. *Epilepsia* **37**, 126–133.

Berg, A. T., Shinnar, S., Hauser, W. A., and Leventhal, J. M. (1990). Predictors of recurrent febrile seizures: A metaanalytic review. *J. Pediatr.* **116**, 329–337.

Berg, A. T., Shinnar, S., Hauser, W. A., Alemany, M., Shapiro, E. D., Salomon, M. E., and Crain, E. F.
    (1992). Predictors of recurrent febrile seizures: A prospective study of the circumstances sur-
    rounding the initial febrile seizure. N. Engl. J. Med. 327, 1122–1127.
Berg, A. T., Shinnar, S., Shapiro, E. D., Salomon, M. E., Crain, E. F., and Hauser, W. A. (1995). Risk
    factors for a first febrile seizure: A matched case-control study. Epilepsia 36, 334–341.
Berg, A. T., Shinnar, S., Darefsky, A. S., Holford, T. R., Shapiro, E. D., Salomon, M. E., Crain, E. F.,
    and Hauser, W. A. (1997). Predictors of recurrent febrile seizures: A prospective cohort study.
    Arch. Pediatr. Adolesc. Med. 151, 371–378.
Berkovic, S., and Scheffer, I. (1998). Febrile seizures: Genetics and relationship to other epilepsy
    syndromes. Curr. Opin. Neurol. 11, 129–134.
Birbeck, G. L. (2000). Seizures in rural Zambia. Epilepsia 41, 277–281.
Bridge, E. M. (1949). "Epilepsy and Convulsive Disorders in Children." McGraw-Hill, New York.
Camfield, P., and Camfield, C. (1995). Febrile seizures. In "Childhood Seizures" (S. Shinnar, N.
    Amir, and D. Branski, eds.), Vol. 6, pp. 32–38. Karger, Basel.
Camfield, P., Camfield, C., Gordon, K., and Dooley, J. (1994). What types of epilepsy are preceded
    by febrile seizures? A population-based study of children. Dev. Med. Child Neurol 36, 887–892.
Cendes, F., Andermann, F., Gloor, P., Lopes-Cendes, I., Andermann, E., Melanson, D., Jones-Got-
    man, M., Robitaille, Y., Evans, A., and Peters, T. (1993). Atrophy of mesial temporal lobe struc-
    tures in patients with temporal lobe epilepsy: Cause or consequence of repeated seizures? Ann.
    Neurol. 34, 795–801.
Chang, Y., Guo, N., Huang, C., Wang, S., and Tsai, J. (2000). Neurocognitive attention and behav-
    ior outcome of school-age children with a history of febrile convulsions: A population study.
    Epilepsia 41, 412–420.
Chiofalo, N., Kirschbaum, A., Fuentes, A., Cordero, M. L., and Madsen, J. (1979). Prevalence of
    epilepsy in children of Melipilla, Chile. Epilepsia 20, 261–266.
Commission on Classification and Terminology of the International League Against Epilepsy
    (1989). Proposal for revised classification of epilepsies and epilepsy syndromes. Epilepsia 30,
    389–399.
Commission on Epidemiology and Prognosis, International League Against Epilepsy (1993).
    Guidelines for epidemiologic studies on epilepsy. Epilepsia 34, 592–596.
Ellenberg, J. H., and Nelson, K. B. (1980). Sample selection and the natural history of disease: Stud-
    ies of febrile seizures. J. Am. Med. Assoc. 243, 1337–1340.
El-Radhi, A. S., Withana, K., and Banejeh, S. (1986). Recurrence rate of febrile convulsion related
    to the degree of pyrexia during the first attack. Clin. Pediatr. 25, 311–313.
Falconer, M. A., Serafetinides, E. A., and Corsellis, J. A. N. (1964). Etiology and pathogenesis of
    temporal lobe epilepsy. Arch. Neurol. 10, 223–248.
Forsgren, L., Sidenvall, R., Blomquist, H. K., and Heijbel, J. (1990). A prospective incidence study
    of febrile convulsions. Acta Paediatr. Scand. 79, 550–557.
Friderichsen, C., and Melchior, J. (1954). Febrile convulsions in children, their frequency and prog-
    nosis. Acta Paediatr. Scand. 43 (Suppl. 100), 307–317.
Germano, I. M., Zhang, Y. F., Sperber, E. F., and Moshe, S. L. (1996). Neuronal migration disorders
    increase seizure susceptibility to febrile seizures. Epilepsia 37, 902–910.
Hackett, R., Hackett, L., and Bhakta, P. (1997). Febrile seizures in a South Indian district: Incidence
    and associations. Dev. Med. Child Neurol. 39, 380–384.
Hamati-Haddad, A., and Abou-Khalil, B. (1998). Epilepsy diagnosis and localization in patients
    with antecedent childhood febrile convulsions. Neurology 50, 917–922.
Hauser, W. A. (1981). The natural history of febrile seizures. In "Febrile Seizures" (K. B. Nelson and
    J. H. Ellenberg, eds.), pp. 5–17. Raven Press, New York.
Hauser, W. A. (1994). The prevalence and incidence of convulsive disorders in children. Epilepsia
    35 (Suppl. 2), S1–S6.

Hauser, W., and Hersdorffer, D. (1990). "Epilepsy: Frequency, Causes and Consequences." Demos, New York.

Hauser, W. A., and Kurland, L. T. (1975). The epidemiology of epilepsy in Rochester, Minnesota, 1935 through 1967. *Epilepsia* 16, 1–66.

Hauser, W., Annegers, J., and Kurland, L. (1993). The incidence of epilepsy and unprovoked seizures in Rochester, Minnesota, 1935–1984. *Epilepsia* 34, 453–468.

Heijbel, J., Blom, S., and Bergfors, P. G. (1980). Simple febrile convulsions: A prospective incidence study and an evaluation of investigations initially needed. *Neuropaediatrie* 11, 45–56.

Hirtz, D. G., Camfield, C. S., and Camfield, P. R. (1997). Febrile convulsions. *In* "Epilepsy: A Comprehensive Textbook" (J. Engel, Jr. and T. A. Pedley, eds.), Vol. 3, pp. 2483–2488. Lippincott-Raven, Philadelphia.

Huang, C., Wang, S., Chang, Y., Huang, M., Chi, Y., and Tsai, J. (1999). Risk factors for a first febrile convulsion in children: A population study in southern Taiwan. *Epilepsia* 40, 719–725.

Knudsen, F. U. (1985). Effective short-term diazepam prophylaxis in febrile convulsions. *J. Pediatr.* 106, 487–490.

Kugler, S. L., and Johnson, W. G. (1998). Genetics of the febrile seizure susceptibility trait. *Brain Dev.* 20, 265–274.

Lennox, W. G. (1953). Significance of febrile convulsions. *Pediatrics* 11, 341–357.

Lennox, W. G. (1960). "Epilepsy and Related Disorders," Vol. 1. Little, Brown and Company, Boston.

Lennox-Buchtal, M. A. (1973). Febrile convulsions: A reappraisal. *Electroencephalogr. Clin. Neurophysiol.* 32 (Suppl.), 1–132.

Lessell, S., Torres, J. M., and Kurland, L. T. (1962). Seizure disorders in a Guamanian village. *Arch. Neurol.* 7, 37–44.

Liu, Z., Mikati, M., and Holmes, G. L. (1995). Mesial temporal sclerosis: Pathogenesis and significance. *Pediatr. Neurol.* 12, 5–16.

Livingston, S. (1958). Convulsive disorders in infants and children. *Adv. Pediatr.* 10, 113–195.

Mathai, K. V., Dunn, D. P., Kurland, L. T., and Reeder, F. A. (1968). Convulsive disorders in the Mariana Islands. *Epilepsia* 9, 77–85.

Michon, P. E., and Wallace, S. J. (1984). Febrile convulsions: Electroencephalographic changes related to rectal temperature. *Arch. Dis. Child.* 59, 371–373.

Millichap, J. G. (1968). "Febrile Convulsions." The Macmillan Company, New York.

Millichap, J. G. (1981). The definition of febrile seizures. *In* "Febrile Seizures" (K. B. Nelson and J. H. Ellenberg, eds.), pp. 1–3. Raven Press, New York.

Monetti, V. C., Granieri, E., Casetta, I., Tola, M. R., Paolino, E., Malagu, S., Govoni, V., and Quatrale, R. (1995). Risk factors for idiopathic generalized seizures: A population-based case control study in Copparo, Italy. *Epilepsia* 36, 224–229.

National Institutes of Health (1980). Febrile seizures: Consensus development conference summary, Vol. 3, no. 2. National Institutes of Health, Bethesda, MD.

Nelson, K. B., and Ellenberg, J. H. (1976). Predictors of epilepsy in children who have experienced febrile seizures. *N. Engl. J. Med.* 295, 1029–1033.

Nelson, K. B., and Ellenberg, J. H. (1978). Prognosis in children with febrile seizures. *Pediatrics* 61, 720–727.

Nelson, K. B., and Ellenberg, J. H. (1981). "Febrile Seizures." Raven Press, New York.

Obi, J. O., Ejeheri, N. A., and Alakija, W. (1994). Childhood febrile seizures (Benin City experience). *Ann. Trop. Paediatr.* 14, 211–214.

Offringa, M., Hazebroek-Kampschreur, A. A. J. M., and Derksen-Lubsen, G. (1991). Prevalence of febrile seizures in Dutch schoolchildren. *Paediatr. Perinat. Epidemiol.* 5, 181–188.

Okan, N., Okan, M., Eralp, O., and Aytekin, A. H. (1995). The prevalence of neurological disorders among children in Gemlik (Turkey). *Dev. Med. Child Neurol.* 37, 597–603.

Pal, D. K. (1999). Methodologic issues in assessing risk factors for epilepsy in an epidemiologic study in India. *Neurology* 53, 2058–2063.

Peterman, M. G. (1952). Febrile convulsions. *J. Pediatr.* 41, 536–540.

Racacho, L. J., McLachlan, R. S., Ebers, G. C., Maher, J., and Bulman, D. E. (2000). Evidence favoring genetic heterogeneity for febrile convulsions. *Epilepsia* 41, 132–139.

Rose, S. W., Penry, J. K., Markush, R. E., Radloff, L. A., and Putnam, P. L. (1973). Prevalence of epilepsy in children. *Epilepsia* 14, 133–152.

Rosman, N. P. (2000). Febrile seizures. *In* "Pediatric Epilepsy: Diagnosis and Therapy" (J. M. Pellock, W. E. Dodson, and B. F. D. Bourgeois, eds.), 2nd Ed., pp. 163–175. Demos, New York.

Rosman, N. P., Labazzo, J. L., and Colton, T. (1993). Factors predisposing to afebrile seizures after febrile convulsions and preventive treatment. *Ann. Neurol.* 34, 452.

Ross, E. M., Peckham, C. S., West, P. B., and Butler, N. R. (1980). Epilepsy in childhood: Findings from the National Child Development Study. *Br. Med. J.* 280, 207–210.

Rossiter, E. J. R., Luckin, J., Vile, A., Ganly, N., Hallowes, R., and Pearson, R. D. (1977). Convulsions in the first three years of life. *Med. J. Austral.* 2, 735–740.

Sander, J. W. A. S., and Shorvon, S. D. (1987). Incidence and prevalence studies in epilepsy and their methodological problems: A review. *J. Neurol. Neurosurg. Psychiatr.* 50, 829–839.

Schuman, S. H., and Miller, L. J. (1966). Febrile convulsions in families: Findings in an epidemiologic survey. *Clin. Pediatr.* 5, 604–608.

Senanayake, N., and Roman, G. C. (1993). Epidemiology of epilepsy in developing countries. *Bull. World Health Org.* 71, 247–258.

Shinnar, S. (1999). Febrile seizures. *In* "Pediatric Neurology Principles and Practice" (K. F. Swaiman and S. Ashwal, eds.), 3rd Ed., Vol. 1, pp. 676–682. Mosby, St. Louis.

Stanhope, J. M., Brody, J. A., Brink, E., and Morris, C. E. (1972). Convulsions among the Chamorro people of Guam, Mariana Islands. *Am. J. Epidemiol.* 95, 299–304.

Stephenson, J. B. P. (1990). "Fits and Faints." MacKeith Press, Oxford.

Sunderland, R., Carpenter, R., and Gardner, A. (1982). Are all born equal? Incidence of febrile convulsions by season of birth. *Br. Med. J.* 284, 624–626.

Tsuboi, T. (1984). Epidemiology of febrile and afebrile convulsions in children in Japan. *Neurology* 34, 175–181.

Tsuboi, T. (1986). Seizures of childhood: A population and clinic based study. *Acta Neurol. Scand. (Suppl.)* 110, 22–29.

Tsuboi, T., and Endo, S. (1991). Genetic studies of febrile convulsions: Analysis of twin and family data. *Epilepsy Res. (Suppl.)* 4, 119–128.

Tsuboi, T., and Okada, S. (1984). Seasonal variation of febrile convulsion in Japan. *Acta Neurol. Scand.* 69, 285–292.

van den Berg, B. J., and Yerushalmy, J. (1969). Studies on convulsive disorders in young children. I. Incidence of febrile and nonfebrile convulsions by age and other factors. *Pediatr. Res.* 3, 298–304.

Verity, C. M., Butler, N. R., and Golding, J. (1985). Febrile convulsions in a national cohort followed up from birth. I. Prevalence and recurrence in the first five years of life. *Br. Med. J.* 290, 1307–1310.

Wallace, S. J. (1974). Recurrence of febrile convulsions. *Arch. Dis. Child.* 49, 763–775.

Wallace, S. J. (1980). They don't do very well. *Pediatrics* 65, 678–679.

Wolf, S. M., and Forsythe, A. (1989). Epilepsy and mental retardation following febrile seizures in childhood. *Acta Paediatr. Scand.* 78, 291–295.

Wolf, S. M., Carr, A., Davis, D. C., Davidson, S., Dale, E. P., Goldenberg, E. D., Hanson, R., Lulejan, G. A., Nelson, M. A., Treiman, P., and Weinstein, A. (1977). The value of phenobarbital in the child who has had a single febrile seizure: A controlled prospective study. *Pediatrics* 59, 378–385.

Zhao, F., Lavine, L., Wang, Z., Cheng, X., Li, S., Emoto, S., Bolis, C. L., and Schoenberg, B. S. (1987). Prevalence and incidence of febrile seizures (FBS) in China. *Neurology* 37 (Suppl. 1), 149.

Zhao, F., Emoto, S. E., Lavine, L., Nelson, K. B., Wang, C., Li, S., Cheng, X., Bolis, C. L., and Schoenberg, B. S. (1991). Risk factors for febrile seizures in the People's Republic of China: A case control study. *Epilepsia* 32, 510–514.

Zielinski, J. J. (1974). Epileptics not in treatment. *Epilepsia* 15, 203–210.

CHAPTER 2

Antecedents and Risk Factors for Febrile Seizures

PETER CAMFIELD, CAROL CAMFIELD, AND KEVIN GORDON
Department of Pediatrics, Dalhousie University and IWK Health Centre, Halifax, Nova Scotia, Canada B3J 3G9

Febrile seizures occur when a susceptible child of a critical age has a fever. The fever is typically higher than in control children with a similar illness. Susceptibility factors have been assessed by population-based studies from California, New York, Wales, Finland, Nova Scotia, the United Kingdom, the United States, and Taiwan. There is compelling evidence that an inherited factor is critical in most cases. A family history of febrile seizures is the most important risk factor, and the more relatives affected the greater the risk. Linkage studies have identified several chromosomal loci that are associated with febrile seizures. Most studies also find that other concomitant brain disorders increase the risk, as does increased exposure to infectious illnesses. Human herpesvirus-6 (HHV-6) infection may be particularly provocative. In the Nova Scotia study, 3% of children had two or more risk factors (a close family history of febrile seizures, slowed development, attendance at day care, and delayed neonatal discharge). Their risk for a first febrile seizure was about 30%, suggesting that anticipatory guidance might be targeted to a small group at especially high risk. © 2002 Academic Press.

I. INTRODUCTION

One child in 28 will have a febrile seizure but the remaining 27 will not (Nelson and Ellenberg, 1976). It would be an enormous clinical boon to be able to predict accurately which child would develop febrile seizures in order to counsel parents and to offer potentially preventive treatment.

Febrile seizures have three critical elements—age, fever, and predisposition. Age and fever are always necessary. A predisposition for febrile seizures is noted in most cases, although it is unclear if it is always required. The critical age is about 6 months to 5 years, although almost all first febrile seizures occur by age 3 years. The febrile seizure tendency, therefore, must be related to a normal stage of brain maturation. There are no current insights into this element of the febrile seizure etiology. It remains unclear why the immature brain is vulnerable to fever.

TABLE 1 Antecedents and Risk Factors for Febrile Seizures[a]

Primary author	Pre- or perinatal factors	Previous fetal death	Feb Sz 1st degree relative	Prior neurological/ dev abn	Increased number of febrile illnesses	Daycare attendence	Temp >39.4°C	HHV-6 or gastro	Maternal smoking
Wallace	+	—	—	—	—	—	—	—	—
Van den Berg*	+	+	—	—	—	—	—	—	—
Verity*	↓bw	—	+	+	—	—	—	—	—
Nelson*	0	0	+	—	—	—	—	—	+
Forsgren*	Only preterm	0	—	—	—	—	—	—	—
Bethune	+	—	+	+	—	+	—	—	—
Rantala	—	—	—	—	—	0	+	HHV-6	—
Berg	0	—	+	—	—	0	+	Gastro	+
Greenwood*	↓bw, ↑maternal BP	0	0	—	—	—	—	—	0
Huang*	0	—	+	—	+	0	+	—	—

[a]Population-based studies are indicated by an asterisk following the name of the primary author. —, Not studied; +, risk factor studied with an association found; 0, risk factor studied with no association found; bw, birthweight; BP, blood preasure; dev abn, developmentally abnormal; temp, temperature; gastro, gastroenteritis.

Second, the child must, by definition, have a febrile illness. Usually the temperature is high, but there has been no published research to indicate that children with febrile seizures are more likely than other children to develop very high temperatures with illness. However, as noted below, children with febrile seizures have a higher temperature compared to febrile controls (Berg *et al.*, 1995). The cause of the fever appears to be nonspecific except that human herpesvirus-6 (HHV6) has more often been implicated as a cause than have other illnesses (Rantala *et al.*, 1995; Barone *et al.*, 1995). It is unclear if HHV-6 has a facilitating role beyond its well-known ability to produce high fever in children (Kondo *et al.*, 1993). There is some suggestion that increased exposure to infectious agents through day care or crowded housing increases the risk of febrile illnesses (Huang *et al.*, 1999).

Third, the child with a febrile seizure is somehow predisposed. There is strong evidence for genetic factors. As well, there is a suggestion that concomitant brain disorders contribute to the risk for a febrile seizure. Presumably, this occurs through a nonspecific reduction in the seizure threshold.

This chapter focuses on the literature that has assessed these three critical factors in comparison with a suitable control group. Particular emphasis is placed on population-based studies because of their lack of selection bias (Tsai *et al.*, 1996). Table 1 summarizes the literature.

II. SUMMARY OF KEY STUDIES

As comprehensively reviewed by Huang *et al.* (1999), there are a significant number of independent risk factors for febrile seizures reported in studies using multivariate analysis. These factors include day care attendance (Bethune *et al.*, 1993), parental education (Hackett *et al.*, 1997), prenatal maternal smoking (Berg *et al.*, 1995; Cassano *et al.*, 1990), maternal alcohol intake (Cassano *et al.*, 1990), late neonatal discharge (Bethune *et al.*, 1993), slow development (Bethune *et al.*, 1993), degree of fever (Berg *et al.*, 1995; Rantala *et al.*, 1995) gastroenteritis (Berg *et al.*, 1995), and family history of febrile seizures (Berg *et al.*, 1995; Bethune *et al.*, 1993; Forsgren *et al.*, 1990). A family history of febrile seizures is identified in every study as an important risk factor. The other factors are not always noted, and in particular pre- or perinatal problems have been less consistently noted. The studies summarized below are ordered by date of publication.

A. WALLACE, 1972—WALES, UNITED KINGDOM

The study by Wallace (1972) assessed 132 children who were admitted to the Royal Hospital for Sick Children in Edinburgh, Scotland for febrile seizures, as compared to their siblings who had not had febrile seizures. Thirty-one children were thought to be neurologically abnormal at the time of admission to hospital. In 122, the admission was for the first seizure. A variety of prenatal and perinatal factors were more common in cases than in the siblings. When these factors were summed, 80 of 132 (60%) cases and 39 of the 180 (22%) siblings had at least one of the "significant" pre- or perinatal adverse events and 23% of the patients but only 3% of their sibs had more than one abnormality.

A number of previous studies also linked the febrile seizure tendency to pre- and perinatal problems. None of the subsequent population-based studies or series of unselected outpatients has come to similar results. We have to assume that somehow this series is unusual.

B. VAN DEN BERG AND YERUSHALMY, 1974—CALIFORNIA

Van den Berg and Yerushalmy (1974) studied a cohort of infants in California who were born and cared for through the Kaiser Foundation healthcare system between 1960 and 1967. Of 7369 infants, 162 had febrile seizures. Controls for cases were chosen at random and matched for several factors, including age and sex. For this study, all mothers had had at least one previous pregnancy. There was an excess of early fetal deaths (<20 weeks) in previous pregnancies of the febrile seizure mothers compared with controls (86/452, or 19.1% of previous pregnancies vs. 55/454, 12.2%, $p < 0.005$). This study has not been clearly replicated but the methodology was careful and the cases unselected except for attendance at a managed care organization at a time when there were few such insurance arrangements. The authors do admit that there was a possibility of recall bias.

C. VERITY *ET AL.*, 1985—UNITED KINGDOM

The study by Verity *et al.* (1985a,b) assessed all children born in the United Kingdom during 1 week (April 5–11, 1970). Of 13,135 parents interviewed 5 years later, 303 children were known to have had at least one febrile seizure. The rate of febrile seizures in girls and boys was identical (2.29% boys, 2.12% girls), although some other studies have noted a slight excess of boys.

For 228 children with febrile seizures, a family history was available and 44 had a first-degree relative with febrile seizures. The rate of positive family history in the rest of the cohort without febrile seizures was not stated.

It was noted that lower birth weight was associated with febrile seizures. Thirty of the 883 (3.4%) with birth weight <2500 g had at least one febrile seizure compared with 270 of the11,872 (2.3%) weighing >2500 g at birth. The excess was made up of those who were known to have neurologic abnormality prior to their first febrile seizure. Therefore, the effect of low birth weight seemed to be the result of a brain injury from complications of prematurity or premature birth in children with existing brain abnormalities. There was a marginal association between febrile seizures and breech birth but not with many other pre- and perinatal factors.

D. NELSON AND ELLENBERG, 1990—UNITED STATES

The National Collaborative Perinatal Project identified about 55,000 children prenatally and followed them to age 7 years (Nelson and Ellenberg, 1990). Cases were consecutive births from several hospitals in large cities in the United States. There were 1706 children who had febrile seizures. The prevalence of many pre- and perinatal factors in the affected children was compared with the remainder of the cohort. There was no clear relationship with any perinatal problems. There was a suggestion that maternal smoking during pregnancy increased the risk of febrile seizures. The strongest association with febrile seizures was a history of febrile seizures in the mother (12.5% of febrile seizure children compared with 0.39% in the remainder of the cohort). The very low rate in mothers of children without febrile seizures raises some question of recall bias.

E. FORSGREN ET AL., 1991—SWEDEN

Forsgren et al. (1991) addressed pre- and perinatal factors as potential risk factors for febrile seizures. They studied children with febrile seizures in the county of Vasterbotten in Sweden. At the time of the study, the county had a population of 245,204. Cases were gathered prospectively by asking nurses and physicians in the region to report all cases over a 20-month period in 1985–1987. The regional EEG laboratory was used to uncover other cases. Case finding was likely complete, because the cumulative risk of a febrile seizure by age 5 years was 4.1%. Cases were compared with two age- and sex-matched controls drawn from the Swedish population register. For most variables studied there were 110 cases and 220 controls. The following factors were not statistically associated with an increased risk of a first febrile seizure: paternal and maternal age, previous maternal reproductive outcome, parity, most prenatal factors except preeclampsia, type of delivery, presentation, fetal heart rate abnormalities, neonatal course, and neonatal hyperbilirubinemia. The only factors associated with febrile seizures were preterm birth (13.6% of cases, 4.2% of controls, $p = 0.01$) and preeclampsia or eclampsia (3.6% vs. 0%, $p = 0.02$). In multivariate analysis only two factors were significantly associated—prematurity and "other than normal mode of presentation at delivery."

F. Bethune *et al.*, 1993—Nova Scotia, Canada

The prospective study by Bethune *et al.* (1993) reported on children presenting with a first febrile seizure to the only pediatric emergency room in a city of about 350,000 (Halifax, Nova Scotia). Seventy-five consecutive children with a first febrile seizure were matched by age and sex to 150 febrile controls and 150 afebrile controls. All controls presented to the emergency department within 10 days of subjects. The authors presumed that all children with a febrile seizure from this community would present to the emergency department. They assumed a 4% incidence that allowed absolute risk estimates. Factors independently associated with febrile seizures were history of febrile seizures in a first- or second-degree relative, attendance at full-time day care, parental perception of slow development in their child, and neonatal discharge after 28 days of age. In the absence of these factors the risk of a febrile seizure was 2.2%. When two or more risk factors were present, the risk of first febrile seizures was 28% (range 20–73%). About 3% of the general population would be expected to have two or more risk factors.

G. Rantala *et al.*, 1995—Oulu, Finland

All children admitted to the Department of Pediatrics, University of Oulu in Oulu, Finland from September, 1986 to May, 1988 with a febrile seizure were matched by age and sex to two other consecutively admitted children who were febrile but without seizures (Rantala *et al.*, 1995). There were 58 patients and 116 controls. Patients were more likely to have exanthem subitum (HHV-6) (5/58 vs. 0/116, $P < 0.05$). Cases were more febrile than controls with an average temperature before admission of 39.4°C vs. 38.8°C ($p < 0.01$).

H. Berg *et al.*, 1995—New York

The case control study by Berg *et al.* (1995) identified 69 children with a first febrile seizure from three inner city hospital emergency departments in New

York. These cases were matched by age and sex with one or two febrile controls (eventually, 99 controls) who received pediatric care at the same institution within 2 weeks. The risk of a febrile seizure nearly doubled for each increase in body temperature in degree Fahrenheit above 101°F. There was a suggestion that febrile seizure patients were more likely to have otitis media and less likely to have gastroenteritis. A family history of febrile seizures in a first-degree relative was noted in 25% of cases and in 5% of controls (OR 7.4). Febrile seizures in more distant relatives and epilepsy in first-degree or more distant relatives were also more common in patients. Prenatal maternal smoking was more common in cases (26% vs 10%) and there was a dose–response curve associating febrile seizures with the number of cigarettes smoked per day. Postnatal exposure to cigarette smoke was not associated with febrile seizures. A variety of other perinatal issues were not related to febrile seizures.

In multivariate analysis, factors remaining significant were temperature, gastroenteritis, family history of febrile seizures in first-degree or second-degree relatives, and any maternal smoking. Day care, shared bedroom, and number of persons in the home were not associated. Sociodemographic factors were not associated; however, because of the matching procedure there was not much opportunity for differences. The lack of association with a family history of epilepsy in the multivariate analysis suggests that the febrile seizure tendency is not just a general susceptibility to seizures but something more specific.

I. GREENWOOD ET AL., 1998—UNITED KINGDOM

The study by Greenwood et al. (1998) examined the prenatal and perinatal records of the children with incident febrile seizures within the British Birth Survey. This cohort was previously studied by Verity with a 5-year follow-up (Verity et al., 1985a,b). In this paper the follow-up was extended to 10 years (94% of the original cohort of 16,163 were reviewed). The number of children with confirmed febrile seizures was 398, accounting for a lifetime incidence of 2.7%.

Multivariate analysis of prenatal and perinatal factors associated with the occurrence of febrile seizures demonstrated progressive associations with highest maternal diastolic pressure and low birth weight and simple associations with one or more maternal prenatal hospital admissions and no breast-feeding. Important nonassociations (with reference to studies noted above) included no association of incident febrile seizures with previous adverse pregnancy outcome (abortions or stillbirths), maternal smoking (nor any trend data), or gestational age.

J. Huang *et al.*, 1999—Taiwan

A very comprehensive survey of all children age 3 years in the Taiwanese city of Taiwan found 256 children with one or more febrile seizures (Huang *et al.*, 1999). Cases were identified by a telephone interview with the families of 10,460 of the 11,129 families with 3-year-old children. They were matched at random with one control from the remainder of the cohort on sex, age, and area of residence. There were no increases in pre- or perinatal problems in cases. Apparently none of the mothers in either group "smoked habitually" during pregnancy, so this factor could not be assessed. Those with febrile seizures were more likely to have delayed development noted prior to the febrile seizure (3.7% vs. 0.4%, $p = 0.05$) and were more likely to have four or more febrile illness/year (33 vs. 23%, $p = 0.02$). Cases were more likely to have at least a first-degree relative with febrile seizures compared to controls (13.8% vs. 4.1%, $p = 0.1$). In a step-wise logistic regression, only family history and number of illnesses remained significant.

III. SYNTHESIS

Based on the literature summarized above, several conclusions seem justified. The most impressive and consistent risk factor for febrile seizures is the presence of a close family history of febrile seizures. The more relatives affected, the greater the risk. Linkage studies have identified at least five different chromosomal loci that are associated with febrile seizures. This is an inherited disorder with a pattern of expression that must be complex! In cohorts of children with a first febrile seizure, the risk that siblings will have febrile seizures is 10–45%, depending on the study (Van Esch *et al.*, 1998). Whether a certain genetic background is necessary for a febrile seizure is not known; however, we suspect that Frantzen (1968) was correct and the disorder is inherited as a dominant with incomplete penetrance (Verity *et al.*, 1985b).

There are a number of factors that may influence the expression of the inherited febrile seizure tendency. Prematurity and delayed neonatal discharge are potential markers for brain injury. Developmental delay also suggests suboptimal brain function. It appears that any acquired or associated brain abnormality further increases the risk of a febrile seizure. It is unclear if such an acquired abnormality is sufficient itself to "cause" a febrile seizure in the absence of a genetic predisposition.

To have a febrile seizure, the child must have a febrile illness. The higher the fever, the higher the risk. HHV-6 appears to be particularly important (Rantala *et al.*, 1995; Barone *et al.*, 1995; Kondo *et al.*, 1995). Gastroenteritis may even be protective in some mysterious fashion (Berg *et al.*, 1995). Children with more frequent infections appear to have more febrile seizures (Huang *et al.*, 1999). There is a substantial literature indicating that children attending day care have increased rates of illness compared to those staying at home (Fleming *et al.*, 1987; Anderson *et al.*, 1988). Attendance at day care in Halifax is probably a way to acquire more infections (Bethune *et al.*, 1993). The density of population in Taiwan may explain why this factor was not present (Huang *et al.*, 1999). Likewise, children in New York may also have increased numbers of infections as a result of the high population density that may have hidden the effect of day care (Berg *et al.*, 1995). Maternal smoking may have an effect similar to that of day care, because there is a correlation between passive smoke exposure and a variety of illnesses in children (Berg *et al.*, 1995; Cassano *et al.*, 1990; Nelson and Ellenberg, 1990). The influence of prenatal versus postnatal cigarette exposure requires more study if there is a need to develop a more compelling argument to stop pregnant women or parents of small children from smoking.

If a child grows through the vulnerable age for febrile seizures without ever having a triggering febrile illness, then an inherited febrile seizure tendency may not be expressed.

IV. HOW DO WE MAKE THIS INFORMATION USEFUL?

The risk factors for febrile seizures reviewed in this chapter are not of much practical value to families. In the Halifax study, a small group of children (about 3% of the population) was identified with a substantial risk of a first febrile seizure (~30%) (Bethune *et al.*, 1993). They had two or more risk factors (first- or second-degree relative with febrile seizures, attendance at day care, slow development, and delayed neonatal hospital discharge). It can be argued that the parents of this small group might benefit from some specific anticipatory guidance, hopefully to reduce the emotional upset of the first febrile seizure. This hypothesis has not been tested directly. Other individual or grouped risk factors are either quite common in the general population or associated with a relatively slight increase in the absolute risk of a febrile seizure (<10%). They are insufficiently predictive to warrant the upset of counselling many families whose children will never have a seizure.

Risk factors provide insight into the pathophysiology of febrile seizures that will eventually yield all the secrets of this common and frightening disorder.

REFERENCES

Anderson L., Parker R., and Strikas R. (1988). Day-care centre attendance and hospitalization for lower respiratory tract illness. *Pediatrics* **82**, 300–308.

Barone, S. R., Kaplan, M. H., and Krilov, L. R. (1995). Human herpesvirus-6 infection in children with first febrile seizures. *J. Pediatr.* 127, 95–97.

Berg, A. T., Shinnar, S., Shapiro, E., Salomon, M. E., Crain, E. F., and Hauser, W. A. (1995). Risk factors for a first febrile seizure: A matched case-control study. *Epilepsia* 36, 334–341.

Bethune, P., Gordon, K. G., Dooley, J. M., Camfield, C. S., and Camfield, P. R. (1993). Which child will have a febrile seizure? *Am. J. Dis. Child.* 147, 35–39.

Cassano, P. A., Koepsell, T. D., and Farwell, J. R. (1990). Risk of febrile seizures in childhood in relation to prenatal maternal cigarette smoking and alcohol intake. *Am. J. Epidemiol.* 132, 462–473.

Fleming, C., Cochi, S., Hightower, A., and Broome, C. (1987). Childhood upper respiratory tract infections: To what degree is incidence affected by day-care attendance? *Pediatrics* 79, 55–60.

Forsgren, L., Sidenvall, R., Blomquist, H. K., Heijbel, J., and Nystrom, L. (1990). An incidence case-referent study of febrile convulsions in children: Genetic and social aspects. *Neuropediatrics* 21, 153–159.

Forsgren, L., Sidenvall, R., Blomquist, H. M., Heijbel, J., and Nystrom, L. (1991). Pre- and perinatal factors in febrile convulsions. *Acta Paediatr. Scand.* 80, 218–225.

Frantzen, E., Lennox-Buchthal, M., Nygaard, A., and Stene, J. (1968). Longitudinal EEG and clinical study of children with febrile convulsions. *Electroencephalogr. Clin. Neurophysiol.* 24, 197–212.

Greenwood, R., Golding, J., Ross, E., and Verity, C. M. (1998). Prenatal and perinatal antecedents of febrile convulsions and afebrile seizures: Data from a national cohort study. *Paediatr. Perinat. Epidemiol.* 12 (Suppl. 1), 76–95.

Hackett, R., Hackett, L., and Bhakta, P. (1997). Febrile seizures in a south Indian district: Incidence and associations. *Dev. Med. Child Neurol.* 39, 380–384.

Huang, C. C., Wang, S. T., Chang, Y. C., Huang, M. C., Chi, Y. C., and Tsai, J. J. (1999). Risk factors for a first febrile convulsion in children: A population study in southern Taiwan. *Epilepsia* 40, 719–725.

Kondo, K., Nagafuji, H., Hata, A., Tomomori, C., and Yamanishi, K. (1993). Association of human herpesvirus 6 infection of the central nervous system with recurrence of febrile convulsions. *J. Infect. Dis.* 167, 1197–1200.

Nelson, K. B., and Ellenberg, J. H. (1976). Predictors of epilepsy in children who have experienced febrile seizures. *N. Engl. J. Med.* 295, 1029–1033.

Nelson, K. B., and Ellenberg, J. H. (1990). Prenatal and perinatal antecedents of febrile seizures. *Ann. Neurol.* 27, 127–131.

Ranatala, H., Uhari, M., and Hietala, J. (1995). Factors triggering the first febrile seizure. *Acta Paediatr.* 84, 407–410.

Tsai, J. J., Huang, M. C., Lung, F. W., Huang, C. C,, and Chang, Y. C. (1996). Differences in factors influencing the familial aggregation of febrile convulsions in population and hospital patients. *Acta Neurol. Scand.* 94, 314–319.

Van den Berg, B. J., and Yerushalmy, J. (1974). Studies on convulsive disorders in young children. *J. Pediatr.* 84, 837–840.

Van Esch, A., Steyerberg, E. W., van Duijin, C. M., Offringa, M., Derksen-Lubsen, G., and van Steensel-Moll, H. A. (1998). Prediction of febrile seizures in siblings: A practical approach. *Neuropediatrics* 157, 340–344.

Verity, C. M., Butler, N. R., and Golding, J. (1985a). Febrile convulsions in a national cohort followed up from birth. I. Prevalence and recurrence in the first five years of life. *BMJ* 290, 1307–1310.

Verity, C. M., Butler, N. R., and Golding, J. (1985b). Febrile convulsions in a national cohort followed up from birth. II. Medical history and intellectual ability at 5 years of age. *BMJ* 290, 1311–1315.

Wallace, S. J. (1972). Aetiological aspects of febrile convulsions. *Arch. Dis. Child.* 47, 171–178.

CHAPTER 3

Recurrent Febrile Seizures

ANNE T. BERG

Department of Biological Sciences, Northern Illinois University,
DeKalb, Illinois 60115

Approximately a third of children who have febrile seizures experience recurrent febrile seizures. Of those who have one recurrence, about half have further recurrences. The first recurrence after an initial febrile seizure usually occurs within a year of the initial seizure. Age is the most important determinant of recurrence risk. The risk is highest in children <12 to 18 months at the time of the initial febrile seizure and decreases as the child gets older. A family history of febrile seizures and a relatively low level of fever are also associated with an increased risk of recurrence. Factors associated with an increased risk of subsequent epilepsy (complex febrile seizures, family history of epilepsy, and neurological abnormalities) are not clearly related to the risk of recurrent febrile seizures per se.

Although complex febrile seizures do not appear to influence the risk of recurrence much if at all, children who have had one prolonged febrile seizure are more likely, if seizures do recur, to have another prolonged febrile seizure. Although treatment is not advocated, especially after a first febrile seizure, the use of abortive therapy (e.g., with diazepam) may be appropriate in children who have experienced a prolonged seizure and who have a high risk of recurrence. © 2002 Academic Press.

I. INTRODUCTION

The good news for families with a child who has experienced a first febrile seizure is that the single most common seizure outcome after a first febrile seizure is not to have another seizure, febrile or otherwise. That having been said, a substantial proportion of children will experience recurrent febrile seizures, and a small percentage will go on to develop unprovoked seizures and epilepsy. The latter group is the subject of Chapter 5. This chapter focuses on the following four issues regarding recurrent febrile seizures:

1. What is the risk that a child will have further febrile seizures and over what time period is this risk the highest?
2. Which factors place a child at high risk of experiencing recurrent febrile seizures?
3. What are the factors associated with having a complex febrile seizure, and do complex features, particularly long duration, tend to recur?
4. What is the value of treatment in reducing recurrence risk?

Throughout this presentation, definitions developed as part of the National Institutes of Health (NIH) Consensus Development Conference on Febrile Seizures (Consensus Development Panel, 1980) and the relevant guidelines of the International League Against Epilepsy (ILAE) (Commission on Classification and Terminology of the International League Against Epilepsy, 1989; Commission on Epidemiology and Prognosis and International League Against Epilepsy, 1993) will be used. Any minor departures or qualifications will be specified.

II. RISK OF A RECURRENT FEBRILE SEIZURE

Numerous studies have examined the question of recurrence risk (Al-Eissa, 1995; Annegers et al., 1990; Berg et al., 1997; El-Radhi, 1998; El-Radhi et al., 1986; Forsgren et al., 1997; Heijbel et al., 1980; Knudsen, 1985a; Kolfen et al., 1998; Nelson and Ellenberg, 1976; Offringa et al., 1992; Rantala and Uhari, 1994; Stanhope et al., 1972; Tarkka et al., 1998; van den Berg, 1974; Verity et al., 1985). For the purposes of obtaining an estimate that can be broadly applicable in the population at large, this presentation deemphasizes results from untreated arms of randomized trials (because the factors that identify children as eligible for or that lead parents to agree to participate in such trials may be related to recurrence risk) and results from studies in which children were all hospitalized (because these generally tend to represent a small proportion of all children with febrile seizures and are likely skewed to represent a more severe outcome). The remaining studies include population-based and birth cohort studies as well as studies that identified and recruited consecutive series of children at the point where they received medical care for the seizure. Taken as a whole, these studies provide a reasonably consistent estimate of the risk of having a first recurrence of between 25 and 40%, with the majority of the estimates hovering within a few points of 35% (Table 1).

The risk of a recurrence varies greatly over time. There are most likely several reasons for this. One of the most obvious is that febrile seizures have a peak occurrence during a developmental window when the brain is most susceptible. The median age at onset for a first febrile seizure is about 18 months. Ap-

TABLE 1   Risk of One or More Febrile Seizure Recurrences in Representative Studies[a]

Study	N	Risk of first recurrence	Risk of second recurrence	Risk of 3+ recurrences
Stanhope et al. (1972)	236	29.2%	NS	NS
van den Berg (1974)	339	38.1%	14.7%	5.0%
Nelson and Ellenberg (1976)	1621	34.1%	16.3%	8.6%
Heijbel et al. (1980)	107	29.9%	14.0%	4.7%
Verity et al. (1985)	290	35.5%	22.1%	13.1%
Annegers et al. (1990)	639	23.2%	*7.0%	*2.8%
Offringa et al. (1992)	155	37.4%	30.3%	25.2%
Berg et al. (1997)	428	31.8%	14.7%	5.8%
Forsgren et al. (1997)	92	42.4%	18.5%	10.9%
Range		23.2–42.4%	7–30.3%	2.8–25.2%
Median		34.1%	15.5%	7.2%
Weighted average		32.2%	15.3%	7.9%

[a]NS, Not stated; *, estimated but not explicitly provided.

proximately 90% of children are under 3 years of age at the time of a first febrile seizure, and it is rare for a first febrile seizure to occur after the age of 5 years (Annegers et al., 1979; Berg et al., 1997; Nelson and Ellenberg, 1976; Nurchi et al., 1982). In fact, some insist that the definition of febrile seizure should preclude seizures with fever occurring after 5 years of age; however, this is by no means universally accepted, and many authors include children with initial onset of febrile seizures after age 5 years (Annegers et al., 1987; Berg et al., 1997; El-Radhi, 1998; Nelson and Ellenberg, 1976; Rantala and Uhari, 1994). The one study to examine this issue did not find evidence to suggest that children who had their febrile seizures after age 5 years, other than being less common, were in fact different from those who had febrile seizures before age 5 years (Webb et al., 1999). For an upper cutoff, it is necessary to refer to the ILAE guidelines (Commission on Classification and Terminology of the International League Against Epilepsy, 1980; Commission on Epidemiology and Prognosis and International League Against Epilepsy, 1993), which define febrile seizures as occurring in childhood. A lower cutoff for adolescence is 10 years of age and thus might be a reasonable upper age cutoff for febrile seizures (Berg et al., 1997, 1999a).

The consequences of the developmental window concept are that, the further away from the initial febrile seizure a child is, and the older he is, the more likely he is to have grown out of the period of susceptibility. Therefore the risk of recurrence decreases with time because of age. Quite consistently across studies, approximately half of all children who have a recurrent febrile seizure do so within the first 6 months of the initial febrile seizure (Annegers *et al.*, 1990; Berg *et al.*, 1997; Offringa *et al.*, 1992, 1994; van den Berg, 1974). Roughly three-quarters of recurrences occur within 1 year, and 90% or more occur within 2 years. These figures are only slightly affected by the fact that follow-up is often truncated after 2 years and frequently is not much more than 3 years. In those studies with follow-up beyond 2 years, the additional risk of recurrence after 2 years is only on the order of a few percent. This represents less than a tenth of the total risk of recurrence.

Of children who have a first recurrence, approximately one-third to one-half will have a second recurrence (Table 1). This represents about 15% of all children with febrile seizures. Another third to a half of those go on to have three or more recurrences. Approximately 10% of children with febrile seizures will have three or more recurrences. As with the first recurrence, the risk of a second recurrence is largely realized within the year immediately following the first recurrence (Annegers *et al.*, 1990; Berg *et al.*, 1997; Offringa *et al.*, 1992, 1994).

III. FACTORS THAT PREDICT A FIRST RECURRENCE

Apart from use of treatment, many factors have been studied as potential predictors of recurrent febrile seizures. The factors that have been examined fall naturally into three categories: (1) factors inherent to the child—age, sex, family history, and neurological/developmental status; (2) factors related to the illness—height of fever, type of illness, and frequency of illness; and (3) the characteristics of the seizure. Although most efforts have addressed prediction of a first recurrence, there is some information about prediction of further recurrences. These two issues will be addressed separately.

A. FACTORS INHERENT TO THE CHILD

1. Age

Age at onset is almost universally found to be associated with the risk of a recurrent febrile seizure (Airede, 1992; Al-Eissa, 1995; Annegers *et al.*, 1990; El-Radhi *et al.*, 1986; Knudsen, 1985b; Laditan, 1994; Nelson and Ellenberg, 1976; Offringa *et al.*, 1992; van den Berg, 1974; van Stuijvenberg *et al.*, 1999; Verity *et al.*, 1985). Specifically, young age at onset is associated with a higher risk of recurrence. Most information is frequently presented in terms of age cutoffs, particularly <12 versus ≥12 months or <18 versus ≥18 months. The risk in the younger group is as much as twice that in the older group (e.g., 40 versus 20%).

In fact, the risk actually seems to decrease continuously with age (Berg *et al.*, 1997; Offringa *et al.*, 1994).

The significance of this finding most likely is a reflection of the fact that children who have their seizure at an early age have more time left during the developmental window of susceptibility in which to have another seizure, compared to children who have their first seizure later in that window. The most informative study to date of this issue is a pooled analysis of five studies that examined the risk of recurrence as a function of attained age; it was found that the risk continuously dropped at a fairly constant rate from about 12 months to 42 months of age and then leveled off thereafter at a very low rate (Offringa *et al.*, 1994). This analysis suggests that a child who had his first febrile seizure at 12 months of age has the same risk of a recurrence once he is (say) 30 months of age as does a child who had his first febrile seizure at 24 months of age.

2. Sex

Although virtually all studies report that male children are more likely to have febrile seizures in the first place, the risk of recurrence once a child has had a febrile seizure is not dependent on the sex of that child (Berg *et al.*, 1997; Offringa *et al.*, 1992, 1994; Rantala and Uhari, 1994; Tarkka *et al.*, 1998).

3. Family History of Febrile Seizures

A history of febrile seizures in a first-degree relative is found by almost all investigators who have examined it to be associated with a 50–100% increase (i.e., up to a doubling) in the risk of recurrent febrile seizures (Annegers *et al.*, 1990; Berg *et al.*, 1997; Offringa *et al.*, 1992, 1994). This finding is of considerable interest because family history of febrile seizures is not predictive of subsequent unprovoked seizures, even though children who have recurrent febrile seizures seem to have an increased risk of developing later unprovoked seizures (Annegers *et al.*, 1979; Berg and Shinnar, 1996b; Nelson and Ellenberg, 1976). In a separate analysis, this paradoxical observation was explored. Children who had recurrent febrile seizures in the absence of factors predictive of recurrence (i.e., were at low risk for febrile seizure recurrence in the first place) were at especially high risk of developing unprovoked seizures. By comparison, those who had recurrent febrile seizures in the presence of risk factors for recurrence (i.e., they were expected to have recurrences) were not at increased risk of having later unprovoked seizures (Berg and Shinnar, 1996b). Among children with febrile seizures, these observations hint at some of the distinctions that we are as yet unable to measure directly. Specifically, they support the notion that some febrile seizures are part of a syndrome quite distinct from epilepsy whereas, in selected cases, febrile seizures may represent the initial expression of epilepsy.

4. Family History of Epilepsy

Relative to family history of febrile seizures, a family history of epilepsy is somewhat less consistently and less strongly associated with the risk of the first febrile seizure recurrence (Berg et al., 1997; Knudsen, 1985a; Offringa et al., 1992, 1994; Rantala and Uhari, 1994; Tarkka et al., 1998). Some studies report no association, others only a modest one. Overall, although some degree of association is not precluded by the available evidence, the prognostic significance of a family history of epilepsy appears to be less than for a family history of febrile seizures for predicting the risk of recurrent febrile seizures; however, as discussed in Chapter 5, this factor is related to subsequent unprovoked seizures and epilepsy.

5. Neurodevelopmental Abnormalities

Children who are recognized as being developmentally delayed or having frank neurological abnormalities may have some increased likelihood of further febrile seizures; however, the data are inconsistent (Berg et al., 1997; Knudsen, 1985b; Nelson and Ellenberg, 1976, 1978; Wolf et al., 1977). More importantly, children with neurological abnormalities are at increased risk of later epilepsy (Annegers et al., 1979; Berg and Shinnar, 1996b; Nelson and Ellenberg, 1976; Tsai and Hung, 1995). For this reason, febrile seizures raise more concerns in a child who is already developmentally compromised.

B. FACTORS ASSOCIATED WITH THE ILLNESS

1. Temperature

The best-studied factor related to the illness is temperature at the time of the initial febrile seizure, which has been found in most studies to be an important predictor of recurrence. Specifically, children whose initial febrile seizure occurred in conjunction with a relatively modest degree of fever are more likely to experience recurrences than are children with more severe fevers. This factor was first reported by El-Radhi and co-workers (1986), who found that the risk of recurrence was several times higher in those whose first febrile seizure occurred in conjunction with a fever <40°C compared to those with higher temperatures. Subsequently, other studies have replicated this general finding (Al-Eissa, 1995; Berg et al., 1997; El-Radhi, 1998; Laditan, 1994; Offringa et al., 1992), although the strength of association has tended to be less dramatic than that initially reported by El-Radhi. In addition, a few studies have not found temperature to be related to recurrence risk (Rantala and Uhari, 1994; Tarkka et al., 1998) or the results have been difficult to interpret (Airede, 1992). Most investigators have considered temperature $<40°C$ versus $\geq40°C$, although one study examined this factor along more of a continuum (Berg *et al.*, 1997) and found that the lower the temperature as measured at or near the time of the initial febrile seizure, the higher the risk of recurrence.

One obvious interpretation of this finding is that children who have seizures in response to a low degree of fever have a lower threshold and therefore have seizures with less provocation than do children who require a higher degree of fever. Fascinating as this appears, it is difficult to study rigorously, because most children's true temperatures are unknown at the time of the seizure and we must rely on either measurements made at home and reported by understandably stressed parents or on measurements made once the child is seen after the seizure. Given the considerable degree of potential error in measuring height of fever at the exact time of the seizure, it is remarkable that this factor is so strongly and consistently associated with recurrence. This suggests the association may be even stronger than it appears.

2. Rate of Rise of Fever

In the past, a rapid onset of fever was thought to be the precipitating factor in febrile seizures, although this is probably not the case (Berg, 1993). This factor is extremely difficult to measure and has not been directly studied in naturally occurring febrile seizures in children. Instead, one study examined the duration of recognized fever prior to the initial febrile seizure (Berg, 1993). A brief period (<1 hour) of recognized fever prior to the initial febrile seizure was associated with a doubling in the risk of recurrent febrile seizures. Of interest, in this study it was the only risk factor identified that was associated with both recurrent febrile and subsequent unprovoked seizures (Berg and Shinnar, 1996b). The significance of this finding is unclear but it may reflect a certain degree of underlying hyperexcitability. Further interpretation should be deferred until others replicate the finding; however, the finding goes against earlier ideas that seizures that occur during the initial onset of temperature are those that are most likely to be the most benign (Livingston *et al.*, 1979).

3. Type of Illness

Most febrile seizures occur in conjunction with a respiratory illness (Berg *et al.*, 1995; Farwell *et al.*, 1994; Nurchi *et al.*, 1982; Rantala and Uhari, 1994; Tarkka *et al.*, 1998). The evidence is conflicting as to whether the type of illness may be associated with whether a febrile seizure occurs or not during a specific illness episode (Berg *et al.*, 1995; Rantala *et al.*, 1995). Only one study has examined whether the risk of recurrence varies with the type of underlying illness for the first febrile seizure. The authors concluded it did not (Rantala *et al.*, 1990).

4. Illness Frequency

It makes sense that a child's risk will be higher if there are more opportunities to have a febrile seizure. Such an association has been reported in at least one study of risk factors for a first febrile seizure (Huang *et al.*, 1999). At least four studies have succeeded in examining illness frequency and its relation to recurrence risk (Knudsen, 1988; Rantala *et al.*, 1995; Tarkka *et al.*, 1998; van Stuijvenberg *et al.*, 1999). All found a very strong effect of the number of subsequent illnesses on the risk of recurrence. One study estimated that each subsequent febrile illness increased the relative risk of recurrence by 18% (Tarkka *et al.*, 1998). Another study found that having four or more subsequent febrile illnesses was associated with more than fourfold increase in the risk of recurrence compared with children who had fewer subsequent febrile illnesses (Knudsen, 1988).

5. Daycare Attendance

Related to illness frequency are social conditions that influence illness frequency. Young children who attend daycare get sick more often than do children who stay at home (Berg *et al.*, 1991). To the extent that daycare attendance has been found to be associated with an increased risk of both the initial febrile seizures (Bethune *et al.*, 1993) and of recurrent febrile seizures (Knudsen, 1985a, 1988), it is most likely because of the increased number of illnesses. It is highly doubtful, based on what is known at this point, that daycare attendance poses any additional risk in and of itself. Other factors, such as crowding in the home, environmental tobacco smoke, and number of children in the home, have not been carefully examined as risk factors for recurrent febrile seizures. Teasing apart the contributions of these and other related factors would be extremely difficult. At the present and based on what we understand, it is reasonable to assume that their influences most likely lie along the same causal pathway as illness frequency.

These observations have some potential public health implications for preventing febrile seizures; however, there are numerous other factors that need to be considered in developing a rational and balanced approach to this issue.

C. Characteristics of the Seizure

There are three characteristics of a febrile seizure that may cause heightened concern: focality, prolonged duration, and recurrence within the same illness episode (typically within 24 hours). Predictors of having a complex recurrence will be discussed separately. With respect to their prognostic value in predicting recurrent febrile seizures, the bulk of the evidence suggests that they have little or no significance for recurrence of febrile seizures. Some studies find no association at all (Berg *et al.*, 1997; Knudsen, 1985b) whereas others find modest associations overall or for selected complex features (Offringa *et al.*, 1994). Complex features are important, however, in predicting later unprovoked seizures and epilepsy (Annegers *et al.*, 1987; Berg and Shinnar, 1996b; Nelson and Ellenberg, 1976; Tsai and Hung, 1995).

1. Prediction of a First Recurrence

With the use of this information, it is possible to estimate the risk that a given child will experience at least one recurrence. This has been done in a few studies with clear distinctions made between children with very low and very high risks of recurrence. For example, if we consider only the three risk factors that have been reasonably well established in the literature, young age at onset (<18 months), lower degree of fever [$<104°F$ ($40°C$)], and a positive family history of febrile seizures, the estimated risk of recurrence is only 15% for children with none of these risk factors and 27, 39, and 65% for children with one, two, and three risk factors (Berg *et al.*, 1997).

2. Subsequent Recurrences

Obviously those children at increased risk of a first recurrence are, by definition, those at increased risk of more than one recurrence. In those studies that have examined factors predictive of a second recurrence conditional on having had a first recurrence, age again seems to play an overwhelming role (Berg *et al.*, 1997; Offringa *et al.*, 1992, 1994). In this case, it is the age at the time of the first recurrence and not at the time of the initial seizure, as suggested above in the discussion of age and first recurrence. Thus, the younger a child at the time of a first recurrence, the higher the risk. Although this is also consistent with closely spaced seizures being a risk factor for subsequent seizures (Berg *et al.*, 2001; Shinnar *et al.*, 2000), the obvious importance of timing within the developmental window of susceptibility cannot be overlooked and is probably the key factor in most children.

3. Family History

A family history of either febrile seizures or of epilepsy may also increase the risk of a second recurrence after a first recurrence (Berg *et al.*, 1997; Offringa *et al.*, 1994). There are few data on this and inconsistencies in what is available.

4. Several Recurrences

Estimation of the risk of having two or three or more recurrent seizures, based on risk factors determined at the time of the initial febrile seizure, has been presented in at least one study (Berg et al., 1997). Based on age (<18 months at first febrile seizure), height of fever (<104°F), and a positive family history, those with no risk factors for recurrence have only a 3% risk of two or more recurrences whereas those with one, two, and three risk factors have risks of 8, 19, and 50%. Three or more recurrences occurred in none of those with no risk factors, and in 3, 9, and 15% of those with one, two, and three risk factors.

IV. COMPLEX FEATURES

Complex features of febrile seizures are important because they are associated with an increased risk of subsequent epilepsy (Annegers et al., 1987; Berg and Shinnar, 1996b; Nelson and Ellenberg, 1976; Tsai and Hung, 1995). The three characteristics of concern are focal seizures, multiple seizures (i.e., seizures that recur within a single illness episode, generally within a 24-hour period), and prolonged seizures.

Very prolonged seizures raise concerns of their own. The definition of "prolonged" varies. A seizure ≥10 minutes in duration is a minimal definition (Annegers et al., 1987; Berg et al., 1997; Wolf et al., 1977). The NIH Consensus Development Conference refers to 15 minutes (Consensus Development Panel, 1980). Other investigators use 20 minutes (Camfield et al., 1994). The proportion of children reported to have a first febrile seizure that is prolonged varies somewhat from study to study. Some of the differences may be due to methods for recruiting patients (i.e., sampling issues). For example, studies that considered only hospitalized patients may be weighted toward those with more severe seizures (e.g., status epilepticus). In addition, however, some of the discrepancies may be due to methodological differences in how seizure information was obtained (i.e., measurement issues) (Berg et al., 1992, 1993). Prospective studies that collected specific information necessary to identify complex features from the parents immediately after the seizure may find a higher rate than studies that relied only on medical chart review. Other factors may also play a role. Overall, and bearing in mind the considerable discrepancies across studies, approximately a quarter to a third of first febrile seizures have one or more complex features.

A few studies have provided information about factors associated with whether the initial febrile seizure is complex or simple (Al-Elissa et al., 1992; Berg and Shinnar, 1996a; Farwell et al., 1994; Verity et al., 1985). All found a tendency for complex features to be present in younger children (generally <12 months). One study found both prolonged and multiple seizures associated with young age (Farwell *et al.*, 1994), whereas another found the association primarily for prolonged seizures with a nonsignificant association for focal seizures (Berg and Shinnar, 1996a). Another group examined the type of underlying illness and reported that it was not associated with whether the initial seizure was simple or complex (Rantala *et al.*, 1990).

The more febrile seizures a child has had the greater the likelihood that one was complex (Berg and Shinnar, 1996a). In addition, it appears that factors associated with having a recurrent febrile seizure (age at onset, family history of febrile seizures, height of fever) did not strongly, if at all, influence the likelihood that the recurrence was complex, either overall or for specific complex features (Berg and Shinnar, 1996a). The most striking finding was that children with an initial prolonged seizure tended, if they had more seizures, to have prolonged recurrences. This tendency for the length of an individual's seizures to be consistent over time has since been examined in greater detail in the context of unprovoked seizures (Shinnar *et al.*, 1997). In addition, several reports have also since found that status epilepticus per se has a tendency to recur (Berg *et al.*, 1999b; Novak *et al.*, 1997; Shinnar *et al.*, 1996, 2001). Finally, one twin study has found a significant concordance for status epilepticus (Corey *et al.*, 1998). Thus, even though the duration of the initial seizure does not appear to influence whether additional seizures occur, if additional seizures do occur, their duration will depend heavily on the duration of the initial seizure.

By combining information about risk factors for recurrence with information about the duration of the initial seizure, children with very low (<5%) and very high (~70%) risk of a subsequent prolonged febrile seizure can be identified (Berg *et al.*, 1997).

V. THE ROLE OF TREATMENT IN REDUCING RISK

In the past, there has been much interest in preventing febrile seizures either by continuous treatment with a drug, typically phenobarbital (Farwell *et al.*, 1990; Wolf *et al.*, 1977), or with intermittent treatment at the time of a recognized illness with a drug such as diazepam (Knudsen, 1985a; Rosman *et al.*, 1993a). Most studies do show some degree of effectiveness of both of these approaches in preventing recurrent febrile seizures, with relative reductions in recurrence risk between 33% (Rosman *et al.*, 1993a) and 75% (Wolf *et al.*, 1977). Neither approach, however, is without side-effects (Camfield *et al.*, 1979), neither is entirely effective, and long-term outcomes such as subsequent epilepsy and educational and neuropsychological outcomes do not seem to be influenced for the better by early treatment and prevention of febrile seizures (Knudsen *et al.*,

TABLE 2   Effect of Treatment on the Risk of Recurrent Febrile Seizures and Subsequent
Unprovoked Seizures or Epilepsy: Data from Three Randomized Clinical Trials

	Recurrent febrile seizures		Later unprovoked seizures/epilepsy	
Study	Treated (%)	Control (%)	Treated (%)	Control (%)
Knudsen (1985b), Knudsen *et al.* (1996)	12	39	3	3
Wolf *et al.* (1977), Wolf and Forsythe (1989)	8	30	5	1
Rosman *et al.* (1993a,b)	21	31	5	5

1996; Rosman *et al.*, 1993b; Wolf and Forsythe, 1989). In fact, three randomized clinical trials have demonstrated substantial reductions in recurrent febrile
seizures as a result of treatment but have also shown that prevention of febrile
seizures does not alter the subsequent risk of later developing unprovoked
seizures or epilepsy (see Table 2).

Several writers in the field have urged that the parental anxiety associated
with having a child with febrile seizures and the fear associated with this should
be treated through education and reassurance, not with drugs prescribed to the
child (Camfield *et al.*, 1995; Freeman, 1990, 1992; Lee, 1994; Newton, 1988;
and see Chapter 20). Although there are certainly some rare exceptions, the preferred approach is currently not to treat children who present with a first febrile
seizure. This topic is discussed in greater detail in Chapter 19.

VI. SUMMARY

Approximately a third of children who have an initial febrile seizure will have
at least one recurrence. Over half of the risk is realized during the first year immediately after the initial febrile seizure. More than 90% of children who recur
do so within 2 years. Age is the single strongest and most consistent determinant of the risk of recurrence. The risk of recurrence drops off continuously as
children get older. Family history of febrile seizures and a relatively low degree
of fever may be associated with a 1.5- to 2-fold increase in risk. Children who
experience many febrile illnesses are also at increased risk because of the greater
opportunity for having a febrile seizure.

A third to a half of those who recur have more than one recurrence. Age appears to be the single most important determinant of multiple recurrences, both
for predicting at the time of the initial febrile seizure and after recurrent
seizures. Additional factors such as a family history of epilepsy may also play a
role in those children who have already experienced at least one recurrence.

Factors that are often discussed but that are not as clearly associated with the risk of febrile seizure recurrence include complex features, neurological abnormalities, and family history of epilepsy. The available data, sometimes substantial, simply do not consistently indicate a strong association, if any, between these factors and recurrence, although they are important for their association with subsequent unprovoked seizures and epilepsy.

After the absolute risk of recurrence, perhaps the next most important piece of information for parents and physicians is that children who have an initial prolonged seizure tend to, if they have further seizures, have prolonged seizures again. Although treatment is generally considered unnecessary, especially after a first seizure, those children who have experienced very prolonged seizures, especially if they are at high risk of recurrent febrile seizures, are those whose parents might be given the option of abortive therapy to be used only in the event of a future seizure.

REFERENCES

Airede, A. I. (1992). Febrile convulsions: Factors and recurrence rate. *Trop. Geogr. Med.* **44**, 233–237.

Al-Eissa, Y. A. (1995). Febrile seizures: Rate and risk factors of recurrence. *J. Child Neurol.* **10**, 315–319.

Al-Elissa, Y. A., Al-Omair, A. O., Al-Herbish, A. S., Al-Jarallah, A. A., and Familusi, J. B. (1992). Antecedents and outcome of simple and complex febrile convulsions among Saudi Children. *Dev. Med. Child Neurol.* **34**, 1085–1090.

Annegers, J. F., Hauser, W. A., Elveback, L. R., and Kurland, L. T. (1979). The risk of epilepsy following febrile convulsions. *Neurology* **29**, 297–303.

Annegers, J. F., Hauser, W. A., Shirts, S. B., and Kurland, L. T. (1987). Factors prognostic of unprovoked seizures after febrile convulsions. *N. Engl. J. Med.* **316**, 493–498.

Annegers, J. F., Blakley, S. A., Hauser, W. A., and Kurland, L. T. (1990). Recurrence of febrile convulsions in a population-based cohort. *Epilepsy Res.* **5**, 209–216.

Berg, A. T. (1993). Are febrile seizures provoked by a rapid rise in temperature? *Am. J. Dis. Child.* **147**, 1101–1103.

Berg, A. T., and Shinnar, S. (1996a). Complex febrile seizures. *Epilepsia* **37**, 126–133.

Berg, A. T., and Shinnar, S. (1996b). Unprovoked seizures in children with febrile seizures: Short-term outcome. *Neurology* **47**, 562–568.

Berg, A. T., Shapiro, E. D., and Capobioanco, L. A. (1991). Group day care and the risk of serious infections illness. *Am. J. Epidemiol.* **133**, 154–163.

Berg, A. T., Steinschneider, M., Kang, H., and Shinnar, S. (1992). Classification of complex features of febrile seizures: Interrater agreement. *Epilepsia* **33**, 661–666.

Berg, A. T., Kang, H., Steinschneider, M., and Shinnar, S. (1993). Identifying complex features of febrile seizures: Medical record review versus medical record plus interview. *J. Epilepsy* **6**, 133–138.

Berg, A. T., Shinnar, S., Shapiro, E. D., Salomon, M. E., Crain, E. F., and Hauser, W. A. (1995). Risk factors for a first febrile seizure: A matched case-control study. *Epilepsia* **36**, 334–341.

Berg, A. T., Shinnar, S., Darefsky, A. S., Holford, T. R., Shapiro, E. D., Salomon, M. E., Crain, E. F., and Hauser, W. A. (1997). Predictors of recurrent febrile seizures: A prospective cohort study. *Arch. Pediatr. Adolesc. Med.* **151**, 371–378.

Berg, A. T., Shinnar, S., Levy, S. R., and Testa, F. M. (1999a). Childhood-onset epilepsy with and without preceding febrile seizures. *Neurology* 53, 1742–1748.

Berg, A. T., Shinnar, S., Levy, S. R., and Testa, F. M. (1999b). Status epilepticus in children with newly diagnosed epilepsy. *Ann. Neurol.* 45, 618–623.

Berg, A. T., Shinnar, S., Levy, S. R., Testa, F. M., Smith-Rapaport, S., and Beckerman, B. (2001). Early development of intractable epilepsy in children: A prospective study. *Neurology* 56, 1445–1552.

Bethune, P., Gordon, K., Dooley, J., Camfield, C., and Camfield, P. (1993). Which child will have a febrile seizure? *Am. J. Dis. Child.* 147, 35–39.

Camfield, C. S., Chaplin, S., Doyle, A., Shapiro, S. H., Cummings, C., and Camfield, P. R. (1979). Side effects of phenobarbital in toddlers; behavioral and cognitive aspects. *J. Pediatr.* 95, 361–365.

Camfield, P., Camfield, C., Gordon, K., and Dooley, J. (1994). What types of epilepsy are preceded by febrile seizures? A population-based study of children. *Dev. Med. Child Neurol.* 36, 887–892.

Camfield, P. R., Camfield, C. S., Gordon, K., and Dooley, J. M. (1995). Prevention of recurrent febrile seizures. *J. Pediatr.* 126, 929–930.

Commission on Classification and Terminology of the International League Against Epilepsy (1989). Proposal for revised classification of epilepsies and epileptic syndromes. *Epilepsia* 30, 389–399.

Commission on Epidemiology and Prognosis, and International League Against Epilepsy (1993). Guidelines for epidemiologic studies on epilepsy. *Epilepsia* 34, 592–596.

Consensus Development Panel (1980). Long-term management of children with fever-associated seizures. *Pediatrics* 66, 1009–1012.

Corey, L. A., Pellock, J. M., Boggs, J. G., Miller, L. L., and DeLorenzo, R. J. (1993). Evidence for a genetic predisposition for status epilepticus. *Neurology* 50, 558–560.

El-Radhi, A. S. (1998). Lower degree of fever at the initial febrile convulsion is associated with an increased risk of subsequent convulsions. *Eur. J. Paediatr. Neurol.* 2, 91–96.

El-Radhi, A. S., Withana, K., and Banajeh, S. (1986). Recurrence rate of febrile convulsion related to the degree of pyrexia during the first attack. *Clin. Pediatr.* 25, 311–313.

Farwell, J. R., Lee, Y. J., Hirtz, D. G., Sulzbacher, S. I., Ellenberg, J. H., and Nelson, K. B. (1990). Phenobarbital for febrile seizures—Effects on intelligence and on seizure recurrence. *N. Engl. J. Med.* 322, 364–369.

Farwell, J. R., Blackner, G., Sulzbacher, S., Adelman, L., and Voeller, M. (1994). First febrile seizures characteristics of the child, the seizure, and the illness. *Clin. Pediatr.* 33, 263–267.

Forsgren, L., Heijbel, J., Nystrom, L., and Sidenvall, R. (1997). A follow-up of an incident case-referent study of febrile convulsions seven years after the onset. *Seizure* 6, 21–26.

Freeman, J. M. (1990). Just say no! Drugs and febrile seizures. *Pediatrics* 86, 624.

Freeman, J. M. (1992). The best medicine for febrile seizures. *N. Engl. J. Med.* 327, 1161–1162.

Heijbel, J., Blom, S., and Bergfors, P. G. (1980). Simple febrile convulsions. A prospective incidence study and an evaluation of investigations intially needed. *Neuropaediatrics* 11, 45–56.

Huang, C.-C., Wang, S.-T., Chang, Y.-C., Huang, M.-C., Chi, Y.-C., and Tsai, J.-J. (1999). Risk factors for a first febrile convulsion in children: A population study in southern Taiwan. *Epilepsia* 40, 719–725.

Knudsen, F. U. (1985a). Effective short-term diazepam prophylaxis in febrile convulsions. *J. Pediatr.* 106, 487–490.

Knudsen, F. U. (1985b). Recurrence risk after a first febrile seizure and effect of short-term diazepam prophylaxis. *Arch. Dis. Child.* 60, 1045–1049.

Knudsen, F. U. (1988). Frequent febrile episodes and recurrent febrile convulsions. *Acta Neurol. Scand.* 78, 414–417.

Knudsen, F. U., Paerregaard, A., Andersen, R., and Andresen, J. (1996). Long term outcome of prophylaxis for febrile convulsions. *Arch. Dis. Child.* 74, 13–18.

Kolfen, W., Pehle, K., and Konig, S. (1998). Is the long-term outcome of children following febrile convulsions favorable? *Dev. Med. Child Neurol.* **40**, 667–671.

Laditan, A. A. O. (1994). Seizure recurrence after a first febrile convulsion. *Ann. Trop. Paediatr.* **14**, 303–308.

Lee, W. L. (1994). Febrile seizures: A new look at an old controversy. *Ann. Acad. Med. Singapore* **23**, 387–390.

Livingston, S., Pauli, L. L., Irving, P., and Kramer, I. (1979). Febrile convulsions: Diagnosis, treatment, and prognosis. *Pediatr. Ann.* **8**, 133–153.

Nelson, K. B., and Ellenberg, J. H. (1976). Predictors of epilepsy in children who have experienced febrile seizures. *N. Engl. J. Med.* **295**, 1029–1033.

Nelson, K. B., and Ellenberg, J. H. (1978). Prognosis in children with febrile seizures. *Pediatrics* **61**, 720–727.

Newton, R. W. (1988). Subsequent management of children with febrile convulsions. *Dev. Med. Child Neurol.* **30**, 402–405.

Novak, G., Maytal, J., Alshansky, A., and Ascher, C. (1997). Risk factors for status epilepticus in children with symptomatic epilepsy. *Neurology* **49**, 533–537.

Nurchi, A. M., Cappai, A., and Repetto, C. (1982). Le convulsioni febbrili—semplici o benigne—valutazioni clinico-statistiche. *Minerva Pediatr.* **34**, 179–183.

Offringa, M., Derksen-Lubsen, G., Bossuyt, P. M., and Lubsen, J. (1992). Seizure recurrence after a first febrile seizure: A multivariate approach. *Dev. Med. Child Neurol.* **34**, 15–24.

Offringa, M., Bossuyt, P. M. M., Lubsen, J., Ellenberg, J. H., Nelson, K. B., Knudsen, F. U., Annegers, J. F., El-Radhi, A., S. M., Habbema, J. D. F., Derksen-Lubsen, G., Hauser, W. A., Kurland, L. T., Banajeh, S. M. A., and Larsen, S. (1994). Risk factors for seizure recurrence in children with febrile seizures: A pooled analysis of individual patient data from five studies. *J. Pediatr.* **124**, 574–584.

Rantala, H., and Uhari, M. (1994). Risk factors for recurrences of febrile convulsions. *Acta Neurol. Scand.* **90**, 207–210.

Rantala, H., Uhari, M., and Tuokko, H. (1990). Viral infections and recurrences of febrile convulsions. *J. Pediatr.* **116**, 195–199.

Rantala, H., Uhari, M., and Hietala, J. (1995). Factors triggering the first febrile seizure. *Acta Paediatr.* **84**, 407–410.

Rosman, N. P., Colton, T., Labazzo, J., Gilbert, P. L., Gardella, N. B., Kaye, E. M., Van Bennekom, C., and Winter, M. R. (1993a). A controlled trial of diazepam administered during febrile illnesses to prevent recurrence of febrile seizures. *N. Engl. J. Med.* **329**, 79–94.

Rosman, N. P., Labazzo, J., and Colton, T. (1993b). Factors predisposing to afebrile seizures after febrile convulsions and preventive treatment. *Ann. Neurol.* **34**, 452.

Shinnar, S., Berg, A. T., Moshe, S. L., O'Dell, C., Alemany, M., Newstein, D., Kang, H., Goldensohn, E. S., and Hauser, W. A. (1996). The risk of seizure recurrence after a first unprovoked afebrile seizure in childhood: An extended follow-up. *Pediatrics* **98**, 216–225.

Shinnar, S., Berg, A. T., Moshe, S. L., O'Dell, C., and Shinnar, R. (1997). How long do seizures last in children with new-onset seizures? *Epilepsia* **38** (Suppl. 8), 225.

Shinnar, S., Berg, A. T., O'Dell, C., Newstein, D., Moshe, S. L., and Hauser, W. A. (2000). Predictors of multiple seizures in a cohort of children prospectively followed from the time of their first unprovoked seizure. *Ann. Neurol.* **48**, 140–147.

Shinnar, S., Berg, A. T., Treiman, D., Hauser, W. A., Hesdorffer, D. C., Sackellares, J. C., Leppik, I., Sillanpaa, M., and Sommerville, K. W. (2001). Status epilepticus and tiagabine therapy: Review of safety data and epidemiologic comparisons. *Epilepsia* **42**, 372–379.

Stanhope, J. M., Brody, J. A., Brink, E., and Morris, C. E. (1972). Convulsions among the Chamorro people of Guam, Mariana Islands. II. Febrile convulsions. *Am. J. Epidemiol.* **95**, 299–304.

Tarkka, R., Rantala, H., Uhari, M., and Pokka, T. (1998). Risk of recurrence and outcome after the first febrile seizure. *Pediatr. Neurol.* **18**, 218–220.

Tsai, M. L., and Hung, K. L. (1995). Risk factors for subsequent epilepsy after febrile convulsions. *J. Formos. Med. Assoc.* **94**, 327–331.

van den Berg, B. J. (1974). Studies on convulsive disorders in young children. III. Recurrence of febrile convulsions. *Epilepsia* **15**, 177–190.

van Stuijvenberg, M., Jansen, N. E., Steyerberg, E. W., Derek-Lubsen, G., and Moll, H. A. (1999). Frequency of fever episodes related to febrile seizure recurrence. *Acta Paediatr.* **88**, 52–55.

Verity, C. M., Butler, N. R., and Golding, J. (1985). Febrile convulsions in a national cohort followed up from birth. I. Prevalence and recurrence in the first five years of life. *Br. Med. J.* **290**, 1307–1310.

Webb, D. W., Jones, R. R., Anzur, A. Y., and Farrell, K. (1999). Retrospective study of late febrile seizures. *Pediatr. Neurol.* **20**, 270–273.

Wolf, S. M., and Forsythe, A. (1989). Epilepsy and mental retardation following febrile seizures in childhood. *Acta. Paediatr. Scand.* **78**, 291–295.

Wolf, S. M., Carr, A., Davis, D. C., Davidson, S., Dale, E. P., Forsythe, A., Goldenberg, E., Hanson, R., Lulejian, G. A., Nelson, M. A., Treitmen, P., and Weinstein, A. (1977). The value of phenobarbital in the child who has had a single febrile seizure: A controlled prospective study. *Pediatrics* **59**, 378–385.

CHAPTER 4

Cognitive Outcome of Febrile Seizures

DEBORAH HIRTZ

National Institutes of Health, Bethesda, Maryland 20852

Febrile seizures were once thought to carry a risk of long-term sequelae with regard to intellectual and behavioral function, but this has not
been borne out by long-term studies of population-based cohorts. Of six
population-based study series of children with febrile seizures, only one
reported an excess of neurological problems. Behavioral sequelae have
not been studied as extensively but appear to be minimal. There seems to
be a tendency for children with febrile seizures to have sleep problems.
Animal models indicate that the immature brain may be relatively resistant to seizure-induced neuronal cell death and/or associated neurological deficits. In general, the susceptibility to seizures that accompany a rise
in body temperature in a toddler or young child is a benign phenomenon
without any adverse long-term effects on cognition and behavior. © 2002
Academic Press.

I. INTRODUCTION

Although at one time febrile seizures were thought to be accompanied by a risk
of later cognitive impairment, the consequences of febrile seizures for a child's
intellectual and behavioral development have now been demonstrated to be
small or nonexistent. Early reports citing a significant risk of intellectual dysfunction after febrile seizures (Aicardi and Chevrie, 1976; Smith and Wallace,
1982; Lennox, 1949; Schiottz-Christensen and Bruhn, 1973) were drawn from
selected referral or hospitalized populations. Subsequent large, population-
based studies have not demonstrated long-term neurologic or behavioral
deficits (Verity *et al.*, 1985a,b, 1988; Ross *et al.*, 1980; Nelson and Ellenberg,
1978; Chang *et al.*, 2000).

II. ANIMAL STUDIES

Febrile seizures occur in 2–4% of young children, are more common than any other seizure disorder of childhood, and indicate an age-related susceptibility. The concern has been that these seizures occur at a key stage of development and therefore may modify brain maturation, leading to neurodevelopmental deficits. Some evidence indicates that certain seizures can cause neuronal injury in the immature brain (Thompson *et al.*, 1998). In one rat model of febrile seizures, transient injury to limbic neuronal populations (Toth *et al.*, 1998) was associated with selective and long-lasting presynaptic increase in inhibitory synaptic transmission in the hippocampus (Chen *et al.*, 1999). However, the consequences of this long-lasting effect in the absence of permanent neuronal damage are not known and may not result in changes in cognition or behavior. Although the authors felt that their data indicated that early-life febrile seizures might lead to persistent effects on neuronal excitability, the mechanisms by which this change may modify subsequent cognitive development are not clear. Other experimental evidence indicates a relative lack of seizure-induced cell death or neuronal injury in the immature brain (Jensen, 1999; Sperber, 1996; Holmes, 1997). It is not known why the immature brain is relatively resistant to seizure-induced neuronal cell death. It is possible that neurotrophic factors present in the developing brain protect against excitotoxic injury (Ghosh *et al.*, 1994; Jensen, 1999).

III. HUMAN STUDIES

A. EARLY EVIDENCE

Earlier series, which found a significant number of children with febrile seizures had later intellectual dysfunction, did not exclude children with prior abnormalities and acute central nervous system (CNS) infection at the time of the seizures. The earliest reports included infantile convulsions of a mixed etiology and type. Neurological status prior to the onset of any febrile convulsions was not known or taken into account, and bias was incurred by examining a selected referral population (Lennox, 1949; Aicardi and Chevrie, 1976; Wallace and Cull, 1979). In a study of monozygotic twins, one of whom had febrile seizures, Schiottz-Christensen and Bruhn (1973) showed and average decrease in IQ score of seven points and more neurological soft signs in the twin who had experienced febrile seizures. There was no relationship to birth factors or to features of the seizure. It was not known if the affected twin had a normal neurodevelopmental examination before any febrile seizure occurred. In a series reported by Smith and Wallace (1982), children with recurrent febrile seizures had lower developmental quotients than those with single febrile seizures, but baseline characteristics were not comparable in the two groups.

Some retrospective reports of highly selected referral groups indicated that mesial temporal sclerosis was associated with a history of prolonged febrile convulsions (Falconer, 1974). In other surgical series (Rasmussen, 1979), when febrile convulsions preceded complex febrile seizures, there was usually an infectious etiology or preexisting neurological disease. For these children, febrile seizures may be the initial manifestation of a seizure disorder, and may be the expression of preexisting brain abnormality, rather than the cause of later brain dysfunction.

B. LARGER POPULATION-BASED SERIES

Although a modest increase in the risk for epilepsy has been documented following convulsions, the absolute risk is still less than 5% (Hirtz, 1997; see also Chapter 5). Almost all of the recent population-based studies did not find an increase in risk of unfavorable neurodevelopmental outcome. In a very large prospective series including 431 sibling pairs with one child with febrile seizures, Ellenberg and Nelson (1978) compared febrile seizure patients with their normal siblings on IQ testing using the Wechsler Intelligence Scales for Children (WISC). Also, the Wide Range Achievement Test (WRAT) was given to determine academic achievement. No difference was noted on IQ or academic performance at age 7 years in those children who had had neither a definite nor a suspected neurodevelopmental abnormality prior to the first febrile seizure. Some deficits were found in children who developed later nonfebrile seizures, particularly in those with later minor motor epilepsy. However, many of these children were developmentally abnormal before any seizure occurred.

In the National Child Development Study in Great Britain (Ross et al., 1980), a large prospective cohort, academic performance was not impaired in children of school age who had a history of febrile convulsions. These children were tested at ages 7 and 11 years. In a subsequent British cohort study, children with febrile convulsions were evaluated at age 5 years and again at age 10 years (Verity et al., 1985b, 1998). For the 5-year outcome, there was no difference in children with and without a history of febrile convulsions in performance on two intellectual tests: the English Picture Vocabulary Test and the Copying Design Score. Children with febrile seizures were more likely to have had speech therapy, but the numbers were too small to be significant. This may have been linked to the fact that there were more children with febrile convulsions suspected of having a hearing problem, and the group was also more likely to have a history suggestive of otitis media. There was no difference in height or head circumference between the two groups. These children were also comprehensively assessed at age 10 years. Sixteen children with documented neurodevelopmental problems before the first febrile convulsion and one atypical case were excluded; 381 children with febrile convulsions were compared at age 10 years to the rest of the cohort on measures of academic progress, intelligence, and behavior. The results of 4 of the 102 measures of academic progress, intelligence, and behavior showed a difference between the febrile seizure group and the entire group, no more than would be expected by chance alone. This result was not affected by whether the convulsions were simple, complex, single, or recurrent.

A Danish cohort of 289 children with febrile seizures randomized in early childhood to two different treatment regimes did not show abnormalities at age 14 years in either group with regard to WISC scores, and a neuropsychological test battery (Knudsen, 1996, 2000). Children with simple and complex febrile seizures had outcomes equally benign (Knudsen, 2000). An additional cohort from Germany (Kolfen *et al.*, 1998) was composed of 80 children ages 6 through 9 years with a history of febrile convulsions. The neuropsychological testing done at ages 6 through 9 years did not reveal differences between the children with a history of febrile convulsions and the controls.

There is one reported population-based study in which long-term follow-up of a population of children with febrile convulsion revealed an excess of neurological problems. Rates for similar problems in a control population were not given. This British cohort study, the National General Practice Study of Epilepsy (NGPSE), identified 220 children with a first febrile convulsion and followed 207 of them for a median of 11.2 years (minimum 8.4 years) (MacDonald *et al.*, 1999). Twelve (6%) of the children developed subsequent epilepsy. Six (3%) had identified neurological problems before any febrile seizure and 20 (10%) developed problems after a first febrile convulsion; of these cases, ten had a clearly defined deficit on long-term follow-up; five had learning difficulties; one was dyspraxic; one was clumsy with abnormal behavior; one had mild cerebral palsy; one had severe general delay and one had mild delay. For the remaining ten children with neurodevelopmental problems, six were referred to psychologists for behavioral problems and four were referred for speech therapy. Eleven percent had received antiepileptic drug therapy.

Another recent population based study from Taiwan offers a more reassuring picture (Chang *et al.*, 2000). The investigators identified 103 children at 3 years of age from a population survey of 4340 live births in Taiwan City, Taiwan between October 1989 and June 1990. The diagnosis was confirmed and the children were followed to age 6 years. Tests of achievement and attention as well as behavioral ratings were given at age 7 years to 87 of the 103 children with febrile seizures and to 87 age-matched randomly selected population-based controls. In this cohort, the children with febrile seizures actually scored higher than the controls in achievement tests and in tests of attention and there were no significant differences in the proportion of children with various behavioral problems in the two groups. The results were not influenced by a young age at first febrile seizure (≤ 1 year), complex features of the febrile seizure, or the number of febrile seizures.

IV. PROLONGED OR COMPLEX FEBRILE SEIZURES

Some of the studies previously mentioned identified an association between prolonged or complex febrile seizures and subsequent neurological disability, but most large prospective population-based studies do not. Complex febrile seizures are generally defined as focal, long lasting, recurring within 24 hours, or associated with focal postictal neurological abnormalities. In the study by Knudsen (1996) of 289 children with a 12-year follow-up, 4 out of 5 children with febrile seizures of very long duration (60–100 minutes) had a normal full-scale IQ and normal academic performance. The fifth child was not tested. There was no difference in the favorable long-term motor, scholastic, and cognitive outcome in children with simple and complex febrile convulsions. In the British Childhood Encephalopathy study, which reported 19 children who had experienced febrile status epilepticus, one child had neurological sequelae (Verity et al., 1993). In a clinic-based study by Maytal and Shinnar (1990), there were no sequelae seen in 44 children with febrile status epilepticus. In the sibling pair study of Nelson and Ellenberg (1978), even in those 27 children who had experienced a febrile seizure lasting 30 minutes or more, the mean full-scale IQ was no different from that of their siblings. The only exception was a child with febrile seizures known to be neurodevelopmentally abnormal before the first seizure occurred. In a retrospective cohort from France (Joannard et al., 1979), there were 318 children who had been hospitalized with febrile seizures; of 5 children who were behind in school, one had experienced a prolonged febrile convulsion.

Several studies have reported an effect of length of seizures or of complex seizures. In one study, children with prolonged febrile convulsions ($n = 80$) had a significantly lower nonverbal intelligence compared to children with simple febrile seizures and to controls (Kölfen et al., 1998). In addition, in this study, children with multiple febrile seizure recurrences performed more poorly in all neurological and neuropsychological tests compared to those with a single febrile seizure or to controls. Smith and Wallace (1982), using the Griffiths Mental Development Scale, found that multiple recurrences were linked to deficits in development. In the NGPSE study, 10 of 43 children who had experienced febrile seizures with complex features required special education, compared to 10 of 177 who had only simple febrile convulsions (MacDonald et al., 1999). This study also reports that having a complex febrile convulsion was associated with a greater risk of having a subsequent neurological abnormality.

V. BEHAVIORAL OUTCOMES

Behavioral outcomes in children who have experienced febrile seizures have not been studied as extensively as intellectual outcomes, but there are some data available from both population-based and selected populations. In a German cohort of 80 children with a history of febrile convulsions, 22% of those evaluated at ages 6 to 9 years exhibited behavioral disturbances [Child Behavior Check-List (CBCL) scores >60], primarily hyperactivity, compared with 6% of the control group (Kölfen et al., 1998). In a randomized study of daily phenobarbital vs. placebo for prevention of febrile seizure recurrence, a control population of age-matched seizure-free children was followed. In this study, children with febrile seizures had more frequent nighttime awakenings than did control children. There was also a slight increase in number of lengthy nighttime awakenings (>1 hour) among febrile seizure children compared to controls (Hirtz et al., 1993).

In the British National cohort study with follow-up at 5 and at 10 years, at 5 years the children with a history of febrile convulsions differed from controls in behavior in only one respect: they were more likely to have sleep problems (Verity et al., 1985a). These consisted mostly of nightmares, night terrors, and difficulty falling asleep, or waking during the night. An extensive series of questions about behavior failed to show any other significant differences. When this cohort was reexamined at age 10 years (Verity et al., 1998), mothers' questionnaires revealed no increase in temper tantrums, or differences with respect to inattentiveness, hyperactivity, clumsiness, or antisocial behavior. Specific questions about sleep problems were not listed as part of the mothers' questionnaire. However, children with febrile seizures were rated as more anxious than control children.

In the population-based study from Taiwan (Chang et al., 2000), no differences were found at age 7 years in the proportion of children with conduct problems, inattention, or hyperactivity or in the hyperactivity index between 87 children with a history of febrile seizures and population-based controls. This study used the Conner's (1989) teacher rating scale.

The above studies suggest generally benign behavioral outcomes. There seems to be a trend toward an increased incidence of more anxious behavior and sleep problems in children with febrile seizures. However, no baseline evaluations of these characteristics of behavior were done before any seizure occurred, thus it is not known whether these behavioral trends are caused by or coexist with the febrile seizures. Another possible explanation could be that the families are more anxious about a child perceived as vulnerable and impact the child's behavior as a result.

VI. BEHAVIORAL AND COGNITIVE SIDE EFFECTS ASSOCIATED WITH ANTIEPILEPTIC DRUGS

Although the majority of children who experience febrile seizures today are not treated with chronic daily medication (see Chapter 19), reports from follow-up studies of children who were enrolled often more than 10 years ago may include a substantial number of treated children. Thus the long-term cognitive outcome reported for some children with febrile seizures may be related to the effects of treatment, notably in cases in which chronic daily phenobarbital was used. In a cohort of 217 children with febrile seizures randomized to daily phenobarbital, 5 mg/kg per day or an identical placebo, a difference in IQ on the Stanford–Binet scales was seen after 2 years of treatment, with those assigned to phenobarbital scoring on average seven points lower. Treatment effects were greatest in children expected to score lowest (Farwell *et al.*, 1990). A nonsignificant difference in IQ was noted 6 months later, as well as on retesting at school age. However, at school age the group that had been assigned to phenobarbital scored lower on reading tests of the Wide Range Achievement Test (WRAT-R) (Sulzbacher, 1999).

Intermittent prophylaxis for febrile seizure recurrences with diazepam does not appear to lead to any long-lasting effects. A hospital-based 12-year follow-up study of 289 children randomized in early childhood to either diazepam prophylaxis at time of fever or at time of seizures assessed intellectual, cognitive, scholastic, and motor function outcome after 12 years. Results of IQ testing did not differ, nor did tests of cognitive abilities, scholastic achievement, or motor function (Knudsen, 1996). These children with febrile seizures had a mean WISC IQ score of 109, which was similar to the IQs found in Danish school children with no history of febrile convulsions (full scale IQ = 110). Thus, neither the seizures nor the treatment regime seem to have affected the children's cognitive development. Other medications such as valproate have not been found useful or have been too toxic to use (Newton, 1988; see also Chapter 19).

VII. CONCLUSION

Although the majority of studies of large, long-term prospectively followed children indicate a benign outcome; there is evidence from a minority of studies that the subset of febrile seizures that are prolonged or are complex may increase the risk of having selected cognitive deficits on follow-up. Even in these subsets, the majority of children do very well. There is no evidence that antiepileptic drug (AED) prophylaxis for recurrences would affect either this possibility or the development of later of epilepsy, and AEDs may have serious medical, cognitive, and behavioral effects far in excess of the risk of febrile seizures (see Chapter 19). Behavioral outcome also seems relatively benign, with the exception that those children with febrile seizures tend to have more problems with sleep and may tend to be more anxious. These characteristics are as likely to have been present before seizures began, as they are to be a result of having had febrile seizures.

The evidence is strong from long-term studies of unselected patients with febrile seizures that there is no impact of febrile seizures on tests of cognitive ability. The age-related susceptibility to seizures accompanying a rise in body temperature constitutes a benign syndrome with a favorable prognosis for cognitive and behavioral outcomes. It would be useful to have results of more research on animal models of febrile seizures, which include paradigms for testing cognitive and behavioral outcomes, so that we can better understand the specific effects on the developing brain in both functional and structural areas.

REFERENCES

Aicardi, J., and Chevrie, J. J. (1976). Febrile convulsions: Neurological sequelae and mental retardation. In "Brain Dysfunction in Infantile Febrile Convulsions" (M. A. B. Brazier and F. Coceani, eds.), pp. 247–257.Raven Press, New York.

Chang, Y.-C., Guo, N.-W., Huang, C.-C., Wang, S.-T., and Tsai, J.-J. (2000). Neurocognitive attention and behavior outcome of school-age children with a history of febrile convulsions: A population study. Epilepsia 41, 412–420.

Chen, K., Baram, T. Z., and Soltesz, I. (1999). Febrile seizures in the developing brain result in persistent modification of neuronal excitability in limbic circuits. Nat. Med. 5, 888–894.

Conners, C. K. (1989). Manual for Conners Rating Scales. Multi Health System. North Tonawanda, New York.

Ellenberg, J. H., and Nelson, K. B. (1978). Febrile seizures and later intellectual performance. Arch. Neurol. 35, 17–21.

Falconer, M. A. (1974). Mesial temporal sclerosis as a common cause of epilepsy: Aetiology, treatment and prevention. Lancet ii, 767–770.

Farwell, J. R., Lee, Y. K. J., Hirtz, D. G., et al. (1990). Phenobarbital for febrile seizures—Effects on intelligence and on seizure recurrence. N. Engl. J. Med. 322, 364–369.

Ghosh, A., Carnahan, J., and Greenberg, M. E. (1994). Requirement for BDNF in activity-dependent survival or cortical neurons. Science 263, 1618–1623.

Hirtz, D. G. (1997). Febrile seizures. Pediatr. Rev. 18 (1), 5–9.

Hirtz, D. G., Chen, T. C., Nelson, K. B., Sulzbacher, S., Farwell, J. R., and Ellenberg, J. H. (1993). Does phenobarbital used for febrile seizure cause sleep disturbances? Pediatr. Neurol. 9 (2), 94–100.

Holmes, G. L. (1997). Epilepsy in the developing brain: Lessons from the laboratory and clinic. Epilepsia 38, 12–30.

Jensen, F. E. (1999). Acute and chronic effects of seizures in the developing brain: Experimental models. *Epilepsia* 40 (Suppl. 1), S51–S58.

Joannard, A., Baum, S., Déchelette, E., Bost, M., and Beaudoing, A. (1979). Evaluation du prognostic a moyen terme des convulsions febriles de l'enfant. *Pédiatrie* 34 (5), 451–459.

Knudsen, F. U. (1996). Febrile seizures—Treatment and outcome. *Brain Dev.* 14, 438–449.

Knudsen, F. U. (2000). Febrile seizures: Treatment and prognosis. *Epilepsia* 41 (1), 2–9.

Kölfen, W., Pehle, K., and König, S. (1998). Is the long-term outcome of children following febrile convulsions favorable? *Dev. Med. Child Neurol.* 40, 667–671.

Lennox, M. A. (1949). Febrile convulsions in childhood. A clinical and electroencephalograghic study. *Am. J. Dis. Child.* 78, 868–82.

MacDonald, B. K., Johnson, A. L., Sander, A. B., and Josemir, W. A. S. (1999). Febrile convulsions in 220 children–Neurological sequelae at 12 years follow-up. *Eur. Neurol.* 41, 179–186.

Maytal, J., and Shinnar, S. (1990). Febrile status epilepticus. *Am. Acad. Pediatr.* 86 (4), 611–616.

Nelson, K. B., and Ellenberg, J. H. (1978). Prognosis in children with febrile seizures. *Pediatrics* 61, 720–7.

Newton, R. W. (1988). Randomized controlled trials of phenobarbital and valproate in febrile convulsions. *Arch. Dis. Child.* 63, 1189–1191.

Rasmussen, T. (1979). Relative significance of isolated infantile convulsions as a primary cause of focal epilepsy. *Epilepsia* 20, 395–401.

Schiottz-Christensen, E., and Bruhn, P. (1973). Intelligence, behavior and scholastic achievement subsequent to febrile convulsions: An analysis of discordant twin pairs. *Dev. Med. Child Neurol.* 15, 565–75.

Smith, J. A., and Wallace, S. J. (1982). Febrile convulsions: Intellectual progress in relation to anticonvulsant therapy and to recurrence of fits. *Arch. Dis. Child.* 57, 104–107.

Sperber, E. F. (1996). The relationship between seizures and damage in the maturing brain. *Epilepsy Res.* S12, 365–376.

Sulzbacher, S., Farwell, J. R., Temkin, N., Lu, A. S., and Hirtz, D. G. (1999). Late cognitive effects of early treatment with phenobarbital. *Clin. Pediatr.* 38, 387–394.

Thompson, K., Holm, A. M., Schousboue, A., Popper, P., Micevych, P., and Wasterlain, C. G. (1998). Hippocampal stimulation produces neuronal death in the immature brain. *Neuroscience* 82, 337–348.

Toth, Z., Yan, X. X., Heftoglu, S., Ribak, C. E., and Baram, T. Z. (1998). Seizure-induced neuronal injury: Vulnerability to febrile seizures in an immature rat model. *J. Neurosci.* 18, 4285–4294.

Verity, C. M., Butler, N. R., and Golding, J. (1985a). Febrile convulsions in a national cohort followed up from birth. I. Prevalence and recurrence in the first five years of life. *Br. Med. J.* 2990, 1307–1310.

Verity, C. M., Butler, N. R., and Golding, J. (1985b). Febrile convulsions in a national cohort followed up from birth. II. Medical history and intellectual ability at 5 years of age. *Br. Med. J.* 290, 1311–1315.

Verity, C. M., Ross, E. M., and Golding, J. (1993). Outcome of childhood status epilepticus and lengthy febrile convulsions: Findings of a national cohort study. *Br. Med. J.* 225–228.

Verity, C. M., Greenwood, R., and Golding, J. (1998). Long-term intellectual and behavioral outcomes of children with febrile convulsions. *N. Engl. J. Med.* 338, 1723–1728.

Wallace, S. J. (1976). Neurological and intellectual deficits: Convulsions with fever viewed as acute indications of life-long developmental defects, *In* "Brain Dysfunction in Infantile Febrile Convulsions" (M. A. B. Brazier and F. Coceani, eds.). Raven Press, New York.

Wallace, S. J., and Cull, A. M. (1979). Long-term psychological outlook for children whose first fit occurs with fever. *Dev. Med. Child Neurol.* 21, 28–40.

CHAPTER 5

Febrile Seizures and the Risk for Epilepsy

DALE C. HESDORFFER* AND W. ALLEN HAUSER*,†

*G.H. Sergievsky Center, Columbia University, New York, New York 10032,
and †Department of Neurology, New York Presbyterian Hospital, New York, New York 10032

Following a first febrile seizure, 2–4% of children experience a subsequent unprovoked seizure, a risk four times the risk in the general population. The increased risk for later unprovoked seizures is substantially greater among children with neurologic abnormalities present from birth than among children without such abnormalities. For most children with febrile seizures (i.e., those with simple febrile seizures), the risk of unprovoked seizure is only slightly increased.

The tendency for recurrent seizures with or without fever is not uniform across all children with febrile seizures. Factors that consistently increase the risk for unprovoked seizures following a first febrile seizure include a family history of epilepsy, complex features of the febrile seizure, and the presence of neurodevelopmental abnormalities present from birth. Increasing duration of fever prior to the first febrile seizure is associated with a reduced risk of developing subsequent unprovoked seizures. These findings suggest that some children may have a low threshold for seizures both with and without fever.

The type of febrile seizure influences the type of unprovoked seizure that may develop. There is an association between complex febrile seizures and partial-onset unprovoked seizures, suggesting an underlying brain pathology common to both, whereas for generalized-onset unprovoked seizures, the tendency to seize repeatedly with fever is most important. Antiepileptic drug treatment, while reducing the risk of recurrent febrile seizures, does not prevent the occurrence of epilepsy among children with febrile seizures. © 2002 Academic Press.

I. INTRODUCTION

Epidemiologic evidence suggests that febrile seizures are associated with subsequent development of unprovoked seizures. For most children with febrile seizures (i.e., those with simple febrile seizures), however, the risk of unprovoked seizure is increased only slightly. This chapter reviews the evidence linking febrile and unprovoked seizures and describes the factors that influence the risk for later unprovoked seizures.

Febrile seizures are distinct from unprovoked seizures. This argument is based on two factors (Berg, 1992). First, the risk of recurrent febrile seizures is far greater than the risk of unprovoked seizures after a febrile seizure. Second, risk factors for recurrent febrile seizures differ from risk factors for subsequent unprovoked seizures. Nonetheless, early investigations of febrile seizures considered some forms of complex febrile seizure as unprovoked seizures unmasked by fever (Livingston, 1954). Although reference is made to these studies, the focus here is on studies that define febrile seizures largely in accordance to the 1980 Consensus Development Panel (NIH, 1980). According to this consensus conference, febrile seizures are convulsions occurring among children with a rectal temperature of at least 101°F, in the absence of a history of seizure or concurrent central nervous system infection. Complex febrile seizures are defined as focal, repeated, or of long duration (variously defined as ≥10 minutes, ≥15 minutes, and ≥30 minutes). Simple febrile seizures are defined as nonfocal, single, and brief.

Our discussion focuses on three approaches to understanding the association between febrile seizures and later unprovoked seizures: the cumulative risk of developing unprovoked seizures; risk factors for the development of unprovoked seizures in children with febrile seizures; and studies of risk factors for epilepsy. Epilepsy is defined as two or more unprovoked seizures.

It is helpful to think of a model to describe the link between febrile seizures and unprovoked seizures. Consider the susceptibility to seize as a bell-shaped curve. In this model, children with the lowest seizure threshold will experience an unprovoked seizure before they are at risk for the development of febrile seizures. Even among children with febrile seizures there will be a range of seizure thresholds, with certain risk factors—such as low temperature at first febrile seizure, neurodevelopmental abnormality (i.e., mental retardation and cerebral palsy), and family history of febrile seizure—serving as indicators for a particularly low seizure threshold in the presence of fever. By extension, the tendency to seize in the absence of fever among children who have experienced a febrile seizure is not uniform. Those children with a particularly low seizure threshold (e.g., due to family history of epilepsy or neurodevelopmental abnormality), even in the absence of fever, are at increased risk for subsequent unprovoked seizures following a febrile seizure.

II. RISK FOR UNPROVOKED SEIZURES FOLLOWING A FIRST FEBRILE SEIZURE

Children with febrile seizures are at a four- to fivefold increased risk for subsequent unprovoked seizures. Earlier studies with different durations of follow-up provide similar estimates of risk (Friderichsen and Melchior, 1954; Frantzen *et al.*, 1968; van den Berg and Yerushalmy, 1969), ranging from 2.5 to 3.2%. The risk for later unprovoked seizures is substantially greater among children with neurologic abnormalities present from birth than among children without such abnormalities.

In the National Collaborative Perinatal Project, children were followed from birth to 7 years of age (Nelson and Ellenberg, 1976). Among the 1706 children who experienced a febrile seizure, 34 developed epilepsy (2%). Epilepsy was defined as recurrent unprovoked seizures where at least one occurred after 48 months of age. In this cohort the underlying risk for epilepsy was 0.5% among neurologically normal children without febrile convulsions, suggesting that febrile seizures increase the risk for epilepsy fourfold.

The British birth survey cohort followed children born during one week in April 1970 until they were 10 years of age (Verity and Golding, 1991). Possible seizures in this study were validated with general practitioners' records or hospital records. Among the 396 children with a first febrile seizure, 17 (4.3%) subsequently experienced an unprovoked seizure. The risk of subsequent unprovoked seizures was substantially reduced for children who were neurologically normal from birth compared to children who were neurologically abnormal from birth. Thirteen of 382 neurologically normal children (3.4%) developed at least one unprovoked seizure and 7 of 382 (1.8%) developed epilepsy following their febrile seizure. The median age at onset of unprovoked seizures was 5 years, 1 month and the median interval from first febrile seizure to first unprovoked seizure was 3 years, 10 months. Among children who were neurologically abnormal from birth and experienced a febrile seizure, 4 of 14 (25%) subsequently developed unprovoked seizures.

Using the Rochester epidemiological project records-linkage system, all children with a first febrile seizure between 1935 and 1979 were identified and followed for subsequent unprovoked seizure (Annegers *et al.*, 1987). Forty-four of the 709 children with a first febrile seizure developed subsequent unprovoked seizures. Again, the risk was lower among children who were neurologically normal from birth (7% by 25 years of age) compared to those who were neurologically abnormal from birth (55%). By 10 years of age, there were fivefold more children with unprovoked seizures than expected in the Rochester population.

After exclusion of the neurologically abnormal children, the cumulative incidence of later unprovoked seizures was 2% by age 5, 4.5% by age 10, 5.5% by age 15, and 7% by age 25, demonstrating a continued increased risk with advancing age. This study demonstrates a continuing increased risk for unprovoked seizure (about threefold) that extends into the third decade of life.

Among a cohort of children identified at 3 years of age with seizures who visited a health center in Tokyo (Tsuboi, 1988) between November 1, 1974 to June 30, 1980, 1406 were identified with febrile seizures. The cumulative risk for subsequent unprovoked seizures was 0.03% by age 3 years and 0.3% by age 14 years, despite a far greater incidence of febrile seizures than that reported elsewhere. This estimate is lower than that from other studies, probably because episodes of febrile seizure and unprovoked seizure were missed in the absence of active surveillance.

In a study of 445 children with a first febrile seizure ascertained from three Bronx hospitals, and the Yale-New Haven Hospital between June 1989 and January 1992, 428 were followed for a maximum of 2 years (Berg and Shinnar, 1996). Children with neurologic abnormalities present from birth were included in this study. The risk of developing an unprovoked seizure was 3.8% by 1 year and 6.2% by 2 years. The risk of epilepsy was 3.0% by 2 years.

III. RISK FACTORS FOR UNPROVOKED SEIZURES AMONG CHILDREN WITH FEBRILE SEIZURES

Consistent risk factors for the development of unprovoked seizures following a first febrile seizure include a family history of epilepsy, complex features of the febrile seizure, and the presence of neurodevelopmental abnormalities present from birth (Annegers *et al.,* 1987; Verity and Golding, 1991; Berg and Shinnar, 1996; Nelson and Ellenberg, 1976). Other risk factors for subsequent unprovoked seizures have been identified in single studies only. We will discuss risk factors for unprovoked seizures in all children with febrile seizures, in neurologically normal children with febrile seizures, and in neurologically abnormal children with febrile seizures. Data are restricted to the four prospective cohort studies employing the consensus conference diagnosis for febrile seizures.

A. ALL CHILDREN WITH FEBRILE SEIZURES

Neurodevelopmental abnormalities present from birth are a strong and consistent risk factor for the development of unprovoked seizure following a febrile seizure (Table 1). The increased risk ranges from 2.1-fold to 13.8-fold, and persists even after adjusting for other risk factors for unprovoked seizure (Berg and Shinnar, 1996). Because other authors have excluded children with neurodevelopmental abnormalities present from birth from more detailed analyses of unprovoked seizure risk, information on other risk factors for unprovoked seizures comes from two studies (Berg and Shinnar, 1996; Nelson and Ellenberg, 1976). These studies suggest that the risk of unprovoked seizures is increased 2-fold by prolonged febrile seizures, 3-fold by a family history of unprovoked seizures, and 1.5-fold for a first complex febrile seizure (Table 1). Interestingly, as the number of hours of fever prior to the febrile seizure increases, the risk of subsequent unprovoked seizures decreases (Berg and Shinnar, 1996). In contrast, the height of the temperature at the first febrile seizure has no effect (Berg and Shinnar, 1996). The inverse relationship between duration of fever prior to a febrile seizure and risk of unprovoked seizure requires confirmation in additional studies, but suggests that following a febrile seizure those children who are at increased risk for subsequent unprovoked seizures have a lower threshold for seizures with and without fever.

Nelson and Ellenberg (1978) examined the combined effects of family history of unprovoked seizures, neurodevelopmental abnormality, and complex febrile seizure on the risk of subsequent unprovoked seizure (Table 2). The combined effect of the risk factors was greater than what would be derived by just adding the risks. Having all three risk factors increased the risk for unprovoked seizures 14-fold, two factors increased the risk 5- to 8-fold, and one factor increased the risk 2- to 3-fold.

B. Neurodevelopmentally Normal Children

The risk for later unprovoked seizures among neurodevelopmentally normal children with a first febrile seizure is greatly increased by a first focal febrile seizure (Verity and Golding, 1991; Annegers et al., 1987), recurrent febrile seizures (Verity and Golding, 1991; Annegers et al., 1987; Berg and Shinnar, 1996), and family history of epilepsy (Verity and Golding, 1991; Annegers et al., 1987;Berg and Shinnar, 1996) (Table 1). Again, this suggests that an underlying seizure diathesis is present in those children who manifest both febrile and unprovoked seizures.

Annegers et al. (1987) examined the combined effects of factors that define complex febrile seizure (i.e., focal, repeated, and prolonged) on the risk of developing unprovoked seizures (Table 2). The combined effect of different combinations of the risk factors was greater than that derived by simply adding the risks. In this model, having all three features of complex febrile seizure increased the risk for unprovoked seizures 20-fold, two factors increased the risk 7- to 9-fold, and one factor increased the risk 2.7- to 4-fold.

There is heterogeneity in risk factors by unprovoked seizure type among children with a febrile seizure (Verity and Golding, 1991; Annegers et al., 1987).

TABLE 1   Risk Factors for the Development of Unprovoked Seizures among Children with Febrile Seizures

	Study[a]							
	Verity and Golding, 1991		Annegers et al., 1987		Berg and Shinnar, 1996		Nelson and Ellenberg, 1976	
Variable	RRu	RRe	RR*	95% CI	RR*	95% CI	RRu	RRe
Neurologically normal children								
First febrile seizure								
Simple	Referent		Referent					Referent
Complex	2.0	2.5	2.8	1.3–6.0			1.8	2.8
Repeated	0.75	1.0						
Prolonged	3.3	3.5						
10–29 minutes	—	—	1.5	0.6–6.1				
≥30 minutes	—	—	2.8	1.0–7.8				
Focal	7.7**	11.5**	3.6	1.4–9.1				
Any febrile seizure								
Simple	Referent							
Complex	9.0	6.0			2.6	0.87–7.6		
Repeated	5.0	4.0						
Prolonged	13.0**	6.0						
Focal	29.0**	29.0**						
Recurrent febrile seizures								
Yes	3.0*		—	—	—	—	—	1.0
Number of febrile seizures								
2 febrile seizures	—	—	1.4	0.6–3.4	1.9	1.3–2.8		
≥3 febrile seizures	—	—	1.8	0.7–4.7				
Family history of unprovoked seizures or epilepsy								
Yes	5.3**	—	1.6	0.5–5.5	2.6	0.59–11.4		—

			95% CI		
Age at first febrile seizure					
<1 year	1.4	0.6–3.4	—	—	—
1–3 years	Referent		—	—	—
>3 years	1.9	0.5–5.5	—	—	—
Duration of fever	—	—	0.67	0.33–1.4	—
Neurodevelopmentally abnormal children					
Duration of fever	—	—	0.10	0.01–0.76	—
Any complex seizure	—	—	5.3	1.03–27.3	—
Number of febrile seizures	—	—	2.6	0.98–6.7	—
Recurrent seizures[c]	—	—	—	—	3.2*
All children					
Neurodevelopmental abnormality	7.4	7.9	13.8	5.6–33.8	2.1	3.2
Number of febrile seizures	—	—	1.6	1.2–2.3	—	3.2
Any complex seizure	—	—	2.7	1.1–6.5	—
First complex seizure	—	—	1.6[b]	0.76–3.5	1.7	1.6
Duration of fever	—	—	0.54	0.28–1.02	—
Seizure ≥30 minutes	—	—	1.9	0.45–8.7	2.7
Family history of afebrile seizures	—	—	3.4[b]	1.03–11.5	2.9*	3.5*
Temperature	—	—	0.84[b]	0.6–1.2	—
Age	—	—	1.1[b]	0.7–1.6	—
Males vs. females	—	—	1.0[b]	0.47–2.3	—
Race/ethnicity					
White	—	—	Referent		—
Black	—	—	0.93[b]	0.29–2.9	—
Hispanic	—	—	1.6[b]	0.66–4.1	—

[a]RRu, Relative risk for an unprovoked seizure; RRe, relative risk for epilepsy; *, adjusted rate ratio for unprovoked seizure; 95% CI, 95% confidence interval; **, $p < 0.05$; —, not reported.

[b]Univariate rate ratio.

[c]Three or more recurrent febrile seizures versus one or two.

TABLE 2 Combined Effect of Characteristics of Febrile Seizures on Risk of Unprovoked Seizures

Variable	Study[a]	
	Annegers et al., 1987	Nelson and Ellenberg, 1978
All children		
Family history of afebrile seizures (factor 1)		5.3%
Neurodevelopmental abnormality (factor 2)		3.3%
Complex first febrile seizure (factor 3)		4.1%
All three factors		23.0%
None of the three factors		1.6%
Family history and neurodevelopmental abnormality (combined factors)		10.3%
Family history and complex febrile seizure (combined factors)		12.6%
Neurodevelopmental abnormality and complex febrile seizure (conbined factors)		8.2%
Neurodevelopmentally normal		
Repeated episodes in 24 hours	9.3%	—
Focal features	8.2%	—
Prolonged	6.5%	—
Repeated and focal	21.3%	—
Repeated and prolonged	16.9%	—
Focal and prolonged	21.5%	—
All three factors	49.0%	—
None of the three factors	2.4%	—

[a]Modeled risk: Based on a multivariate model for unprovoked seizures following febrile seizures.

Verity and Golding (1991) observed that among the 13 children with unprovoked seizures, 9 had a complex febrile seizure, of whom 6 developed unprovoked complex partial seizures (66.7%). Five of the 6 children with unprovoked complex partial seizures had focal features during their febrile seizure. All of the 4 children with simple febrile seizures who developed unprovoked seizures had generalized tonic–clonic unprovoked seizures. Thirty-two children experienced an unprovoked seizure in the Rochester, Minnesota, cohort (Annegers et al., 1987); half were generalized-onset and half were partial-onset. Individual components of complex febrile seizures (focal, repeated, prolonged) increased the risk for partial-onset unprovoked seizure but not for generalized-onset unprovoked seizure. Late age at onset and at least three recurrent febrile seizures increased the risk for generalized-onset unprovoked seizures but not for partial-onset unprovoked seizures. Thus, there is an association between complex febrile seizures and partial-onset unprovoked seizures, suggesting an underlying brain pathology common to both. The tendency to seize repeatedly with fever appears the most important risk factor for generalized-onset unprovoked seizures. Because the tendency to experience repeated febrile seizures appears to have a genetic component (Rich *et al.*, 1987), subsequent generalized-onset unprovoked seizures in these children may be part of this genetic predisposition.

C. Neurodevelopmentally Abnormal Children

Two studies have examined the risk factors for later unprovoked seizures among neurodevelopmentally abnormal children who experience a febrile seizure (Berg and Shinnar, 1996; Nelson and Ellenberg, 1976). Both found an increased risk of later unprovoked seizures or epilepsy associated with febrile seizure recurrence (Table 1). Berg and Shinnar (1996) found that the risk for unprovoked seizure was increased fivefold by a complex febrile seizure (Table 1). Increasing duration of fever prior to the first febrile seizure was associated with a reduced risk of developing later unprovoked seizures (Berg and Shinnar, 1996). Thus, increasing duration of fever appears to decrease the risk of unprovoked seizure in all children, but this is due to a very strong inverse relationship between these factors in neurodevelopmentally abnormal children. Even in children who are neurodevelopmentally abnormal prior to their first febrile seizure, the tendency to develop later unprovoked seizures seems related to possible underlying brain pathology manifested by the tendency to experience complex febrile seizures, and by a low threshold for febrile seizure manifested by a tendency toward recurrent febrile seizures and a tendency to seize after a short duration of fever.

D. General Seizure Susceptibility among Children with Febrile Seizures

In the model of seizure susceptibility described above, the tendency for recurrent seizures with or without fever is not uniform across all children with febrile seizures. Another analysis of the study by Berg *et al.* (1998) further illustrates this point. This analysis shows that among children with febrile seizures, further seizures with fever can occur even after the development of unprovoked seizures. After adjusting for previously identified risk factors for recurrent febrile seizures, Berg *et al.* (1998) found that unprovoked seizures increased the risk for recurrent febrile seizures 3.5-fold (95% CI = 1.3–5.8). This reinforces the contention that children who experience both febrile and unprovoked seizures have a low seizure threshold in general and are prone to recurrent episodes.

IV. FEBRILE SEIZURES IN COHORTS WITH EPILEPSY

Febrile seizures have been examined as an antecedent of unprovoked seizures in incidence cohorts of epilepsy. Incidence cohorts include individuals with newly diagnosed epilepsy. Antecedent febrile seizures occur in 13–18% of children with new-onset epilepsy (Berg *et al.*, 1999; Camfield *et al.*, 1994; Rwiza *et al.*, 1992). In Rochester, Minnesota, prior febrile seizures occurred in 19% of children and adults with generalized tonic–clonic seizures at any age (Rocca *et al.*, 1987a), in 18% with complex partial seizures (Rocca *et al.*, 1987b), and in 21% with generalized absence seizures (Rocca *et al.*, 1987c). Estimates are much higher in clinical series of individuals evaluated for epilepsy surgery (Davies *et al.*, 1996; Harvey *et al.*, 1995; Cendes *et al.*, 1993). However, these series suffer from recall bias of past febrile seizures, selection bias, and an overrepresentation of intractable epilepsy.

In case-control studies of epilepsy, the strength of the relationship between prior febrile seizures and epilepsy is strong for prevalent epilepsy (Pal, 1999; Gracia *et al.*, 1990). Cohorts of prevalent epilepsy include individuals who have had epilepsy for many years as well as some newly diagnosed cases. In a case-control study of children with prevalent epilepsy in India (Pal, 1999), prior febrile seizures were 6.5-fold more common among cases compared to controls (95% CI = 1.5–28.7). Another prevalent case-control study from the Republic of Panama (Gracia *et al.*, 1990) found that children with epilepsy were 5.6-fold more likely than controls to have had prior febrile seizures (95% CI = 1.2–29.1).

Three parallel case-control studies of incident unprovoked seizure among children and adults in Rochester, Minnesota evaluated prior febrile seizures as a risk factor separately for absence seizures, generalized tonic–clonic seizures, and complex partial seizures (Rocca *et al.*, 1987a–c). Cases were residents of Rochester at the time of their first unprovoked seizures and had been born in Rochester. Two controls born in Rochester were selected for each case and were matched on date of birth, hospital of birth, gender, and residency in Rochester on the date of the case's first unprovoked seizure. Prior febrile seizures were associated with absence seizures (OR $= 12.0$, $p = 0.007$), generalized tonic–clonic seizures (OR $= \infty$), and complex partial seizures (OR $= 15.3$, $p < 0.0001$). The association between febrile seizures and complex partial seizures was further explored, by examining characteristics of the febrile seizures. Febrile seizures before the age of 2 years increased the risk for complex partial seizures 30.5-fold ($p < 0.0001$) and complicated febrile seizures increased the risk 26.5-fold.

Further epidemiologic evidence for an association between characteristics of febrile seizures and epilepsy comes from cohort studies of childhood epilepsy. In a cohort of incident childhood-onset epilepsy, complex febrile seizures were associated with a younger age of onset of epilepsy (Berg et al., 1999). There was no association between focal or prolonged febrile seizures and localization-related epilepsy or temporal lobe epilepsy. Camfield et al. (1994) studied all children of age 1 month to 16 years with a new diagnosis of epilepsy in Nova Scotia, Canada between 1977 and 1985. Excluded from this cohort were children with minor motor seizures, generalized absence, progressive brain disease, severe myoclonic epilepsy of childhood, febrile seizures following unprovoked seizures, and unknown history of prior febrile seizures. The association between febrile seizure characteristics and epilepsy was examined in 489 children with epilepsy. Intractable seizures were defined as at least one seizure every 2 months during the last year of follow-up despite trials of at least three different antiepileptic medications. Similar to the results of Berg et al. (1999), age of onset of epilepsy was significantly lower for children with prior febrile seizures (67.8 months) than for children without prior febrile seizures (82.9 months). Prior febrile seizures were 2.1-fold more common among children with generalized-onset seizures compared to those with partial-onset seizures. Although preceding prolonged febrile seizures were associated with prior neurodeficit and intractable seizures, they were not associated with epilepsy seizure type. Prior prolonged febrile seizures were 8.8-fold more common among children with intractable epilepsy compared to those without intractable epilepsy. However, intractable complex partial seizures were uncommon after prolonged febrile seizures, occurring in only 12.5% of children.

Although febrile seizures are a consistent risk factor for subsequent unprovoked seizures, they are present in only 13–19% of incident epilepsy. An antecedent febrile seizure increases the risk for subsequent epilepsy 5- to 15-fold in case-control studies, regardless of the seizure type of the individual with epilepsy. The onset of epilepsy tends to be earlier if there has been an antecedent febrile seizure. Further, associations have been reported between complex febrile seizures and complex partial epilepsy and between prolonged febrile seizures and intractable epilepsy.

V. DO ANTIEPILEPTIC DRUGS PREVENT UNPROVOKED SEIZURES FOLLOWING FEBRILE SEIZURES?

Although studies have not been designed to answer this question directly, some data are available from studies designed to determine whether antiepileptic drugs prevent recurrent febrile seizures. These studies find that prophylactic anticonvulsants, while reducing the risk of recurrent febrile seizures (see Chapters 3, 7, and 19), do not prevent the occurrence of subsequent unprovoked seizures (Knudsen, 1985).

VI. CONCLUSIONS

Children with febrile seizures are at a 4- to 5-fold increased risk for subsequent unprovoked seizures—a risk of 2.5–3.2%. The risk for later unprovoked seizures is substantially greater among children with neurologic abnormalities present from birth than among children without such abnormalities. Antecedent febrile seizures occur in 13–18% of children with new-onset epilepsy. Prophylactic anticonvulsants do not alter this risk.

Consistent risk factors for the development of unprovoked seizures following a first febrile seizure include a family history of epilepsy, complex features of the febrile seizure, and the presence of neurodevelopmental abnormalities present from birth. Other risk factors for subsequent unprovoked seizures, such as duration of febrile illness prior to the febrile seizure, have been identified in single studies only.

ACKNOWLEDGMENT

This work was funded in part by 1 R01 HD36867–01 from the National Institute of Child Health and Human Development.

REFERENCES

Annegers, J. F., Hauser, W. A., Shirts, S. B., and Kurland, L. T. (1987). Factors prognostic of unprovoked seizures after febrile convulsions. *N. Engl. J. Med.* **316**, 493–498.
Berg, A. T. (1992). Febrile seizures and epilepsy: The contribution of epidemiology. *Paediatr. Perinatal Epidemiol.* **6**, 145–152.
Berg, A. T., and Shinnar, S. (1996). Unprovoked seizures in children with febrile seizures: Short-term outcome. *Neurology* **47**, 562–568.
Berg, A. T., Darefsky, A. S., Holford, T. R., and Shinnar, S. (1998). Seizures with fever after unpro-

voked seizures: An analysis in children followed from the time of a first febrile seizure. *Epilepsia* **39**, 77–80.

Berg, A. T., Shinnar, S., Levy, S. R., and Testa, F. M. (1999). Childhood-onset epilepsy with and without preceding febrile seizures. *Neurology* **53**, 1742–1748.

Camfield, P., Camfield, C., Gordon, K., and Dooley, J. (1994). What types of epilepsy are preceded by febrile seizure? A population-based study of children. *Dev. Med. Child Neurol.* **36**, 887–892.

Cendes, F., Andermann, F., Gloor, P., Lopes-Cendes, I., Andermann, E., Melanson, D., Jones-Gotman, M., Robitaille, Y., Evans, A., and Peters, T. (1993). Atrophy of mesial structure in patients with temporal lobe epilepsy: Cause of consequence of repeated seizures? *Ann. Neurol.* **34**, 795–801.

Davies, K. G., Hermann, B. P., Dohan, F. C., Foley, K. T., Bush, A. J., and Wyler, A. R. (1996). Relationship of hippocampal sclerosis to duration and age of onset of epilepsy, and childhood febrile seizures in temporal lobectomy patients. *Epilepsy Res.* **24**, 119–126.

Frantzen, E., Lennox-Buchthal, M., and Nygaard, A. (1968). Longitudinal EEG and clinical study of children with febrile convulsions. *Electroencephalogr. Clin. Neurophysiol.* **24**, 197–212.

Friderichsen, C., and Melchior, J. (1954). Febrile convulsions in children, their frequency and prognosis. *Acta Paediatr.* **29** (Suppl. 100), 110–113.

Gracia, F., Loo de Lao, S., Castillo, L., Larreategui, M., Archbold, C., Brenes, M. M., and Reeves, W. C. (1990). Epidemiology of epilepsy in Guaymi Indians from Bocas del Toro Province, Republic of Panama. *Epilepsia* **31**, 718–723.

Harvey, A. S., Grattan-Smith, J. D., Desmond, P. M., Chow, C. W., and Berkovic, S. F. (1995). Febrile seizures and hippocampal sclerosis: Frequent and related findings in intractable temporal lobe epilepsy of childhood. *Pediatr. Neurol.* **12**, 210–216.

Knudsen, F. U. (1985). Effective short-term diazepam prophylaxis in febrile convulsions. *J. Pediatr.* **106**, 487–490.

Livingston, S. (1954). *In* "The Diagnosis and Treatment of Convulsive Disorders in Children," p. 314. Charles C. Thomas, Springfield, IL.

National Institutes of Health (1980). Febrile seizures: Long-term management of children with fever-associated seizures. *Br. Med. J.* **281**, 277–279.

Nelson, K. B., and Ellenberg, J. H. (1976). Predictors of epilepsy in children who have experienced febrile seizures. *N. Engl. J. Med.* **295**, 1029–1033.

Nelson, K. B., and Ellenberg, J. H. (1978). Prognosis in children with febrile seizures. *Pediatrics* **61**, 720–7.

Pal, D. (1999). Methodological issues in assessing risk factors for epilepsy in an epidemiologic study in India. *Neurology* **53**, 2058–2063.

Rich, S. S., Annegers, J. F., Hauser, W. A., and Anderson, V. E. (1987). Complex segregation analyses of febrile convulsions. *Am. J. Hum. Genet.* **41**, 249–257.

Rocca, W. A., Sharbrough, F. W., Hauser, W. A., Annegers, J. F., and Schoenberg, B. S. (1987a). Risk factors for generalized tonic-clonic seizures: A population-based case-control study in Rochester, Minnesota. *Neurology* **37**, 1315–1322.

Rocca, W. A., Sharbrough, F. W., Hauser, W. A., Annegers, J. F., and Schoenberg, B. S. (1987b). Risk factors for complex partial seizures: A population-based case-control study. *Ann. Neurol.* **21**, 22–31.

Rocca, W. A., Sharbrough, F. W., Hauser, W. A., Annegers, J. F., and Schoenberg, B. S. (1987c). Risk factors for generalized absence seizures: A population-based case-control study in Rochester, Minnesota. *Neurology* **37**, 1309–1314.

Rwiza, H. T., Kilonzo, G. P., Haule, J., Matuja, W. B. P., Mteza, M. I., Mbena, P., Kilima, P. M., Mwaluko, G., Mwang'ombola, R., Mwaijande, F., Rweyemamu, G., Matowo, A., and Jilek-Aall, L. M. (1992). Prevalence and incidence of epilepsy in Ulanga, a rural Tanzanian district: A community-based study. *Epilepsia* **33**, 1051–1056.

Tsuboi, T. (1988). Prevalence and incidence of epilepsy in Tokyo. *Epilepsia* **29**, 103–110.

van den Berg, B. J., and Yerushalmy, J. (1969). Studies on convulsive disorders in young children: I. Incidence of febrile and non-febrile convulsions by age and other factors. *Pediatr. Res.* **3**, 298–304.

Verity, C. M., and Golding, J. (1991). Risk of epilepsy after febrile convulsions: A national cohort study. *Br. Med. J.* **303**, 1373–1376.

CHAPTER 6

Do Febrile Seizures Promote Temporal Lobe Epilepsy? Retrospective Studies

FERNANDO CENDES AND FREDERICK ANDERMANN

Department of Neurology and Neurosurgery, Montreal Neurological Institute and Hospital, McGill University, Montreal, Quebec, Canada H3A 2B4

The sequence of febrile seizures followed by intractable temporal lobe epilepsy (TLE) is rarely seen from a population perspective. However, several studies have shown a significant relationship between a history of prolonged febrile seizures in early childhood and mesial temporal sclerosis (MTS). The interpretation of these observations remains quite controversial. One possibility is that the early febrile seizure damages the hippocampus and is therefore a cause of MTS. Another possibility is that the child has a prolonged febrile seizure because the hippocampus was previously damaged due to a prenatal or perinatal insult or due to a genetic predisposition. Recent imaging studies have shown that prolonged and focal febrile seizures can produce acute hippocampal injury that evolves to hippocampal atrophy and that complex febrile seizures can actually originate in the temporal lobes in some children. There are now also several lines of evidence indicating that genetic predisposition is an important causal factor of both febrile seizures and MTS. In view of recent clinical and molecular genetic studies, it appears that the relationship between febrile seizures and later epilepsy is frequently genetic and there are a number of syndrome-specific genes for febrile seizure.

MTS most likely has different causes. A number of retrospective studies indicate that complex febrile seizures are a causative factor for the later development of MTS and TLE. However, there are also some contradictory results from several prospective and retrospective studies. Most likely the association between febrile seizures and TLE results from complex interactions between several genetic and environmental factors. © 2002 Academic Press.

I. STUDIES

The sequence of febrile seizures followed by intractable temporal lobe epilepsy (TLE) is rare, seen from a population perspective (Camfield *et al.*, 1994). However, several studies have shown a significant relationship between a history of prolonged febrile seizures in early childhood and mesial temporal sclerosis (MTS), as determined by magnetic resonance imaging (MRI) or postoperative histopathology (Abou-Khalil *et al.*, 1993; Cendes *et al.*, 1993a; Falconer, 1971, 1974; Falconer *et al.*, 1964; Kuks *et al.*, 1993; Maher and McLachlan, 1995; Ounstead *et al.*, 1966; Trenerry *et al.*, 1993; Zimmerman, 1940). Nelson and Ellenberg (1976) studied 1706 children who had experienced at least one febrile seizure and were followed to the age of 7 years. Epilepsy developed in only 2% of them. However, in children with prior abnormal development and whose first febrile seizure was complex (longer than 15 minutes, multiple or focal) epilepsy developed at a rate 18 times higher than in children with no febrile seizure, and 8 times higher than in children with simple febrile seizure.

The interpretation of these observations remains quite controversial (Abou-Khalil *et al.*, 1993; Berg *et al.*, 1998; Doose, 1998; Maher and McLachlan, 1995; Shinnar, 1998; Sloviter and Pedley, 1998). One possibility is that the early febrile seizure damages the hippocampus and is therefore a cause of hippocampal sclerosis (Abou-Khalil *et al.*, 1993; Hamati-Haddad and Abou-Khalil, 1998; Kanemoto *et al.*, 1998; VanLandingham *et al.*, 1998). Another possibility is that the child has a prolonged febrile seizure because the hippocampus was previously damaged due to a prenatal or perinatal insult or due to a genetic predisposition (Cendes *et al.*, 1995; Davies *et al.*, 1996; Fernandez *et al.*, 1998; Kobayashi *et al.*, 2000; Sloviter and Pedley, 1998). The finding that hippocampal sclerosis is associated more frequently with developmental anomalies such as focal cortical dysplasia and heterotopia than with other structural lesions may support the second explanation (Cendes *et al.*, 1995; Raymond *et al.*, 1994; Sloviter and Pedley, 1998; Watson *et al.*, 1997). An MRI study of individuals from families with febrile seizures has shown subtle hippocampal abnormalities even among asymptomatic individuals, also suggesting preexisting damage leading to febrile seizures and/or to mesial TLE (Fernandez *et al.*, 1998).

A retrospective study of a series of 167 consecutive patients with lesional epilepsy (Cendes *et al.*, 1995) supports the concept of prolonged febrile seizure leading to MTS in a predisposed hippocampus. A history of prolonged febrile seizure in early childhood was significantly more frequent in those patients who had coexistent hippocampal atrophy than in those without dual pathology (20% versus 3%). In addition, Hamati-Haddad and Abou-Khalil (1998) showed that patients with TLE had a significantly higher incidence of febrile seizure in infancy than those with extratemporal epilepsy.

A related question is whether hippocampal sclerosis is the cause of repeated seizures or their consequence. Several investigations have shown that no significant relationship exists between atrophy of mesial temporal lobe structures and the duration and frequency of seizures (Cendes *et al.*, 1993a,b, 1995; Davies *et al.*, 1996; Kuks *et al.*, 1993; Trenerry *et al.*, 1993). These studies, along with the previously mentioned febrile seizure studies, suggest that hippocampal sclerosis is caused by an insult occurring early in life and that it remains relatively stable. Each subsequent seizure does not appear to cause significant additional neuronal cell loss or progressive worsening of hippocampal atrophy. Other studies have produced seemingly conflicting results, indicating progressive hippocampal damage with more severe or more prolonged epilepsy (Garcia *et al.*, 1997; Kalviainen *et al.*, 1998; Mouritzen Dam, 1982; Pitkanen *et al.*, 1996; Tasch *et al.*, 1999). Some studies propose an intermediate view, suggesting that hippocampal sclerosis is caused for the most part by an "initiating precipitating event" on top of which further progressive damage is superimposed over time (Mathern *et al.*, 1995a,b; Tasch *et al.*, 1999; Theodore *et al.*, 1999; Van Paesschen *et al.*, 1997). The discrepancies among these different studies may be explained, in part, by differences in the methods used, and also by the fact that TLE is a heterogeneous condition, with varying types of underlying pathological abnormalities. Thus, depending on the patient population studied, a significant correlation between atrophy and duration of epilepsy may or may not be present (Berg and Shinnar, 1997; Sloviter and Pedley, 1998; Theodore and Wasterlain, 1999).

Classical hippocampal sclerosis has all the earmarks of an inert lesion acquired in the remote past. This raises the question as to what type of acute insult has caused the sclerosis. A fresh lesion with a distribution characteristic of hippocampal sclerosis was found in the hippocampi of children between the ages of 3 months and 7 years who died during status epilepticus, often but not necessarily associated with a febrile illness (Ounstead *et al.*, 1966; Zimmerman, 1940). Status epilepticus is often followed by extensive neuronal damage involving the hippocampus, as well as other limbic, neocortical, and subcortical structures (Hauser, 1988; Meldrum and Brierley, 1973).

It is therefore possible that the classical lesion of hippocampal sclerosis is the consequence of a prolonged seizure or status epilepticus occurring in a period of childhood when the hippocampus is particularly vulnerable to convulsion-induced excitotoxic damage (Gloor, 1991). A plausible pathogenetic mechanism is that the excitotoxic damage involves sectors of the hippocampus rich in kainate or N-methyl-D-aspartate (NMDA) receptors that lack protection against Ca^{2+} overload (Ben-Ari, 1985; Collingridge and Bliss, 1987; Geddes and Cotman, 1986; Gloor, 1991; Kudo and Ogura, 1986; Miller, 1991; Sloviter *et al.*, 1991; Zimmerman, 1940).

This pathogenetic explanation fails, however, to explain why hippocampal sclerosis is frequently unilateral. Is it possible that both prolonged febrile seizures (which are often predominantly unilateral) and the resultant damage may have been primed by some preexisting hippocampal abnormality? This merits consideration in view of the high incidence of hippocampal sclerosis found at autopsy in infants (including stillborn fetuses) with evidence for pre- and perinatal conditions that may lead to hypoxic or hypoglycemic brain damage (Meencke and Veith, 1991; Veith, 1970). Although these children obviously had pathologies severe enough to lead to death and therefore represent a highly selected group, they may represent only the tip of the iceberg; milder forms of such pathology may be a factor rendering infants susceptible to develop prolonged convulsions during a febrile illness. Among the group of patients with chronic epilepsy that came to autopsy and were studied by Veith (1970), those who had no significant pathology other than hippocampal sclerosis had similarly high incidence of pre- and perinatal factors predisposing to hypoxic and hypoglycemic brain damage. Even though these individuals did not represent a typical cross-section of those with epilepsy, because they had a high incidence of mental retardation, the findings are nevertheless of interest because (1) they reinforce the notion that some preexisting damage may be present in patients with hippocampal sclerosis following prolonged febrile seizures and (2) the disorders most commonly encountered, hypoxia and hypoglycemia, may produce a profile of hippocampal damage similar to that caused by prolonged seizures, presumably by the same glutamate-mediated excitotoxic mechanism (Meldrum and Garthwaite, 1990). The high incidence of MTS in autopsies of patients with West syndrome and Lennox–Gastaut syndrome (Jellinger, 1987; Meencke and Janz, 1984; Meencke and Veith, 1991) may be related to the pathogenic factors identified in Veith's study (1970).

The findings of VanLandingham et al. (1998) are in agreement with these hypotheses. They performed magnetic resonance imaging (MRI) studies after complex febrile seizures in 27 infants and found definite imaging abnormalities in 6 of the 15 infants with focal or lateralized febrile seizures but in none of the 12 who had generalized febrile seizures. The MRIs showed preexisting bilateral hippocampal atrophy consistent with the history of perinatal insults in 2 of the 6 infants with lateralized febrile seizures. The remaining 4 infants who had MRI abnormalities and lateralized febrile seizures had had significantly longer seizures than the others. Their MRI changes suggested acute edema with increased hippocampal T2-weighted signal intensity and increased volume predominantly in the hippocampus of the hemisphere where seizures originated. Of those with acute edema, one had temporal electrographic seizure activity (during the febrile seizure) and another had a cyst in the choroid fissure displacing the affected hippocampus. Both these infants had follow-up MRIs showing subsequent hippocampal atrophy. These findings confirm that prolonged and focal febrile seizures can occasionally produce acute hippocampal injury that evolves to atrophy and that complex febrile seizures can actually originate in the temporal lobe in some children (VanLandingham et al., 1998).

Genetic predisposition, as suggested by Schmidt et al. (1985), appears to be an important causal factor in patients with MTS and antecedent prolonged febrile seizures. We have shown a high incidence of febrile seizures and/or epilepsy in the families of these patients (Abou-Khalil *et al.*, 1993). We found a higher incidence of gestational or birth complications (mostly minor) in those TLE patients who had had prolonged febrile seizures. This suggests that such perinatal or other preexisting factors may make it more likely for a febrile seizure to be prolonged or complex in children who have a genetic predisposition for febrile seizure. Such perinatal or preexisting factors may in themselves not be sufficient to produce TLE, but the subsequent prolonged and often lateralized febrile seizures could lead to hippocampal sclerosis and focal temporal epileptogenicity.

Additional clinical and molecular genetic studies show that there is some specificity in the types of epilepsy that follows febrile seizures, rather than the febrile seizure being a nonspecific marker of a lowered seizure threshold (Berkovic and Scheffer, 1998). The relationship between febrile seizures and later development of epilepsy is frequently genetic and there are a number of syndrome-specific genes for febrile seizures (Berkovic and Scheffer, 1998).

In a study of familial temporal lobe epilepsy, 41% of our patients with familial TLE had seizures refractory to anticonvulsant medication. Eleven of the 18 (61%) patients with an available MRI had findings compatible with MTS, and 8 had seizures severe enough to require surgical treatment (Cendes *et al.*, 1998). Five of 36 (14%) patients had antecedents of complex febrile seizures and 3 had simple febrile seizures. In one of the five patients with a history of complex febrile seizures in childhood, attacks stopped at 12 years of age and there was no MRI scan available. The remaining four patients with complex febrile seizures had moderate to severe degrees of hippocampal atrophy as seen by MRI; three of these patients underwent surgery, and histopathological examination confirmed MTS. Conversely, all three patients who had single febrile seizures, of short duration and without focal signs, had either no further seizures or a benign course of their epilepsy, with seizures stopping by 12 years of age (Cendes *et al.*, 1998).

In another study (Kobayashi *et al.*, 2000), we evaluated 98 affected individuals from 22 families in whom more than two patients had TLE. Sixty-eight individuals fulfilled the clinical and electroencephalogram (EEG) criteria for mesial temporal lobe epilepsy. History of earlier febrile seizures was positive in only 4 of these 68 (6%). Three of these patients had good seizure control on medication, one who had had simple febrile seizures and two who had had recurrent complex febrile seizures. Only one patient had refractory seizures and antecedent complex febrile seizures. Eleven of the 98 (11%) individuals evaluated had only febrile seizures in childhood and did not fulfill the criteria for mesial TLE. Febrile seizures were recurrent in five patients: three had simple and two had complex febrile seizures. Detailed qualitative analysis of high-resolution MRIs from these patients with familial mesial TLE showed abnormalities suggestive of MTS in 57% of them, despite their heterogeneous clinical presentation. The hippocampal abnormalities ranged from an abnormal shape or axis of the hippocampi to severe hippocampal atrophy with hyperintense T2 signal. The distribution of hippocampal atrophy according to the seizure outcome groups was as follows: 6 of 13 (46%) of patients with seizure remission, 16 of 31 (51%) of those with good seizure control receiving medication, and all 16 patients with refractory mesial TLE. Hippocampal atrophy was also found in patients who did not fulfill the criteria for mesial TLE: 6 of 10 (60%) of patients with recurrent generalized tonic–clonic seizures, 1 of 4 (25%) of those with a single partial seizure, and 3 of 10 (30%) of patients who had only simple febrile seizures in childhood. These findings may suggest that hippocampal abnormalities are probably not the sole consequence of repeated seizures and that genetically determined mechanisms might play an important role in the development of hippocampal damage, at least in these familial cases (Kobayashi et al., 2000).

It has been widely accepted, based on large series of surgical patients, that there is a strong correlation between MTS and the severity of the epilepsy. In addition, MTS identified by MRI has been associated with poor control of seizures by antiepileptic medication. However, our findings of MRI abnormalities in patients with good outcome or seizure remission indicate that MTS is found not only in patients with medically refractory TLE (Kobayashi et al., 2000). Evidence for this has already been hinted at in the literature, including descriptions of sporadic patients with MTS who do not have medically refractory epilepsy (Franceschi et al., 1989; Kim et al., 1999). Despite the frequent hippocampal abnormalities, a history of febrile seizures was uncommon among our patients with familial mesial TLE. This is similar to the previous report of familial TLE (Berkovic et al., 1994, 1996) and different from most other series of patients with TLE (Cendes et al., 1993b; Falconer, 1971; Gloor, 1991; Maher and McLachlan, 1995; Sagar and Oxbury, 1987). This suggests that the development of hippocampal pathology in familial mesial TLE is not necessarily linked to prolonged febrile episodes early in life.

II. CONCLUSIONS

The causes of MTS are unknown. Although there is a high incidence of complex febrile seizures among patients with MTS (Abou-Khalil et al., 1993; Cendes et al., 1993a; Falconer, 1971), it is still not clear whether complex febrile seizures are an epiphenomenon or a causative factor (Berg et al., 1998; Shinnar, 1998). Recognition of the incidence of positive family history in patients with mesial TLE and the more recent studies of familial TLE indicate a strong genetic role in the development of MTS (Berkovic et al., 1994, 1996; Cendes et al., 1998; Gambardella et al., 2000; Kobayashi et al., 2000). In view of the seemingly contradictory findings obtained in several studies, it is likely that the association of simple or complex febrile seizures with TLE results from complex interactions with genetic or environmental modifiers, or both.

REFERENCES

Abou-Khalil, B., Andermann, E., Andermann, F., Olivier, A., and Quesney, L. F. (1993). Temporal lobe epilepsy after prolonged febrile convulsions: Excellent outcome after surgical treatment. *Epilepsia* 34, 878–883.

Ben-Ari, Y. (1985). Limbic seizures and brain damage produced by kainic acid: Mechanisms and relevance to human temporal epilepsy. *Neuroscience* 14, 375–403.

Berg, A. T., and Shinnar, S. (1997). Do seizures beget seizures? An assessment of the clinical evidence in humans. *J. Clin. Neurophysiol.* 14, 102–110.

Berg, A. T., Darefsky, A. S., Holford, T. R., and Shinnar, S. (1998). Seizures with fever after unprovoked seizures: An analysis in children followed from the time of a first febrile seizure. *Epilepsia* 39, 77–80.

Berkovic, S. F., and Scheffer, I. E. (1998). Febrile seizures: Genetics and relationship to other epilepsy syndromes. *Curr. Opin. Neurol.* 11, 129–134.

Berkovic, S. F., Howell, R. A., and Hopper, J. L. (1994). Familial temporal lobe epilepsy: A new syndrome with adolescent/adult onset and a benign course. *In* "Epileptic Seizures and Syndromes" (P. Wolf, ed.), pp. 259–265. John Libbey, London.

Berkovic, S. F., Mcintosh, A., Howell, R. A., Mitchell, A., Sheffield, L. J., and Hopper, J. L. (1996). Familial temporal lobe epilepsy—A common disorder identified in twins. *Ann. Neurol.* 40, 227–235.

Camfield, P., Camfield, C., Gordon, K., and Dooley, J. (1994). What types of epilepsy are preceded by febrile seizures? A population-based study of children. *Dev. Med. Child Neurol.* 36, 887–892.

Cendes, F., Andermann, F., Dubeau, F., Gloor, P., Evans, A., Jones-Gotman, M., Olivier, A., Andermann, E., Robitaille, Y., Lopes-Cendes, I., Peters, T., and Melanson, D. (1993a). Early childhood prolonged febrile convulsions, atrophy and sclerosis of mesial structures and temporal lobe epilepsy: An MRI volumetric study. *Neurology* 43, 1083–1087.

Cendes, F., Andermann, F., Gloor, P., Lopes-Cendes, I., Andermann, E., Melanson, D., Jones-Gotman, M., Evans, A., and Peters, T. (1993b). Atrophy of mesial structures in patients with temporal lobe epilepsy: Cause or consequence of repeated seizures? *Ann. Neurol.* 34, 795–801.

Cendes, F., Cook, M. J., Watson, C., Andermann, F., Fish, D. R., Shorvon, S. D., Bergin, P., Free, S., Dubeau, F., and Arnold, D. L. (1995). Frequency and characteristics of dual pathology in patients with lesional epilepsy. *Neurology* 45, 2058–2064.

Cendes, F., Lopes-Cendes, I., Andermann, E., and Andermann, F. (1998). Familial temporal lobe epilepsy: A clinically heterogeneous syndrome. *Neurology* 50, 554–557.

Collingridge, G. L., and Bliss, T. V. P. (1987). NMDA-receptors—Their role in long-term potentiation. *Trends Neurosci.* 10, 288–293.

Davies, K. G., Hermann, B. P., Dohan, F. C., Foley, K. T., Bush, A. J., and Wyler, A. R. (1996). Relationship of hippocampal sclerosis to duration and age of onset of epilepsy, and childhood febrile seizures in temporal lobectomy patients. *Epilepsy Res.* 24, 119–126.

Doose, H. (1998). Contradictory conclusions about the possible effects of prolonged febrile convulsions [letter]. *Epilepsia* 39, 108–110.

Falconer, M. A. (1971). Genetic and related aetiological factors in temporal lobe epilepsy. A review. *Epilepsia* 12, 13–31.

Falconer, M. A. (1974). Mesial temporal (Ammon's horn) sclerosis as a common cause of epilepsy. Aetiology, treatment, and prevention. *Lancet* 2, 767–770.

Falconer, M. A., Serafetinides, E. A., and Corselis, J. A. N. (1964). Etiology and pathogenesis of temporal lobe epilepsy. *Arch. Neurol.* **10**, 233–248.

Fernandez, G., Effenberger, O., Vinz, B., Steinlein, O., Elger, C. E., Dohring, W., and Heinze, H. J. (1998). Hippocampal malformation as a cause of familial febrile convulsions and subsequent hippocampal sclerosis. *Neurology* **50**, 909–917.

Franceschi, M., Triulzi, F., Ferini-Strambi, L., Giusti, M. C., Minicucci, F., Fazio, F., Smirne, S., and Del Maschio, A. (1989). Focal cerebral lesions found by magnetic resonance imaging in cryptogenic nonrefractory temporal lobe epilepsy patients. *Epilepsia* **30**, 540–546.

Gambardella, A., Messina, D., Le Piane, E., Oliveri, R. L., Annesi, G., Zappia, M., Andermann, E., Quattrone, A., and Aguglia, U. (2000). Familial temporal lobe epilepsy autosomal dominant inheritance in a large pedigree from southern Italy. *Epilepsy Res.* **38**, 127–132.

Garcia, P. A., Laxer, K. D., van der Grond, J., Hugg, J. W., Matson, G. B., and Weiner, M. W. (1997). Correlation of seizure frequency with N-acetyl-aspartate levels determined by ^{1}H magnetic resonance spectroscopic imagining. *Magn. Reson. Imaging* **15**, 475–478.

Geddes, J. W., and Cotman, C. W. (1986). Plasticity in hippocampal excitatory amino acid receptors in Alzheimer disease. *Neurosci. Res.* **3**, 672–678.

Gloor, P. (1991). Mesial temporal sclerosis: Historical background and an overview from a modern perspective. In "Epilepsy Surgery" (H. Luders, ed.), pp. 689–703. Raven Press, New York.

Hamati-Haddad, A., and Abou-Khalil, B. (1998). Epilepsy diagnosis and localization in patients with antecedent childhood febrile convulsions. *Neurology* **50**, 917–922.

Hauser, A. W. (1988). Status epilpeticus: Frequency, etiology, and neurological sequelae. *Adv. Neurol.* **34**, 3–14.

Jellinger, K. (1987). Neuropathological aspects of infantile spasms. *Brain Dev.* **9**, 349–357.

Kalviainen, R., Salmenpera, T., Partanen, K., Vainio, P., Riekkinen, P., and Pitkanen, A. (1998). Recurrent seizures may cause hippocampal damage in temporal lobe epilepsy. *Neurology* **50**, 1377–1382.

Kanemoto, K., Takuji, N., Kawasaki, J., and Kawai, I. (1998). Characteristics and treatment of temporal lobe epilepsy with a history of complicated febrile convulsion. *J. Neurol. Neurosurg. Psychiatry* **64**, 245–248.

Kim, W. J., Park, S. C., Lee, S. J., Lee, J. H., Kim, J. Y., Lee, B. I., and Kim, D. I. (1999). The prognosis for control of seizures with medications in patients with MRI evidence for mesial temporal sclerosis. *Epilepsia* **40**, 290–293.

Kobayashi, E., Lopes-Cendes, I., Guerreiro, C. A. M., Sousa, S. C., Guerreiro, M. M., and Cendes, F. (2000). Hippocampal atrophy in familial mesial temporal lobe epilepsy and its relationship with seizure outcome. *Neurology (in press).*

Kudo, Y., and Ogura, A. (1986). Glutamate-induced increase in intracellular Ca^{++} concentration in isolated hippocampal neurones. *Br. J. Pharmacol.* **89**, 191–198.

Kuks, J. B., Cook, M. J., Fish, D. R., Stevens, J. M., and Shorvon, S. D. (1993). Hippocampal sclerosis in epilepsy and childhood febrile seizures. *Lancet* **342**, 1391–1394.

Maher, J., and McLachlan, R. S. (1995). Febrile convulsions. Is seizure duration the most important predictor of temporal lobe epilepsy? *Brain* **118**, 1521–1528.

Mathern, G. W., Babb, T. L., Vickrey, B. G., Melendez, M., and Pretorius, J. K. (1995a). The clinical-pathogenic mechanisms of hippocampal neuron loss and surgical outcomes in temporal lobe epilepsy. *Brain* **118**, 105–118.

Mathern, G. W., Pretorius, J. K., and Babb, T. L. (1995b). Influence of the type of initial precipitating injury and at what age it occurs on course and outcome in patients with temporal lobe seizures. *J. Neurosurg.* **82**, 220–227.

Meencke, H. J., and Janz, D. (1984). Neuropathological findings in primary generalized epilepsy: A study of eight cases. *Epilepsia* **25**, 8–21.

Meencke, H. J., and Veith, G. (1991). Hippocampal sclerosis in epilepsy. In "Epilepsy Surgery" (H. Luders, ed.), pp. 705–715. Raven Press, New York.

Meldrum, B. S., and Brierley, J. B. (1973). Prolonged epileptic seizures in primates. Ischemic cell change and its relation to ictal physiological events. Arch. Neurol. 28, 10–17.

Meldrum, B., and Garthwaite, J. (1990). Excitatory amino acid neurotoxicity and neurodegenerative disease. [Review]. Trends Pharmacol. Sci. 11, 379–387.

Miller, R. J. (1991). The revenge of the kainate receptor. Trends Neurosci. 14, 477–479.

Mouritzen Dam, A. M. (1982). Hippocampal neuron loss in epilepsy and after experimental seizures. Acta Neurol. Scand. 66, 601–642.

Nelson, K. B., and Ellenberg, J. H. (1976). Predictors of epilepsy in children who have experienced febrile seizures. N. Engl. J. Med. 295, 1029–1033.

Ounstead, C., Lindsay, J., and Norman, R. (1966). "Biological Factors in Temporal Lobe Epilepsy." Willian Heinemann Medical Books, London.

Pitkanen, A., Laakso, M., Kalviainen, R., Partanen, K., Vainio, P., Lehtovirta, M., Riekkinen, P., and Soininen, H. (1996). Severity of hippocampal atrophy correlates with the prolongation of MRI T-2 relaxation in temporal lobe epilepsy but not in Alzheimer's disease. Neurology 46, 1724–1730.

Raymond, A. A., Fish, D. R., Stevens, J. M., Cook, M. J., Sisodiya, S. M., and Shorvon, S. D. (1994). Association of hippocampal sclerosis with cortical dysgenesis in patients with epilepsy. Neurology 44, 1841–1845.

Sagar, H. J., and Oxbury, J. M. (1987). Hippocampal neuron loss in temporal lobe epilepsy: Correlation with early childhood convulsions. Ann. Neurol. 22, 334–340.

Schmidt, D., Tsai, J. J., and Janz, D. (1985). Febrile seizures in patients with complex partial seizures. Acta Neurol. Scand. 72, 68–71.

Shinnar, S. (1998). Prolonged febrile seizures and mesial temporal sclerosis [editorial; comment]. Ann Neurol. 43, 411–412.

Sloviter, R. S., and Pedley, T. A. (1998). Subtle hippocampal malformation: Importance in febrile seizures and development of epilepsy [editorial; comment]. Neurology 50, 846–849.

Sloviter, R. S., Sollas, A. L., Barbaro, N. M., and Laxer, K. D. (1991). Calcium-binding protein (calbindin-D-28K) and parvalbumin immunocytochemistry in the normal and epileptic human hippocampus. J. Comp. Neurol. 308, 381–396.

Tasch, E., Cendes, F., Li, L. M., Dubeau, F., Andermann, F., and Arnold, D. L. (1999). Neuroimaging evidence of progressive neuronal loss and dysfunction in temporal lobe epilepsy [see comments]. Ann. Neurol. 45, 568–576.

Theodore, W., and Wasterlain, C. G. (1999). Do early seizures beget epilepsy? [editorial; comment]. Neurology 53, 898–899.

Theodore, W. H., Bhatia, S., Hatta, J., Fazilat, S., DeCarli, C., Bookheimer, S. Y., and Gaillard, W. D. (1999). Hippocampal atrophy, epilepsy duration, and febrile seizures in patients with partial seizures. Neurology 52, 132–136.

Trenerry, M. R., Jack, C. R., Jr., Sharbrough, F. W., Cascino, G. D., Hirschorn, K. A., Marsh, W. R., Kelly, P. J., and Meyer, F. B. (1993). Quantitative MRI hippocampal volumes: Association with onset and duration of epilepsy, and febrile convulsions in temporal lobectomy patients. Epilepsy Res. 15, 247–252.

VanLandingham, K. E., Heinz, E. R., Cavazos, J. E., and Lewis, D. V. (1998). Magnetic resonance imaging evidence of hippocampal injury after prolonged focal febrile convulsions. Ann. Neurol. 43, 413–426.

Van Paesschen, W., Connelly, A., King, M. D., Jackson, G. D., and Duncan, J. S. (1997). The spectrum of hippocampal sclerosis: A quantitative magnetic resonance imaging study. Ann. Neurol. 41, 41–51.

Veith, G. (1970). Anatomische Studie uber die Ammonshornsklerose im Epileptikergehirn. *Dtsch. Z. Nervenheilk* **197**, 293–314.

Watson, C., Jack, C. R., Jr., and Cendes, F. (1997). Volumetric magnetic resonance imaging. Clinical applications and contributions to the understanding of temporal lobe epilepsy. *Arch. Neurol.* **54**, 1521–1531.

Zimmerman, H. M. (1940). The histopathology of convulsive disorders in children. *J. Pediatr.* **13**, 359–390.

CHAPTER 7

Do Febrile Seizures Lead to Temporal Lobe Epilepsy? Prospective and Epidemiological Studies

SHLOMO SHINNAR

Departments of Neurology and Pediatrics, and Comprehensive Epilepsy Management Center, Montefiore Medical Center, Albert Einstein College of Medicine, Bronx, New York 10467

Retrospective studies from tertiary epilepsy centers report that many adults with intractable temporal lobe epilepsy have a history of prolonged or atypical febrile seizures in childhood. However, epidemiological studies do not support a causal association between febrile seizures and epilepsy in general and temporal lobe epilepsy in particular. This is true for both simple and complex febrile seizures. It is clear that febrile seizures, particularly complex febrile seizures, are associated with an increased risk of epilepsy, though not necessarily of temporal lobe epilepsy. However, the epidemiological data are best explained by considering febrile seizures as a marker of susceptibility to seizures and future epilepsy, rather than as a cause. In other words, children with an underlying predisposition to seizures based on either genetic or anatomical abnormalities, will in the developmental age window of susceptibility to febrile seizures also be more likely to experience febrile seizures. Furthermore, children with underlying brain abnormalities may be more susceptible to have febrile seizures that are both long and complex. It is clear from imaging studies that very prolonged seizures lasting an hour or more can be associated with acute hippocampal injury that may progress to mesial temporal sclerosis (MTS) in some cases. The frequency with which this occurs even in cases of febrile status epilepticus is unknown. Cases of this nature are sufficiently rare that even large series of febrile seizures or of childhood-onset epilepsy will contain only a few cases and therefore the problem needs to be addressed combining epidemiological methods with imaging studies and other techniques. Although there is strong evidence supporting the occurrence of seizure-induced injury with very prolonged febrile seizures, the epidemiological data do not support an association between less prolonged seizures, even if complex, and temporal lobe epilepsy. It is also clear that the majority of cases of temporal lobe epilepsy and even of MTS are not associated with prior febrile seizures, thus febrile seizure-induced injury cannot account for the majority of patients with temporal lobe epilepsy or MTS. Further studies are needed to identify those children who are at risk for seizure-induced injury from prolonged febrile seizures and the necessary conditions for such injury to occur. © 2002 Academic Press.

I. INTRODUCTION

Retrospective studies (see Chapter 6, this volume) from tertiary epilepsy centers report that many adults with intractable temporal lobe epilepsy have a history of prolonged or atypical febrile seizures in childhood (Abou-Khalil et al., 1993; Bruton, 1988; Cendes et al., 1993a,b; Falconer et al., 1964; Falconer, 1971; French et al., 1993; Margerison and Corsellis, 1966; Mathern et al., 1995a,b; Sagar and Oxbury, 1987). Animal models of febrile seizures indicate that prolonged febrile seizures may be associated with long-term changes in hippocampal excitability (Dube et al., 2000; Toth et al., 1998) (see Chapters 9 and 15) and that brains with preexisting abnormalities may be more predisposed to both seizures and seizure-induced injury (Germano et al., 1996) (see Chapter 10). However, population-based studies have failed to find this association, as have prospective studies of febrile seizures. This chapter will review the data from epidemiological and prospective studies of febrile seizures and epilepsy regarding the association between febrile seizures, particularly prolonged febrile seizures and subsequent temporal lobe epilepsy.

II. PROSPECTIVE EPIDEMIOLOGICAL STUDIES OF FEBRILE SEIZURES

Data from five large cohorts of children with febrile seizures indicate that 2–10% of children who have febrile seizures will subsequently develop unprovoked seizures or epilepsy (Annegers et al., 1979, 1987; Berg and Shinnar, 1996b; Nelson and Ellenberg, 1978; van den Berg and Yerushalmi, 1969; Verity and Golding, 1991). Note that the higher number comes from the study of Annegers et al., (1987), which had the longest follow-up period. In most studies, the risk of developing epilepsy after a single simple febrile seizure is only mildly elevated over the risk in the general population (Annegers et al., 1979, 1987; Berg and Shinnar, 1996b; Nelson and Ellenberg, 1976, 1978; van den Berg and Yerushalmi, 1969; Verity and Golding, 1991). The risk factors for developing epilepsy after febrile seizures are reviewed in Chapter 5.

Complex febrile seizures are clearly associated with an increased risk of subsequent epilepsy. There is some controversy whether the number of complex features affect the risk of later epilepsy. Two studies have examined this issue in detail. Both found that very prolonged febrile seizures (i.e., febrile status epilepticus) were associated with an increased risk of subsequent epilepsy, above that of a complex febrile seizure that was less prolonged (Annegers *et al.*, 1987; Berg and Shinnar, 1996b). However, the study of Annegers *et al.* (1987) found that having two complex features (e.g., prolonged and focal) further increased the risk of subsequent epilepsy; this association was not found in the study of Berg and Shinnar (1996b).

The types of epilepsy developed are variable. Annegers *et al.* (1987) report that usually those with generalized febrile seizures will develop generalized epilepsies whereas those with focal febrile seizures will develop focal epilepsies. This suggests that the febrile seizures may be an age-specific expression of seizure susceptibility in patients with an underlying seizure diathesis (Annegers *et al.*, 1987; Shinnar and Moshe, 1991). In general, as discussed below, the types of epilepsy that occur in children with prior febrile seizures are varied and not very different than that which occur in children without such a history (Berg *et al.*, 1996b; Camfield *et al.*, 1994; Sofianov *et al.*, 1983). Also of note is that populations with a cumulative incidence of febrile seizures of 10%, such as in Tokyo, Japan, do not have an increased incidence of epilepsy (Tsuboi, 1984; Tsuboi *et al.*, 1991). The weight of the epidemiological data is against a causal association in the majority of cases.

A significant limitation of all these prospective studies is that there are no data provided on the specific epilepsy syndrome (Commission, 1989) in any of the prospective cohort studies of febrile seizures (Annegers *et al.*, 1979, 1987; Berg *et al.*, 1996b; Nelson and Ellenberg, 1976, 1978; Tsuboi *et al.*, 1991; Verity *et al.*, 1991, 1993; van den Berg and Yerushalmi, 1969). All focus on risk factors for epilepsy, as discussed in detail in Chapter 5, but only a few (Annegers *et al.*, 1979, 1987; Berg and Shinnar, 1996b) even tell us whether the epilepsy was focal or generalized. Thus, other data must be examined to address the relationship between febrile seizures and temporal lobe epilepsy.

III. PROSPECTIVE RANDOMIZED THERAPEUTIC TRIALS OF FEBRILE SEIZURES

If febrile seizures are causally related to epilepsy in general and temporal lobe epilepsy in particular, then preventing them should reduce the risk of subsequent epilepsy. There have been three well-designed randomized clinical trials for preventing febrile seizure recurrence (see Chapters 3 and 19) that have also assessed the risk of subsequently developing epilepsy (Knudsen *et al.*, 1996;

Rosman *et al.*, 1993; Wolf and Forsythe, 1989). In two of these studies, follow-ups of 10 or more years were available (Knudsen *et al.*, 1996; Wolf and Forsythe, 1989). Despite the fact that the treatment arm was effective in reducing the risk of recurrent febrile seizures in all three studies, there was no difference in the rate of developing epilepsy in any of the three studies. In general, there is no evidence from prospective randomized trials that treating febrile seizures or any other form of acute symptomatic seizures prevents subsequent epilepsy (Berg and Shinnar, 1997; Shinnar and Berg, 1996). Unfortunately, as was the case with studies of febrile seizures discussed previously, no information is given regarding specific epilepsy syndromes, including temporal lobe epilepsy. These studies included a substantial number of children with complex febrile seizures, but the number who actually had febrile status epilepticus in each series was quite small.

IV. PROSPECTIVE STUDIES OF FEBRILE STATUS EPILEPTICUS

If febrile seizures cause temporal lobe epilepsy, a good place to study this association would be in very prolonged febrile seizures or febrile status epilepticus. Febrile status epilepticus, which is the extreme end of complex febrile seizures, accounts for approximately 5% of all febrile seizures (Berg and Shinnar, 1996a). However, it accounts for approximately one-quarter of all pediatric status epilepticus (Dodson *et al.*, 1993; Maytal *et al.*, 1989) and for approximately two-thirds of status epilepticus in the second year of life (Shinnar *et al.*, 1997). The data from retrospective studies presented in Chapter 6 and from imaging studies presented in Chapter 8 are most convincing with regard to the association between febrile status epilepticus and mesial temporal sclerosis and temporal lobe epilepsy. The data from prospective outcome studies of febrile status epilepticus are intriguing but far from definitive.

Studies of the outcomes of febrile seizures that specifically analyzed the risk of epilepsy after febrile status epilepticus (Annegers *et al.*, 1987; Berg and Shinnar, 1996b; Verity *et al.*, 1993) all report a much higher risk of epilepsy following febrile status epilepticus. As was the case with the overall studies, the specific epilepsy syndromes are not listed. Studies of childhood status epilepticus that included children with febrile status generally report only short-term outcomes of morbidity and mortality and, with few exceptions. do not report the risk for subsequent epilepsy (Shinnar and Babb, 1997). In those that do (Maytal and Shinnar, 1990) the duration of follow-up is only a few years and the epilepsy syndromes are not specified. In a reported cohort of 180 children with febrile status epilepticus prospectively recruited between 1984 and 1996 (Shinnar *et al.*, 2001) the risk of epilepsy to date after a mean of 10 years is approximately 20% (S. Shinnar, unpublished data), but the specific epilepsy syndromes have not yet been ascertained.

The most interesting data in this regard are the prospective studies of febrile status epilepticus that have imaged the children within 72 hours of the seizure (vanLandingham *et al.*, 1998); these are discussed in detail in Chapter 8. Of note is that only those children whose seizures were both focal and prolonged developed either acute changes or mesial temporal sclerosis (MTS). Also, to date, only one of the children who developed MTS has gone on to have temporal lobe epilepsy. Long-term follow-up of such cohorts utilizing both clinical and imaging data may provide more answers as to how often this phenomenon actually occurs.

V. EPIDEMIOLOGICAL STUDIES OF EPILEPSY

The retrospective studies (Abou-Khalil *et al.*, 1993; Bruton, 1988; Cendes *et al.*, 1993a,b; Falconer *et al.*, 1964; Falconer, 1971; French *et al.*, 1993; Margerison and Corsellis, 1966; Mathern *et al.*, 1995a,b; Sagar and Oxbury, 1987) reviewed in Chapter 6 are mostly from selected populations with refractory mesial temporal lobe epilepsy undergoing evaluations for epilepsy surgery. In this section we will review the data from population-based studies of epilepsy. In epidemiological studies of childhood-onset epilepsy, 10–20% of people with epilepsy or unprovoked seizures have a history of prior febrile seizures (Berg *et al.*, 1999d; Camfield *et al.*, 1994; Sofianov *et al.*, 1983). This is a much higher rate of febrile seizures than the 2–4% rate reported in the general population in North America (Shinnar, 1999) (see Chapter 1). However, an association between febrile seizures and temporal lobe epilepsy or even with complex partial seizures is not found in these studies.

Sofianov *et al.* (1983) examined 846 children with epilepsy seen between 1968 and 1976, in a clinic where the majority of children with seizures in that district in Yugoslavia were seen. Of these 846 children 172 (20%) had a history of prior febrile seizures, including 61 children with simple febrile seizures and 111 with complex febrile seizures. The type of epilepsy was classified according to the earlier classification of Gastaut (1969) and the results are not listed in detail. They do report that the great majority of children with prior febrile seizures had secondarily generalized seizures. There were no statistically significant differences in the types of epilepsy among children with and without prior febrile seizures. There were also no differences in remission rates in the children with epilepsy with and without a history of prior febrile seizures.

Camfield *et al.* (1994) examined all children in Nova Scotia with onset of epilepsy between 1977 and 1985. After excluding those with minor motor seizures and those with absence seizures they found that 73 (15%) of 489 children with epilepsy had prior febrile seizures. Generalized tonic–clonic seizures were more frequently preceded by febrile seizures (26 of 119; 22%) than were complex partial seizures (16 of 126; 14%) or partial seizures with secondary generalization (24 of 179; 13%). Prior febrile seizures were more common in those with definite generalized seizures (26 of 93; 28%) than in those with definite partial seizures (45 of 293; 15%, $p < 0.03$).

In the study of Camfield et al. (1994), 17 children had prolonged febrile seizures defined as lasting 20 minutes or more. The mean duration of these was 68.5 minutes with a range of 20 to 120 minutes. Prolonged febrile seizures were more likely to occur in children with neurological disability. However, they were not clearly associated specifically with any one seizure type occurring in 2% (2 of 126) of children with tonic–clonic seizures, 6% (8 of 129) with complex partial seizures, and 4% (7 of 184) with partial seizures with secondary generalization. However, in this study, prolonged febrile seizures were associated with the development of intractable epilepsy. When followed up in 1989–1990, 39 of 482 subjects with adequate data were defined as intractable, including 7 (41%) of 17 with prolonged febrile seizures versus 32 (7%) of 433 with no history of prolonged febrile seizures ($p = 0.0002$), whether or not they had a history of other febrile seizures. Although prolonged febrile seizures were strongly associated with the development of intractable epilepsy, the association with intractable temporal lobe epilepsy in this study is much weaker. Of the 39 children with intractable epilepsy, 16 had complex partial seizures. Only 2 of these had prior prolonged febrile seizures in the absence of other identifiable causes for their intractable seizures. One of these underwent temporal lobectomy and the pathology was mesial temporal sclerosis.

Berg et al. (1999b) prospectively recruited a community-based cohort of 613 children with newly diagnosed epilepsy in Connecticut between 1993 and 1997. Seventy-three (14%) of the 524 children with age of onset above 1 year for whom a history was available had a prior history of febrile seizures, including 33 with complex febrile seizures (Berg et al., 1999d). These included focal seizures in 17, multiple seizures in 19, and prolonged seizures (≥ 10 minutes) in 9 children, 7 of whom had febrile status epilepticus (≥ 30 minutes). There was no association between febrile seizures and either complex partial seizures or temporal lobe epilepsy. A history of febrile seizures was less common in children with absence seizures (6%, $p = 0.003$) and simple partial seizures (6%, $p = 0.04$) but was no different in those with complex partial seizures (15%), either with or without secondary generalization. There was no difference in the rate of prior febrile seizures between children with localization-related epilepsies (45 of 322; 14%) and generalized epilepsies (13 of 140; 9%). Within the localization-related epilepsies, there were no differences in the rate of prior febrile seizures among those with temporal lobe epilepsy (10 o 79; 13%) and those with extratemporal epilepsy (9 of 66; 14%).

If one limits the analysis to complex febrile seizures the results are not very different. There is still no association between prior complex febrile seizures and either temporal lobe epilepsy or complex partial seizures (Berg *et al.*, 1999d). Focal febrile seizures were equally likely in those with idiopathic and symptomatic localization-related epilepsy. Prolonged febrile seizures were somewhat more common in those with symptomatic localization-related epilepsy (5 of 24; 21%) as defined by the International League Against Epilepsy (ILAE) (Commission, 1989; Berg *et al.*, 1999a,b) than in those with cryptogenic (1 of 15; 7%) or idiopathic (0 of 6; 0%) localization-related epilepsies, but this did not reach statistical significance ($p = 0.18$) (Berg *et al.*, 1999d). The one clear association was that, on multivariable analysis, those with complex febrile seizures had an earlier age of onset of epilepsy compared to those with no history of prior febrile seizures (odds ratio 0.8 per year increase in age, $p = 0.002$) or those with only simple febrile seizures. This finding is of particular interest because, in surgical series, MTS is associated with a younger age of onset of epilepsy (Abou-Khalil *et al.*, 1993; Bruton, 1988; Cendes *et al.*, 1993a,b; Davies *et al.*, 1996; French *et al.*, 1993; Margerison and Corsellis, 1966; Sagar and Oxbury, 1987). Davies *et al.* (1996) report that the association between MTS and febrile seizures in their series of surgical cases was largely explained by the age of onset of the epilepsy. Both MTS and a history of febrile seizures were associated with a younger age of onset. Once the effects of age of onset were controlled for, neither febrile seizures nor prolonged febrile seizures were significantly associated with MTS.

In the Connecticut study of newly diagnosed childhood epilepsy, neuroimaging was available in 488 (80%) of the 613 children, including MRIs in 388 (Berg *et al.*, 2000). There were 3 cases of MTS based on the initial MRI and none of them had a prior history of febrile seizures of any type (Berg *et al.*, 1999d, 2000). Of note is that in the Connecticut study to date, 64 (11%) of 599 children followed for more than 18 months have met the criteria for intractability, defined as failing to respond to two or more antiepileptic drugs and an average of one or more seizure per month for 18 months (Berg *et al.*, 2001a,b). There was no association between prior febrile seizures, either simple or complex, and early development of intractability in this study.

The only population-based studies of epilepsy that include adults and specifically address the issue of prior febrile seizures are from the Rochester, Minnesota patient registry of the Mayo Clinic (Rocca *et al.*, 1987a,b,c). The results are reported by seizure type (Commission, 1981) and not by epilepsy syndrome (Commission, 1989). Of 82 subjects with complex partial seizures, 16 (20%) had a history of febrile seizures compared with 2% of control subjects without epilepsy ($p < 0.0001$). On the other hand, this rate is not very different than the 10–20% rate reported in patients with all forms of epilepsy in the studies of childhood-onset seizures previously discussed (Berg *et al.*, 1999d; Camfield *et* al., 1994; Sofianov et al., 1983). In fact, these same authors also separately published studies of risk factors for absence (Rocca et al., 1987b) and generalized tonic–clonic seizures (Rocca et al., 1987c) from the same database. Prior febrile seizures were present in 6 (20%) of 30 patients with absence seizures and 10 (20%) of 53 cases of generalized tonic–clonic seizures. The rate of prior febrile seizures in all three groups was much higher than the 2% rate seen in controls without epilepsy but was not different in patients with complex partial seizures than in those with other seizure types. What was different was the distribution of the types of febrile seizures seen. In the 16 subjects with complex partial seizures who had prior febrile seizures, 14 (88%) had febrile seizures with one or more complex features, including 9 with focal seizures, 9 with more than one seizure in 24 hours, and 9 with seizures lasting longer than 15 minutes.

Hamati Haddad and Abou-Khalil (1998) studied patients presenting to a seizure clinic and reported that 133 (13%) of 1005 subjects had a history of prior febrile seizures. This study did examine epilepsy syndromes and reported that 78 (25%) of 310 subjects with temporal lobe epilepsy had a history of prior febrile seizures, compared with 12 (6%) of 216 with extratemporal partial epilepsy ($p < 0.0001$) and 16 (11%) of 146 subjects with generalized epilepsy ($p < 0.001$). Subjects with temporal lobe epilepsy were also more likely to have a history of prolonged febrile seizures. Although the population in this study was less selected than that reported in surgical series, it was still a population referred to a seizure clinic at a tertiary care hospital, and as such would be a more select group than the subjects in population- and community-based studies, which makes the interpretation of the findings more difficult.

VI. LIMITATIONS OF PROSPECTIVE AND POPULATION-BASED STUDIES

Epidemiological studies have changed our understanding of the incidence, prevalence and natural history of febrile seizures and of epilepsy (Berg and Shinnar, 1994) There are, however, several limitations to the prospective and population-based studies, only some of which are avoidable. The lack of classification of outcome by epilepsy syndrome in the published studies is unfortunate though not fully avoidable. Many of these studies were done prior to the new guidelines for epidemiological research in epilepsy (Commission, 1993) and even prior to the current classification scheme of epilepsy syndromes (Commission, 1989; Roger et al., 1992). In addition, the data necessary to classify syndromes are not always available in such observational studies. However, the definition of temporal lobe epilepsy has not changed much over the years, though our diagnostic ability to recognize it has improved. Furthermore, several epidemiological studies of seizures have shown that it is possible in most cases to identify epilepsy syndromes in newly diagnosed cases (Berg et al., 1999a,b) and to go back and classify syndromes in previously recruited cohorts (Shinnar et al., 1999; Sillanpaa et al., 1999), so that this should be feasible in principle.

A more serious limitation is the duration of follow-up needed to define the association. In retrospective studies (reviewed in Chapter 6), the latency period between the febrile seizures and the subsequent development of recognizable temporal lobe epilepsy is quite long, with latency periods averaging 8 to 11 years (French et al., 1993; Mathern et al., 1995a,b). Therefore, prospective studies of febrile seizures would have to have follow-up periods of more than 10 years to identify properly the evolution of febrile seizures to temporal lobe epilepsy. Of the prospective studies of febrile seizures, only the study of Tsuboi et al. (1991) has a 16-year follow-up of a clinic-based cohort of children with febrile seizures. The other studies (Berg et al., 1996b; Nelson and Ellenberg, 1976, 1978; Verity and Golding, 1991) all have follow-ups of less than 10 years and focus on short-term risks. The study with the longest duration of follow-up (Annegers et al., 1987) is based on a chart review of the Mayo Clinic data, and although population based is not a prospective study. Prospective follow-up studies of many years are very difficult and expensive to do and none of the available studies is ideal for studying the specific outcome of febrile seizures leading to temporal lobe epilepsy.

An additional severe limitation of epidemiological studies is the relative rarity, at least in the human, of the target event (febrile seizures causing temporal lobe epilepsy). If one looks at the imaging studies discussed in Chapter 8 and particularly at the series examining the relationship between prolonged febrile seizures and MTS (Fernandez et al., 1998; Maher and McLachlan, 1995; van-Landingham et al., 1998), they report that the mean duration of the febrile seizure in those cases was 90 to 100 minutes. It is clear that not all cases of MTS are associated with refractory temporal lobe epilepsy (Kim et al., 1999; Kobayashi et al., 2001). It is also clear that only a minority of cases of MTS or temporal lobe epilepsy are associated with prior febrile seizures, whether causally or otherwise (Abou-Khalil et al., 1993; Berg et al., 1999d, 2000; Bruton, 1988; Camfield et al., 1994; Cendes et al., 1993a,b; Falconer et al., 1964; Falconer, 1971; French et al., 1993; Margerison and Corsellis, 1966; Mathern et al., 1995a,b; Rocca et al., 1987a; Sagar and Oxbury, 1987; Sofianov et al., 1983). Even if all cases of MTS were associated with refractory temporal lobe epilepsy, we would be chasing the proverbial needle in a haystack. Approximately 5% of cases of febrile seizures last 30 or more minutes, meeting the criteria for status epilepticus (Berg and Shinnar, 1996a). Of children with febrile status epilepticus, approximately 40% of seizures last 60 minutes or more and 18% last 120 minutes or more (Shinnar et al., 2001). If one adds the requirement that the febrile seizure be focal, which was also a requirement for acute hippocampal injury (vanLandingham *et al.*, 1998), that occurs in approximately 40% of febrile status epilepticus (Chevrie and Aicardi, 1975; Shinnar *et al.*, 2001). Therefore, approximately one in six cases of febrile status epilepticus will be focal and last more than 60 minutes. This would translate into less than 1% of febrile seizures. Because acute injury and/or subsequent MTS do not occur in all cases, the numbers needed to find an effect using only epidemiological techniques are huge and well beyond the numbers seen in any of the published epidemiological series of the outcome of febrile seizures.

Similar problems arise in the population-based studies of epilepsy. In the entire cohort of 613 children with newly diagnosed epilepsy in Connecticut, 56 (9%) had a history of status epilepticus by the time of diagnosis but only 8 (1%) had a history of prior febrile status epilepticus (Berg *et al.*, 1999c) . Similarly, in the study of childhood epilepsy in Nova Scotia, a history of prolonged febrile seizures (>20 minutes) was present in 17 (3%) of 489 subjects (Camfield *et al.*, 1994). Given the large number of children with epilepsy who have prior febrile seizures (10–20%), which in the majority of cases are not causally related, epidemiological techniques are unlikely to find an association even if a causal relation was present in a small subgroup of cases.

One should remember that, in general, epidemiological studies demonstrate an association and not a cause-and-effect relationship. When that relationship is strong and particularly when one can show a dose-dependent effect, and a temporal relationship exists, a causal relationship is often inferred, though other criteria may be needed to prove it. However, in the case of febrile seizures, when the actual event (a febrile seizure) is common but there is a high threshold for an adverse effect to occur and the outcome studied (epilepsy or temporal lobe epilepsy) is also not rare, with a multifactorial etiology, epidemiological techniques in isolation may not be the optimal way to approach the problem.

VII. FEBRILE SEIZURES AND TEMPORAL LOBE EPILEPSY: CAUSAL RELATIONSHIP OR EARLY MARKER FOR SUBSEQUENT TEMPORAL LOBE EPILEPSY?

In the epidemiological studies of febrile seizures, there is an increased risk of subsequent epilepsy in children with febrile seizures, particularly complex febrile seizures (see Chapter 5). In addition, there is a much higher rate of prior febrile seizures in studies of epilepsy of all types (Berg *et al.*, 1999d; Camfield *et al.*, 1994; Hamati-Haddad and Abou-Khalil, 1998; Rocca *et al.*, 1987a,b,c; Sofianov *et al.*, 1983), including both generalized and partial epilepsies. The epidemiological data are much more consistent with febrile seizures being a marker of increased seizure susceptibility than being causally related to epilepsy in general and temporal lobe epilepsy in particular (Berg *et al.*, 1999d; Camfield *et al.*, 1994; Shinnar and Moshe, 1991; Rocca *et al.*, 1987a,b,c; Sofianov *et al.*, 1983). Those with generalized febrile seizures are more likely to develop a generalized epilepsy whereas those with focal febrile seizures are more likely to develop a partial epilepsy (Annegers *et al.*, 1987). There is also an association between prolonged febrile seizures and partial epilepsy (Annegers *et al.*, 1987). However, it is confounded by the fact that prolonged febrile seizures are also more likely to be focal (Berg and Shinnar, 1996a; Chevrie and Aicardi, 1975). One should note that although the epidemiological data do not support a causal relationship between febrile seizures and temporal lobe epilepsy, neither do they rule out the possibility that a causal relationship exists in a small proportion of the cases. Of particular interest are the data from the study of Camfield *et al.* (1994) that prolonged febrile seizures were associated with intractable seizures, although this was not the case in the study of newly diagnosed childhood-onset epilepsy in Connecticut (Berg *et al.*, 2001b).

In the past few years, the focus of debate on this issue has shifted. As the review of the retrospective data in Chapter 6 demonstrates, the association between febrile seizures and temporal lobe epilepsy is a complex one that is clearly not always causal. Conversely, the imaging studies reviewed in Chapter 8, and in particular the elegant study of vanLandingham *et al.* (1998), provide strong evidence that the association is causal at least in some cases. Therefore, the focus of the current debate is on how often the association is a causal one (Shinnar, 1998; Sloviter and Pedley, 1998), and what are the other factors—such as preexisting brain abnormalities, genetic predisposition, and the type of precipitating illness—that determine when febrile seizures will cause injury (Berkovic and Jackson, 2000; Kanemoto *et al.*, 2000; Shinnar, 1998). The imaging studies may also explain why epidemiological studies do not suggest a causal relationship between prolonged febrile seizures and temporal lobe epilepsy. In these studies, which examined MTS as a surrogate for temporal lobe epilepsy (Fernandez *et al.*, 1998; Maher and McLachlan, 1995; vanLandingham *et al.*, 1998), the mean seizure duration associated with either acute hippocampal edema or subsequent MTS was 90 to 100 minutes. This is well beyond what is seen with most complex febrile seizures and is prolonged even for cases of febrile status epilepticus (Maytal *et al.*, 1989; Shinnar *et al.*, 2001). In addition, the clinical (Fernandez *et al.*, 1998; Maher and McLachlan, 1995; vanLandingham *et al.*, 1998) and animal (Germano *et al.*, 1996) data suggest that children with preexisting brain abnormalities may be more predisposed both to having prolonged seizures and to seizure-induced injury. There is a high frequency of subtle cortical dysplasia (Hardiman *et al.*, 1988; Mathern *et al.*, 1995a,b) or other preexisting hippocampal abnormalities in patients with evidence of MTS. In epidemiological studies the existence of a cortical dysplasia or other abnormality would lead to the classification of both the prolonged febrile seizure and the temporal lobe epilepsy as being caused by the preexisting abnormality, unless there was clear and convincing proof, such as an acute imaging study, of seizure-induced injury. Given the high noise level of prior febrile seizures in patients with epilepsy, where the febrile seizures clearly are a marker for increased seizure susceptibility, it is not surprising that epidemiological studies have not detected the relatively small number of cases in which a causal relationship exists.

REFERENCES

Abou-Khalil, B., Andermann, E., Andermann, F., Olivier, A., and Quesney, L. F. (1993). Temporal lobe epilepsy after prolonged febrile convulsions: Excellent outcome after surgical treatment. *Epilepsia* 34, 878–883.

Annegers, J. F., Hauser, W. A., Elveback, L. R., and Kurland, L. T. (1979). The risk of epilepsy following febrile convulsions. *Neurology* 29, 297–303.

Annegers, J. F., Hauser, W. A., Shirts, S. B., and Kurland, L. T. (1987). Factors prognostic of unprovoked seizures after febrile convulsions. *N. Engl. J. Med.* 316, 493–498.

Berg, A. T., and Shinnar, S. (1994). The contributions of epidemiology to the understanding of childhood seizures and epilepsy. *J. Child Neurol.* 9 (Suppl. 2), S19–S26.

Berg, A. T., and Shinnar, S. (1996a). Complex febrile seizures. *Epilepsia* 37, 126–133.

Berg, A. T., and Shinnar, S. (1996b). Unprovoked seizures in children with febrile seizures: Short term outcomes. *Neurology* 47, 562–568.

Berg, A. T., and Shinnar, S. (1997). Do seizures beget seizures? An assessment of the clinical evidence in humans. *J. Clin. Neurophysiol.* 14, 102–110.

Berg, A. T., Levy, S. R., Testa, F. M., and Shinnar, S. (1999a). Classification of childhood epilepsy syndromes in newly diagnosed epilepsy: Interrater agreement and reasons for disagreement. *Epilepsia* 40, 439–444.

Berg, A. T., Shinnar, S., Levy, S. R., and Testa, F. M. (1999b). Newly diagnosed epilepsy in children: Presentation and diagnosis. *Epilepsia* 40, 445–452.

Berg, A. T., Shinnar, S., Levy, S. R., and Testa, F. M. (1999c). Status epilepticus in children with newly diagnosed epilepsy. *Ann. Neurol.* 45, 618–623.

Berg, A. T., Shinnar, S., Levy, S. R., and Testa, F. M. (1999d) Childhood-onset epilepsy with and without preceding febrile seizures. *Neurology* 53, 1742–1748.

Berg, A. T., Testa, F. M., Levy, S. R., and Shinnar, S. (2000). Neuroimaging in children with newly diagnosed epilepsy: A community-based study. *Pediatrics* 106, 527–532.

Berg, A. T., Shinnar, S., and Levy, S. R., *et al.* (2001a). Defining early seizure outcomes in pediatric epilepsy: The good, the bad, and the in-between. *Epilepsy Res.* 43, 75–84.

Berg, A. T., Shinnar, S., Levy, S. R., Testa, F. M., Smith-Rapaport, S., and Beckerman, B. (2001b). Early development of intractable epilepsy in children: A prospective study. *Neurology* 56, 1445–1452.

Berkovic, S. F., and Jackson, G. D. (2000). The hippocampal sclerosis whodunit: Enter the genes. *Ann. Neurol.* 47, 571–574.

Briellmann, R. S., Jackson, G. D., Torn-Broers, B. A., and Berkovic, S. F. (2001). Causes of epilepsies: Insights from discordant twin pairs. *Ann. Neurol,* 49, 45–52.

Bruton, C. J. (1998). "The Neuropathology of Temporal Lobe Epilepsy" pp. 1–158. Oxford University Press, New York.

Camfield, C. S., Camfield, P. R., Dooley, J. M., and Gordon, K. (1994). What type of afebrile seizures are preceded by febrile seizures?—A population-based study of children. *Dev. Med. Child Neurol.* **36**, 887–892.

Cendes, F., Andermann, F., Dubeau, F., *et al.* (1993a). Early childhood prolonged febrile convulsions, atrophy and sclerosis of mesial structures, and temporal lobe epilepsy: An MRI volumetric study. *Neurology* **43**, 1083–1087.

Cendes, F., Andermann, F., Gloor, P., *et al.* (1993b). Atrophy of mesial structures in patients with temporal lobe epilepsy: Cause or consequence of repeated seizures. *Ann. Neurol.* **34**, 795–801.

Chan, S., Chin, S. S. M., Kartha, K., *et al.* (1996). Reversible signal abnormalities in the hippocampus and neocortex after prolonged seizure. *AJNR Am. J. Neuroradiol.* **17**, 1725–1731.

Chevrie, J. J., and Aicardi, J. (1975). Duration and lateralization of febrile convulsions. Etiological factors. *Epilepsia* **16**, 781–789.

Commission on Classification and Terminology of the International League Against Epilepsy (1981). Proposal for revised clinical and electrographic classification of epileptic seizures. *Epilepsia* **22**, 489–501.

Commission on Classification and Terminology of the International League Against Epilepsy (1989). Proposal for revised classification of epilepsies and epileptic syndromes. *Epilepsia* **30**, 389–399.

Commission on Epidemiology and Prognosis, International League Against Epilepsy (1993). Guidelines for epidemiologic studies on epilepsy. *Epilepsia* **34**, 592–596.

Davies, K. G., Hermann, B. P., Dohan, F. C., Foley, K. T., Bush, A. J., and Wyler, A. R. (1996). Relationship of hippocampal sclerosis to duration and age of onset of epilepsy, and childhood febrile seizures in temporal lobectomy patients *Epilepsy Res.* **24**, 119–126.

Dodson, W. E., DeLorenzo, R. J., Pedley, T. A., Shinnar, S., Treiman, D. M., and Wannamaker, B. B. (1993). The treatment of convulsive status epilepticus: Recommendations of the Epilepsy Foundation of America's Working Group on Status Epilepticus. *JAMA J. Am. Med. Assoc.* **270**, 854–859.

Dube, C., Chen, K., Eghbal-Ahmadi, M., Brunson, K., Soltesz, I., and Baram, T. Z. (2000). Prolonged febrile seizures in the immature rat model enhance hippocampal excitability long term. *Ann. Neurol.* **47**, 336–344.

Falconer, M. (1971). Genetic and related etiological factors in temporal lobe epilepsy: A review. *Epilepsia* **12**, 13–31.

Falconer, M. A., Serafetinides, E. A., and Corsellis, J. A. N. (1964). Etiology and pathogenesis of temporal lobe epilepsy. *Arch. Neurol.* **10**, 233–248.

Fernandez, G., Effenberger, O., Vinz, B., *et al.* (1993). Hippocampal malformation as a cause of familial febrile convulsions and subsequent hippocampal sclerosis. *Neurology* **50**, 909–917.

French, J. A., Williamson, P. D., Thadani, M., *et al.* (1993). Characteristics of medial temporal lobe epilepsy: I. Results of history and physical examination. *Ann. Neurol.* **34**, 774–780.

Gastaut, H. (1969). Classifiacation of the epilepsies. *Epilepsia* **10** (Suppl.), 14–21.

Germano, I. M., Zhang, Y. F., Sperber, E., and Moshe, S. (1996). Neuronal migration disorders increase susceptibility to hyperthermia induced seizures in developing rats. *Epilepsia* **37**, 902–910.

Hamati-Haddad, A., and Abou-Khalil, B. (1998). Epilepsy diagnosis and localization in patients with antecedent childhood febrile convulsions. *Neurology* **50**, 917–922.

Hardiman, O., Burke, T., Phillips, J., *et al.* (1988). Microdysgenesis in resected temporal neocortex: Incidence and clinical significance in focal epilepsy. *Neurology* **38**, 1041–1047.

Kanemoto, K., Kawasaki, J., Miyamoto, T., Obayashi, H., and Nishimura, M. (2000). Interleukin (IL) 1beta, IL-1alpha, and IL-1 receptor antagonist gene polymorphisms in patients with temporal lobe epilepsy. *Ann. Neurol.* **47**, 571–574.

Kim, W. J., Park, S. C., Lee, S. J., *et al.* (1999). The prognosis for control of seizures with medications in patients with MRI evidence for mesial temporal sclerosis. *Epilepsia* **40**, 290–293.

Knudsen, F. U., Paerregaard, A., Andersen, R., and Andresen, J. (1996). Long term outcome of pro-phylaxis for febrile convulsions. *Arch. Dis. Child.* **74**, 13–18.

Kobayashi, E., Lopes-Cendes, I., Guerreiro, C. A. M., Sousa, S. C., Guerreiro, M. M., and Cendes, F. (2001). Seizure outcome and hippocampal atrophy in familial mesial temporal lobe epilepsy. *Neurology* **56**, 166–172.

Maher, J., and McLachlan, R. S. (1995). Febrile convulsions: Is seizure duration the most impor-tant predictor of temporal lobe epilepsy? *Brain* **118**, 1521–1528.

Margerison, J. H., and Corsellis, J. A. N. (1966). Epilepsy and the temporal lobes. *Brain* **89**, 499–530.

Mathern, G. W., Babb, T. L., Vickrey, B. G., Melendez, M., and Pretorius, J. K. (1995a). The clini-cal-pathologic mechanisms of hippocampal neuronal loss and surgical outcomes in temporal lobe epilepsy. *Brain* **118**, 105–118.

Mathern, G. W., Pretorius, J. K., and Babb, T. L. (1995b). Influence of the type of initial precipitat-ing injury and at what age it occurs on course and outcome in patients with temporal lobe seizures. *J. Neurosurg.* **82**, 220–227.

Maytal, J., and Shinnar, S. (1990). Febrile status epilepticus. *Pediatrics* **86**, 611–616.

Maytal, J., Shinnar, S., Moshe, S. L., and Alvarez, L. A. (1989). Low morbidity and mortality of sta-tus epilepticus in children. *Pediatrics* **83**, 323–331.

Nelson, K. B., and Ellenberg, J. H. (1976). Predictors of epilepsy in children who have experienced febrile seizures. *N. Engl. J. Med.* **295**, 1029–1033.

Nelson, K. B., and Ellenberg, J. H. (1978). Prognosis in children with febrile seizures. *Pediatrics* **61**, 720–727.

Rocca, W. A., Sharbrough, F. W., Hauser, W. A., Annegers, J. F., and Schoenberg, B. S. (1987a). Risk factors for complex partial seizures: A population-based case-control study. *Ann. Neurol.* **21**, 22–31.

Rocca, W. A., Sharbrough, F. W., Hauser, W. A., Annegers, J. F., and Schoenberg, B. S. (1987b). Risk factors for absence seizures: A population-based case-control study in Rochester, Minnesota. *Neurology* **37**, 1309–1314.

Rocca, W. A., Sharbrough, F. W., Hauser, W. A., Annegers, J. F., and Schoenberg, B. S. (1987c). Risk factors for generalized tonic-clonic seizures: A population-based case-control study in Rochester, Minnesota. *Neurology* **37**, 1315–1322.

Roger, J., Bureau, M., Dravet, C., *et al.*, eds. (1992). "Epileptic Syndromes in Infancy, Childhood and Adolescence," 2nd Ed. John Libbey & Co., London.

Rosman, N. P., Labazzo, J. L., and Colton, T. (1993). Factors predisposing to afebrile seizures after febrile convulsions and preventive treatment. *Ann. Neurol.* **34**, 452.

Sagar, H. J., and Oxbury, J. M. (1987). Hippocampal neuron loss in temporal lobe epilepsy: Corre-lation with early childhood convulsions. *Ann. Neurol.* **22**, 334–340.

Shinnar, S. (1998). Prolonged febrile seizures and mesial temporal sclerosis. *Ann. Neurol.* **43**, 411–412.

Shinnar, S. (1999). Febrile seizures. *In* "Pediatric Neurology: Principles and Practice," 3rd. Ed., pp. 676–682 (K. E. Swaiman and S. Ashwal, eds.). Mosby, St. Louis, MO.

Shinnar, S., and Babb, T. L. (1997). Long-term sequelae of status epilepticus. *In* "Epilepsy: A Com-prehensive Textbook" (J. Engel, Jr. and T. A. Pedley, eds.), pp. 755–763. Lippincott-Raven, Philadelphia.

Shinnar, S., and Berg, A. T. (1996). Does antiepileptic drug therapy prevent the development of "chronic" epilepsy? *Epilepsia* **37**, 701–708.

Shinnar, S., and Moshe, S. L. (1991). Age specificity of seizure expression in genetic epilepsies. *In* "Genetic Strategies in Epilepsy Research" (V. E. Anderson, W. A. Hauser, I. E. Leppik, J. L. Noebels, and S. S. Rich, eds.), pp. 69–85. Raven Press, New York.

Shinnar, S., Pellock, J. M., Moshe, S. L., *et al.* (1997). In whom does status epilepticus occur: Age-related differences in children. *Epilepsia* **38**, 907–914.

Shinnar, S., O'Dell, C., and Berg, A. T. (1999). Distribution of epilepsy syndromes in a cohort of children prospectively monitored from the time of their first unprovoked seizure. *Epilepsia* **40**, 1378–1383.

Shinnar, S., Pellock, J. M., Berg, A. T., *et al.* (2001). Short term outcomes of children with febrile status epilepticus *Epilepsia* **42**, 47–53.

Sillanpaa, M., Jalava, M., and Shinnar, S. (1999). Epilepsy syndromes in patients with childhood-onset epilepsy. *Pediatr. Neurol.* **21**, 533–537.

Sloviter, R. S., and Pedley, T. A. (1998). Subtle hippocampal malformation: Importance in febrile seizures and development of epilepsy. *Neurology* **50**, 846–849.

Sofianov, N., Sadikario, A., Dukovski, M., and Kuturec, M. (1983). Febrile convulsions and later development of epilepsy. *Am. J. Dis. Child.* **137**, 123–126.

Toth, Z., Yan, X. X., Haftoglou, S., Ribak, C. E., and Baram, T. Z. (1998). Seizure-induced neuronal injury: Vulnerability to febrile seizures in immature rat model. *J. Neurosci.* **18**, 4285–4294.

Tsuboi, T. (1984). Epidemiology of febrile and afebrile convulsions in children in Japan. *Neurology* **34**, 175–181.

Tsuboi, T., Endo, S., and Iida, N. (1991). Long-term follow-up of a febrile convulsion cohort. *Acta Neurol. Scand.* **84**, 369–373.

van den Berg, B. J., and Yerushalmi, J. (1969). Studies on convulsive disorders in young children, I. Incidence of febrile and nonfebrile convulsions by age and other factors. *Pediatr. Res.* **3**, 298–304.

vanLandingham, K. E., Heinz, E. R., Cavazos, J. E., and Lewis, D. V. (1998). MRI evidence of hippocampal injury after prolonged, focal febrile convulsions. *Ann. Neurol.* **43**, 413–426.

Verity, C. M., and Golding, J. (1991). Risk of epilepsy after febrile convulsions: a national cohort study. *Br. Med. J.* **303**, 1373–1376.

Verity, C. M., Ross, F. M., and Golding, J. (1993). Outcome of childhood status epilepticus and lengthy febrile convulsions: Findings of national cohort study. *Br. Med. J.* **307**, 225–228.

Wolf, S. M., and Forsythe, A. (1989). Epilepsy and mental retardation following febrile seizures in childhood. *Acta Paediatr. Scand.* **78**, 291–295.

CHAPTER 8

Do Prolonged Febrile Seizures Injure the Hippocampus? Human MRI Studies

TERESA V. MITCHELL* AND DARRELL V. LEWIS[†]

Departments of *Radiology and [†]Pediatrics, Duke University Medical Center, Durham, North Carolina 27710

Whether prolonged febrile seizures produce lasting injury to the hippocampus is a critical question concerning the etiology of temporal lobe epilepsy. Clinical retrospective evidence from epilepsy surgery centers suggests that prolonged febrile seizures can cause hippocampal sclerosis and temporal lobe epilepsy. However, epidemiological follow-up studies of infants with febrile seizures do not find an increased incidence of temporal lobe epilepsy. By using magnetic resonance imaging (MRI) to detect acute hippocampal injury following febrile seizures, this controversy may be resolved. The MRI data may reveal if and how often hippocampal injury occurs during febrile seizures and whether it evolves into hippocampal sclerosis and temporal lobe epilepsy. In addition, MRI may uncover predisposing conditions that make the hippocampus more susceptible to injury and epileptogenesis. Preliminary MRI data suggest that hippocampal sclerosis can result from prolonged and focal febrile seizures in infants who otherwise appear clinically normal both before and after the injury. © 2002 Academic Press.

I. INTRODUCTION

A febrile seizure has been defined as a seizure occurring in childhood after age 1 month, associated with a febrile illness in the absence of an infection of the central nervous system (CNS) or other acute cause and with no history of previous afebrile seizures (Commission on Epidemiology and Prognosis, International League Against Epilepsy, 1993). Febrile seizures are classified as complex febrile seizures if they satisfy one or more of the following criteria: (1) duration is longer than fifteen minutes, (2) more than one episode occurs in a 24-hour period, or (3) seizure manifestations are focal or lateralized. Finally, a single seizure that lasts longer than 30 minutes, or a series of seizures lasting longer than 30 minutes without interictal recovery, is classified as febrile status epilepticus (Maytal and Shinnar, 1990; Commission on Epidemiology and Prognosis, International League Against Epilepsy, 1993).

For many years, neurologists have hypothesized that complex febrile seizures injure the hippocampus, resulting in permanent hippocampal sclerosis and predisposing the individual to temporal lobe epilepsy (TLE) in adulthood (see Chapter 6). Although prospective epidemiological studies have revealed no links between febrile seizures and later development of TLE, retrospective data from epilepsy surgery centers show that from 30% (Harvey *et al.*, 1997; Cendes *et al.*, 1993; Mathern *et al.*, 1995a) to as high as 70% (Williamson *et al.*, 1993; Davidson and Falconer, 1975) of patients with TLE due to hippocampal sclerosis have histories of prolonged febrile seizures in early childhood. Prospectively, however, very few young children who experience complex febrile seizures go on to develop TLE. This mismatch between prospective and retrospective data may be explained in several ways. First, actual hippocampal injury during a complex febrile seizure resulting in subsequent hippocampal sclerosis and TLE may be rare and therefore difficult to detect in epidemiological studies, whereas within a sample of intractable TLE patients this event may be much more common. Second, hippocampal sclerosis will not be detected in epidemiological studies that cannot employ magnetic resonance imaging (MRI) because hippocampal sclerosis typically remains subclinical for between 8 (French *et al.*, 1993) and 11 (Mathern *et al.*, 1995b) years before TLE emerges. Finally, there may be other mitigating factors that interact with complex febrile seizures to place the child at higher risk for later TLE, such as remote injury during birth or preexisting pathology such as subtle focal cortical dysgenesis (Fernandez *et al.*, 1998).

The advent of MRI technology has allowed epileptologists to describe *in vivo* the extent and nature of hippocampal abnormalities that accompany TLE in adults (Jack, Jr. *et al.*, 1990; Jackson *et al.*, 1990; Lencz *et al.*, 1992). MRI has proved very valuable in lateralizing the side of onset of temporal lobe seizures in patients coming to temporal lobectomy (Spencer *et al.*, 1993). MRI data from children with typical TLE have likewise documented that some also have typical hippocampal sclerosis early in the course of their seizure disorders (Harvey *et al.*, 1995).

High-resolution MRI has also provided convincing evidence that prolonged seizures can produce acute brain injury that often appears to be limited to the hippocampal region. The abnormal scans acquired shortly after prolonged seizures or status epilepticus have revealed an increased hippocampal T2 signal. This increased signal is likely due to edema, although accompanying volume measurements to assess hippocampal swelling have been done in only a minority of these case reports. In some cases the hippocampal abnormalities have resolved on follow-up scans (Chan *et al.*, 1996; DeCarolis *et al.*, 1991) and in others follow-up has demonstrated hippocampal sclerosis (Nohria *et al.*, 1994; Stafstrom *et al.*, 1996). Thus, it appears that MRI not only detects chronic hippocampal sclerosis, but also is sensitive to recent hippocampal injury.

The application of MRI to the question of acute hippocampal injury in complex febrile seizures is just beginning. Just how often hippocampal abnormalities will be seen, what the evolution of the MRI abnormalities will be, what the clinical risk factors are, and what the mechanisms are that cause hippocampal injury all remain to be determined. In this chapter, we first describe the retrospective MRI studies linking TLE and hippocampal sclerosis to complex febrile seizures and then the current prospective studies involving MRIs done acutely following complex febrile seizures. Finally, we speculate about the mechanisms of injury based on the available MRI data and address issues in the methodology of MRI studies of hippocampal injury in complex febrile seizures.

II. RETROSPECTIVE MRI STUDIES EXAMINING THE LINK OF COMPLEX FEBRILE SEIZURES TO HIPPOCAMPAL INJURY

A. Adults with TLE

The key retrospective link established between complex febrile seizures and TLE is that adults with TLE associated with hippocampal sclerosis commonly have histories of prolonged febrile seizures in infancy. Prior to specialized hippocampal MRI studies, pathological examination of hippocampi resected at surgery had suggested that hippocampal sclerosis was more severe in adults with histories of infantile convulsions than in patients with hippocampal sclerosis but no history of infantile convulsions (Sagar and Oxbury, 1987). More recently, measurements of hippocampal volume using MRI have also been done to test this association. Trenerry *et al.* (1993) used MRI hippocampal volumetry of TLE patients with hippocampal sclerosis and found atrophy and volume asymmetry was greater in those with a history of complex febrile seizures compared to patients with hippocampal sclerosis but no such history. Cendes *et al.* (1993) measured amygdalar and hippocampal atrophy in nonlesional TLE patients using MRI volumetry and also found greater atrophy in those with histories of prolonged febrile seizures.

Kuks *et al.* (1993) used hippocampal volumetry and detected asymmetric hippocampal atrophy in 45 of 107 patients with medically intractable epilepsy. Complex febrile seizures had occurred in 3 of 12 (25%) patients with focal hippocampal atrophy and in 13 of 19 (68%) patients with diffuse but unilateral hippocampal atrophy. Complex febrile seizures had occurred in only 1 of 25 patients with normal MRIs and in 3 of 37 (8%) of patients with small focal lesions such as dysplasia or benign tumors. Thus in this sample, complex febrile seizures were more common events in the histories of epileptic patients with hippocampal atrophy, and most frequent in those with diffuse hippocampal atrophy.

Jackson and colleagues (1998) analyzed MRIs from three pairs of adult monozygotic twins in which only one twin of each pair had been diagnosed with TLE. This methodology was used to assess the genetic vs. environmental contributions to the etiology of hippocampal sclerosis. By MRI criteria, each of the twins with TLE had hippocampal sclerosis. In two of the twin pairs, both sibs had had multiple febrile seizures as infants, although in each case, only the sib with hippocampal sclerosis had a documented prolonged (45 to 60 minutes) febrile seizure preceding the onset of TLE. In the third pair, the unaffected sib had no history of febrile seizures. Although none of the twins had MRI evidence of cortical or hippocampal dysgenesis, two of the twins with hippocampal sclerosis had slightly smaller hemispheres ipsilateral to the hippocampal sclerosis compared to their sib controls. Perinatal difficulties did not seem to play a role because they were actually more common in the unaffected sibs and no other insults were known. The authors concluded that there was no evidence for a genetic basis for hippocampal sclerosis in their sample and that it was likely an acquired injury from prolonged childhood febrile seizures.

B. CHILDREN WITH TLE

Gratten-Smith *et al.* (1993) conducted a systematic MRI study of children diagnosed with TLE to assess whether the incidence of hippocampal sclerosis in this population was similar to that in adults. Previous reports had suggested that hippocampal sclerosis occurred much less frequently in children with TLE than in adults with TLE, lending credence to the hypothesis that hippocampal sclerosis develops as a result of recurrent temporal lobe seizures across a number of years. Fifty-three children with intractable TLE were studied, ranging in age from 2 to 17 years. Overall, the incidence of hippocampal sclerosis in the sample was 57%, comparable to the adult incidence of 65% (Babb and Brown, 1987). MRI demonstrated hippocampal sclerosis in 76% of these children who had preceding neurological insults and only in 21% of those without preceding insults (Harvey *et al.*, 1995). Of 22 children with histories of complex febrile seizures, 17 had hippocampal sclerosis on MRI. On the other hand, age at onset of TLE and duration of TLE did not correlate with presence of hippocampal sclerosis on MRI, giving no support to the hypothesis that hippocampal sclerosis develops as a result of recurrent temporal lobe seizures across a number of years. Cross *et al.* (1993) also examined MRIs from epileptic children ages 1 to 15 years and they too found hippocampal abnormalities were much more frequent in those with histories of severe infantile convulsions.

Using magnetic resonance spectroscopy, Holopainen *et al.* (1998) examined the mesial temporal areas including the hippocampi of 13 children with epilepsy and temporal lobe spike foci on electroencephalography. They found magnetic resonance spectroscopy changes indicative of hippocampal sclerosis in 4 of 7 with historical complex febrile seizures and in 1 of 6 without.

C. Children with Complex Febrile Seizures

Szabó *et al.* (1999) measured hippocampal volumes in five infants with complex febrile seizures and compared them to hippocampal volumes in control patients. Although one infant was scanned acutely 2 days after the complex febrile seizure, the other four were performed 2 to 46 months after the complex febrile seizures and would therefore be beyond the period of acute changes. None of the complex febrile seizures exceeded 20 minutes in duration. Control volumes were obtained from patients with normal MRIs and clinical symptoms that were determined to be "neurologically insignificant." None of the 11 control patients had first-degree relatives with epilepsy. Although this control group is not as carefully selected as in some studies (Giedd *et al.*, 1996a), it provides important data with which to compare results from the five patients with complex febrile seizures. The results from the control group were that total hippocampal volume increased linearly with age (38 mm^3 per month), whereas the ratio of right hippocampal volume to left hippocampal volume (mean value, 1.03) decreased with age. In comparison, complex febrile seizure patients had a tendency toward smaller overall hippocampal volume and a larger right-to-left ratio than did controls, but neither effect was statistically significant. This study clearly indicates that large samples will be necessary to determine whether differences in hippocampal volume between complex febrile seizure patients and their age mates are reliable. The authors concluded that their findings could represent some developmental abnormality, but that more studies would be required to make any conclusions.

III. PROSPECTIVE MRI STUDIES IN CHILDREN
WITH PROLONGED SEIZURES

The ideal prospective MRI study of infants with seizures would be impossible because it would require that a control MRI be done prior to the first seizure. However, some data are now becoming available from infants who have been identified as study subjects and imaged within days following their initial seizures and who have had follow-up MRIs to measure subsequent hippocampal growth.

A. STATUS EPILEPTICUS

A pediatric case study clearly demonstrated that status epilepticus in the absence of fever in an infant could damage the hippocampus and cause hippocampal sclerosis. Nohria et al. (1994) collected serial MRI scans on a young developmentally delayed child within 1 day of her first seizure at age 32 months, after another seizure 6 weeks later, and again 13 months after the first seizure. Both seizures had left-lateralized body signs, lasted 45 to 50 minutes, and were during bouts of otitis media, although afebrile. MRIs were high-resolution, T2-weighted fast spin echo sequences that allowed for volumetric as well as T2 intensity measurements. Results from the first MRI showed high T2 signal intensity of the right hippocampus that was reduced on the second scan and minimal by the third. The ratio of right-to-left hippocampal volumes was 0.94, 0.87, and 0.72 on the first, second, and third scans, respectively. The appearance of the right hippocampus on the third scan was identical to that of hippocampal sclerosis as seen on fast spin echo MRIs from TLE patients (Tien et al., 1993). The patient developed intractable complex partial seizures and underwent a right temporal lobectomy at age 51 months. Although hippocampal tissue was not available for examination, the specimens of temporal lobe neocortex showed microdysgenesis with increased numbers of neurons in the white matter and occasional clustering of large neurons in the deep cortical layers. This may be a human example of a preexisting dysgenesis rendering a hippocampus more susceptible to injury during status epilepticus, as suggested by animal models (Germano et al., 1996).

In a very similar instance, Perez et al. (2000) reported an infant who presented with afebrile repetitive seizures at 3 months of age in the setting of microcephaly, developmental delay, and a sibling with cryptogenic mental retardation. MRI within 24 hours of seizure onset showed left hippocampal swelling and subependymal nodular heterotopia. At 6 months, repetitive seizures occurred again, this time from the right brain with T2 hyperintensity of the right fusiform gyrus white matter. Follow-up at 11 months during a seizure-free period showed bilateral hippocampal atrophy. Thus, acute and chronic hippocampal damage can clearly result from status epilepticus.

B. Prolonged Complex Febrile Seizures and MRI Evidence of Hippocampal Injury

Additional MRI data suggest that severe complex febrile seizures both cause acute injury and can result in hippocampal sclerosis. VanLandingham *et al.* (1998) collected MRIs with fast spin echo oblique coronal views of the hippocampi from 27 complex febrile seizure patients 8 to 34 months of age. Eighteen of these infants were entered into this study on presentation with their complex febrile seizure, and 9 were identified retrospectively by record review. The majority of subjects, 23 of 27, had postictal MRIs obtained within 6 days of the ictus. MRIs were read by a radiologist blind to the clinical information and classified as normal, definitely abnormal, or possibly abnormal. Definite abnormalities were defined as marked or very obvious visually, or in the case of volume changes, corroborated by volumetry. Possible abnormalities were subtle changes in T2 or volume not corroborated by volumetry. Abnormalities were classed as acute if both increased volume and signal were present and as chronic if there was decreased volume with or without signal abnormalities.

Complex febrile seizures were classed as either lateralized or generalized. The lateralizing feature used in most patients was focal clonic jerking of an upper or lower extremity or both, but in a few subjects head and eye deviation were the only indicators of lateralization. Only one was noted to have a Todd's paresis after the complex febrile seizure. In each case, the hemisphere of origin of the seizure is assumed to be contralateral to the clinically lateralizing features.

MRI abnormalities were frequent in the 15 subjects with lateralized complex febrile seizures. Six of 15 had definite and 3 had possible abnormalities. Four patients with lateralized complex febrile seizures showed both increased hippocampal volume and T2 signal, indicating acute injury. This change was predominately unilateral in 3 patients, as shown in subject 8 of the original study in Figure 1A, and located in the hippocampus on the side of the seizure origin, whereas the fourth subject had bilateral hippocampal edema, worse on the side of seizure origin. The definite chronic abnormalities in the other two, both of whom had histories of perinatal insults, were decreased volume and increased signal in both hippocampi and mild periventricular leukomalacia. Three patients had possible MRI abnormalities. In two the changes were of a chronic nature and consisted of a visually apparent reduction of volume of the hippocampus ipsilateral to the seizure, not confirmed by volume measurements.

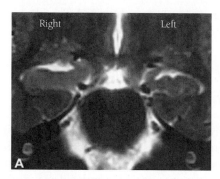 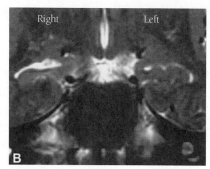

FIGURE 1   Fast spin echo oblique coronal sections through the head of the hippocampi of subject 8. (A) MRI done 2 days after the patient had a 72-minute-long complex febrile seizure with focal left-sided jerking. Note the increased size and signal in the right hippocampal head (on the left
side of the MRI). (B) Follow-up MRI done 1 year later showing the subsequent decrease in size of
the right hippocampus but the remaining increased signal. Adapted from MRI evidence of hippocampal injury after prolonged, focal febrile convulsions. K. E. VanLandingham, E. R. Heinz, J. E.
Cavazos, and D. V. Lewis; *Ann Neurol.* Copyright © 1998, John Wiley & Sons, Inc.

One had a possible acute abnormality consisting of a subtle increase in T2 signal in a portion of the hippocampus ipsilateral to the seizure origin with no apparent volume abnormality.

In contrast, in the 12 patients with generalized complex febrile seizures only
1 had a possible abnormality. That MRI showed subtle T2 signal increase and
volume increase in both hippocampi, although the hippocampus volumes by
measurement were not abnormal.

The histories of all subjects were reviewed for potential risk factors predisposing to complex febrile seizures. Four of the 15 lateralized subjects had a
history of perinatal difficulties, including the two with definite chronic MRI
abnormalities who had required perinatal extracorporeal membrane oxygena-
tion. Only one of the patients with acute hippocampal edema had a significant
history and she had undergone uneventful open-heart surgery for pulmonary
valvular stenosis 9 months prior to her complex febrile seizure. In the generalized group, two were born prematurely without known neurological complications and one had had open-heart surgery, but both had normal MRIs.

A number of clinical parameters were analyzed for correlation with MRI abnormalities, including lateralized vs. generalized classification, rectal temperature at presentation, total duration of seizures, number of seizures, and age. The
lateralized group had a significantly higher incidence of abnormal MRIs compared to the generalized group and, in addition, the four subjects with acute
edema had significantly longer total seizure duration compared to the rest of
the subjects, with an average duration of 99 minutes. Temperature, number of
seizures, and age did not correlate with MRI abnormalities.

Hippocampal volumetry was performed on all subjects and on seven control infants. There was no apparent difference in the distribution of hippocampal volumes between the controls and the complex febrile seizure subjects. However, when ratios of hippocampal volume on the side of seizure origin to the hippocampal volume on the contralateral side were measured for each subject in the lateralized complex febrile seizure group, the ratios were significantly greater in the four patients with visually apparent hippocampal edema. At the time of the publication, follow-up MRIs had been performed on two of the patients with definite edema and both had developed hippocampal sclerosis characterized by atrophy of the previously swollen hippocampus with residual abnormal T2 signal (Figures 1B and 2).

This study is still ongoing and now consists of a cohort of 58 infants with complex febrile seizures, 44 of whom had febrile status epilepticus. The incidence of definite acute hippocampal abnormalities in the febrile status epilepticus group is 4 of 44, or 9%. Follow-up MRIs have now been performed on all four patients in the original group who demonstrated definite hippocampal edema and on five additional subjects whose postictal scans were judged to be normal or possibly abnormal. The three subjects with predominantly unilateral hippocampal edema have developed unilateral hippocampal sclerosis and the subject with bilateral swelling has developed bilateral hippocampal sclerosis,

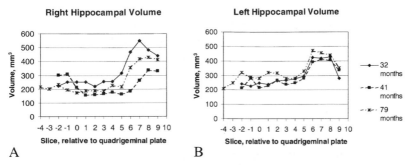

FIGURE 2 Graphical representation of the volumes of the right (A) and left (B) hippocampi of subject 8 at the time of the original complex febrile seizure (32 months of age) and at two subsequent follow-up MRIs at 41 and 79 months of age. The volumes (in mm^3) for each 3-mm-thick slice of the hippocampus from the head (on the right side of the graphs) to the tail (on the left side) are plotted. The slices are numbered with respect to the slice containing the outline of the quadrigeminal plate (designated as slice 0). Note that the head of the right hippocampus was initially most swollen and then at 41 months showed a striking decline in volume, with partial recovery by 79 months. The left hippocampus showed an arguable slight decline in volume at 41 months and a definite increase in volume by 79 months. Both hippocampi appeared to increase in length by 79 months by the addition of more posterior slices.

worse on the side of maximal swelling. In contrast, none of the five subjects with normal or possibly abnormal scans following their complex febrile seizures has shown atrophy on follow-up MRIs. As in the original group, the two clinical parameters that still seem significantly associated with acute T2 hyperintensity are lateralization and prolonged duration, reinforcing the impression that hippocampal injury is most likely with prolonged focal febrile seizures.

C. Long-Term Outcome of Infants with Hippocampal Sclerosis Identified by MRI

Prior to the advent of MRI studies of hippocampal injury in infants, hippocampal sclerosis was identified only after it had been announced by the onset of TLE. The clinical correlates of hippocampal sclerosis alone without TLE are therefore unknown. How often hippocampal sclerosis leads to TLE is likewise completely unknown and subclinical hippocampal sclerosis has been described in autopsy studies of individuals without epilepsy (Meencke and Veith, 1991). Developmental defects as severe as autism have been reported in infants with bilateral hippocampal sclerosis (DeLong and Heinz, 1997; Gross and Andermann, 1998); however it is unclear whether unilateral hippocampal sclerosis affects development. These questions can be resolved by following cohorts of infants with MRI-documented hippocampal sclerosis.

Although there are insufficient data to determine the clinical manifestations and outcome of children with MRI-documented hippocampal sclerosis, we do have follow-up information on the four infants identified in our original group. Of these four infants with acquired hippocampal sclerosis, one (subject 8 of VanLandingham et al., 1998) has developed complex partial seizures that, on videoelectroencephalography, clinically and electrically appear to be coming from the right temporal lobe, where the hippocampal sclerosis is located, although the interictal spikes are right central–parietal and therefore the localization is not entirely clear. The other three infants with acquired hippocampal sclerosis have not developed epilepsy. The follow-up periods for these four infants are now 3 to 5 years. The subjects with hippocampal sclerosis clearly vary in their developmental progress. Two are apparently normal in their elementary school performance, one has been diagnosed with attention deficit disorder, and the one with epilepsy has a marked language delay. This small group clearly suggests that, without a consistent clinical signature prior to the development of TLE, hippocampal sclerosis will be difficult to detect in epidemiological studies of complex febrile seizures without imaging. Follow-up will continue on these children, including psychometric testing and repeat MRIs to determine the long-term prognosis of hippocampal sclerosis.

IV. MRI STUDIES AND POTENTIAL MECHANISMS OF HIPPOCAMPAL INJURY

Although there are very few MRI data on hippocampal injury in complex febrile seizures, review of these data may suggest possible clinical risk factors and predisposing abnormalities that may contribute to hippocampal injury. Some previously mentioned potentially important risk factors are seizure duration, age of the subject, focality due to presence of subtle dysgenesis or other preexisting lesions, possibly focal encephalitis, and genetic predisposition.

A. SEIZURE DURATION

The limited human MRI data are in agreement with the experimental literature (Gruenthal, 1998; Vicedomini and Nadler, 1987; Meldrum and Brierley, 1973), which suggests that seizure duration may be a critical factor in determining whether MRI evidence of hippocampal injury will be seen following febrile seizures. In the study of Szabó et al. (1999) none of the complex febrile seizures exceeded 20 minutes in duration and no evidence of hippocampal sclerosis was reported on follow-up MRIs. On the other hand, the infant described by Nohria et al. (1994), although afebrile, had a 50 minute long seizure in the setting of otitis media and exhibited acute hippocampal swelling on MRI. Finally, the average total seizure duration in the infants with acute hippocampal edema in the study of VanLandingham et al. (1998) was 99 minutes compared to a mean of 41 minutes in the lateralized complex febrile seizure infants without edema, and 46 minutes in the entire generalized group. The MRI studies thus agree with the retrospective (Annegers et al., 1987; Maher and McLachlan, 1995) and prospective (Verity et al., 1993) cohort studies that did not use MRI in which seizure duration was a clear risk factor for later development of complex partial seizures.

B. AGE AND SUSCEPTIBILITY TO HIPPOCAMPAL INJURY

Animal data have suggested that age is an important factor in determining the nature and extent of hippocampal injury as a result of seizures. Compared to adult rats, 10- to 20-day-old infants rats show little or no neuronal death in the hippocampus following limbic status epilepticus induced by kainic acid (Sperber et al., 1991; Nitecka et al., 1984; Cavalheiro et al., 1987), although this observation is in dispute because other models of limbic status epilepticus do show hippocampal injury in infant animals (Thompson et al., 1998; Thompson and Wasterlain, 1997; Baram and Ribak, 1995). Like the infant rat data, an effect of age on hippocampal vulnerability is also unclear in retrospective data from patients with hippocampal sclerosis and TLE. A number of clinical investigators (Sagar and Oxbury, 1987; Cendes *et al.*, 1993) have concluded that hippocampal injury is more likely when convulsions occur in patients younger than 3 to 4 years of age as compared to older patients. On the other hand, Mathern *et al.* (1995a) conclude that there is no evidence of an age dependence of hippocampal vulnerability, but that hippocampal sclerosis due to prolonged seizures is just as severe when the prolonged seizures occur in older children as when they occur in young infants.

It may be important that the period of most rapid postnatal hippocampal growth is between birth and 24 to 36 months of age (Lange *et al.*, 1997; Utsunomiya *et al.*, 1999). This closely corresponds to the period during which infants are most susceptible to febrile status epilepticus, with 95% of cases occurring prior to 36 months of age in one large series (Maytal and Shinnar, 1990). Because neurogenesis and maturation of dendritic trees is ongoing in the human dentate gyrus during at least the first year of life (Seress, 1992), febrile seizures occur at a time when developmental programs might well be interfered with or altered by seizure activity. This suggests that injury to the hippocampus during this time could have significant consequences for later development and functioning. The data from VanLandingham *et al.* (1998) and the follow-up on those infants allow us to say that acute hippocampal edema can progress to hippocampal sclerosis in infants aged 15 to 32 months at the time of the febrile status epilepticus. However, additional MRI data will clearly be needed to enable us to assess age as a risk factor in the occurrence of hippocampal sclerosis.

C. LATERALIZED VS. GENERALIZED SEIZURES AND HIPPOCAMPAL INJURY

The only MRI study of complex febrile seizures comparing the incidence of hippocampal injury in focal or lateralized seizures versus generalized seizures was that of VanLandingham *et al.* (1998). In that study, MRI abnormalities and hippocampal injury were clearly more frequent in patients with lateralized seizures. There are reasons to suspect that, independent of duration, focal complex febrile seizures are more likely to be associated with hippocampal injury than are generalized convulsions. Focality of complex febrile seizures has more than once emerged as a risk factor for later focal epilepsy (Nelson and Ellenberg, 1976; Annegers *et al.*, 1987; Sagar and Oxbury, 1987; Abou-Khalil *et al.*, 1993; Wallace, 1982). Presently, it is unclear whether focality and long duration are independent risk factors. Berg and Shinnar (1996) found a high association between the two. Annegers *et al.* (1987) concluded that although duration and focality are associated, they are independent and additive risk factors.

In a completely normal, symmetric brain, it is not clear why febrile seizures would be lateralized. It is also not clear why a prolonged lateralized seizure would be more likely to produce hippocampal injury than would an equally prolonged generalized seizure, although the MRI data suggest that this is the case. However, it is reasonable to suspect that a lateralized seizure indicates an underlying lateralized brain abnormality and there is evidence that preexisting abnormalities such as cortical dysgenesis may be not only a nidus for the development of seizure activity during a febrile illness, but may also increase the propensity for seizure- or hyperthermia-induced neuronal injury. For example, rat pups with induced cortical dysgenesis are more susceptible to hyperthermia-induced seizures and hyperthermia-induced hippocampal neuronal death than are controls (Germano et al., 1996). The interesting observation that hyperthermic seizures in a febrile seizure model in normal rats begin in the amygdala or hippocampus or both (Baram et al., 1997) suggest that structural asymmetries of the limbic circuitry could determine on which side a febrile seizure begins.

The common coexistence of hippocampal sclerosis and asymmetric cortical dysgenesis (Hardiman et al., 1988; Ho et al., 1998) in TLE also argues for a causal connection of cortical dysgenesis and hippocampal injury. In the case of Nohria et al. (1994) subtle neocortical dysgenesis was found on the side of the injured hippocampus at temporal lobectomy. More recently, dysgenesis of the hippocampus has been suggested as a possible etiology for febrile seizures. MRI studies of two families with genetically determined unilateral hippocampal dysgenesis demonstrated that only family members with the malformation had febrile seizures (Fernandez et al., 1998). It is puzzling, however, that the febrile seizures in these family members were generalized by history, although historical data, particularly if obtained long after seizures, may be often unreliable regarding the duration and exact nature of febrile seizures. Nevertheless, one subject in each family had developed hippocampal sclerosis and TLE following multiple, brief, apparently generalized febrile seizures.

Lesions other than cerebral dysgenesis may also set the stage for lateralized seizures and for hippocampal injury during the seizures. One of the infants with lateralized seizures and acute hippocampal injury reported by VanLandingham et al. (1998) had a choroid fissure cyst compressing the injured hippocampus and another infant had had open-heart surgery at 6 months, which could conceivably have caused a subclinical hippocampal injury, predisposing her to the complex febrile seizure at 15 months.

The concept of two insults leading to hippocampal sclerosis, one preceding a severe seizure and serving as a nidus of hyperexcitability accounting for the focality of the seizure and the second insult due to and occurring during the severe seizure, is becoming more popular. Perhaps MRI studies of infants with febrile seizures, with careful attention to brain (and especially hippocampal) morphology, and a careful search for previous insults may support this hypothesis.

D. Focal Encephalitis, Complex Febrile Seizures, and Hippocampal Injury?

An additional potential mechanism of complex febrile seizures and hippocampal injury is limbic encephalitis. The 6-month-old male infant reported by Perez *et al.* (2000) may have had focal encephalitis, causing the lateralized complex febrile seizures and right hippocampal swelling seen on MRI. If that infant's seizures were due to exanthum subitum, as was suggested by the rash that appeared late in the illness, then a human herpes virus (HHV) would be the likely agent. Studies of infants presenting with febrile seizures indicate that a significant percentage of them suffer from initial infections with HHV6 (Hall *et al.*, 1994) and many of these have HHV6 DNA in their cerebrospinal fluid (Caserta *et al.*, 1994). HHV7 has also been associated with febrile seizures, exanthum subitum, and neurological dysfunction (van den Berg *et al.*, 1999). One report even suggests that febrile seizures during HHV6 primary infections may be more severe than with other etiologies (Suga *et al.*, 2000). There has been an isolated case report of suspected HHV6 encephalitis in a bone marrow transplant recipient, producing hippocampal swelling on MRI (Tsujimura *et al.*, 1998) similar to that seen after some complex febrile seizures, and we have observed several bone marrow transplant recipients with asymmetric hippocampal swelling on MRI studies, limbic seizures, and HHV6 DNA in their cerebrospinal fluid (M. Wainwright *et al.*, unreported observations) who ultimately developed hippocampal sclerosis. Enterovirus has also been found in the cerebrospinal fluid (CSF) in the setting of febrile seizures (Hosoya *et al.*, 1997), and rotavirus has been found in CSF in afebrile benign seizures in infants with gastrointestinal symptoms (Nishimura *et al.*, 1993). It is reasonable to hypothesize that if viral invasion of the nervous system is common in febrile seizures, then in rare instances focal limbic encephalitis could occur and account for an unknown fraction of cases of prolonged complex febrile seizures and hippocampal injury.

E. Using MRI-Based Studies to Screen for Genes Affecting Susceptibility to Seizure-Induced Hippocampal Sclerosis

Genetic modifiers of response to injury can be investigated in cohorts identified during MRI-based studies of hippocampal injury in complex febrile seizures, afebrile prolonged seizures, and head trauma. For instance, by banking cells for genetic analysis on subjects receiving acute and follow-up MRIs after these insults, one could define the portion of the cohort that developed hippocampal sclerosis and then screen those subjects for candidate genes that might make them more susceptible to the development of hippocampal sclerosis. For example, it has been suggested that genes coding for interleukin receptor antagonists might determine susceptibility to hippocampal sclerosis following hippocampal insult (Kanemoto *et al.*, 2000). In addition, a genetic predisposition to status epilepticus has been suggested as well (Corey *et al.*, 1998) and cohorts of subjects with prolonged seizures from MRI-based studies might be screened for candidate genes regulating seizure duration. Finally, a number of genetic loci associated with febrile seizures are being characterized (Racacho *et al.*, 2000) and one could determine whether specific loci might be associated with complex febrile seizures or hippocampal injury.

V. CONSIDERATIONS IN MRI METHODOLOGY FOR DETECTING HIPPOCAMPAL INJURY FOLLOWING COMPLEX FEBRILE SEIZURES

The methods and criteria for detecting and diagnosing hippocampal sclerosis in MRI studies of adults with TLE have been well documented (Jackson *et al.*, 1990; Jack, Jr. *et al.*, 1992; Spencer *et al.*, 1993). However, the detection of hippocampal injury and the evolution of this injury in childhood pose several additional challenges.

A. Unknown Time Course and Nature of Hippocampal Signal Changes Following Prolonged Seizures

When, following a complex febrile seizure, is the best time to perform an imaging study and what is the most sensitive imaging modality to use to detect hippocampal injury? Animal studies have evaluated the usefulness of MRI, magnetic resonance spectroscopy, and diffusion-weighted imaging in detecting hippocampal injury following limbic status epilepticus. Although T2-weighted images have typically been used to detect seizure-induced injury clinically, animal studies show robust postictal changes in N-acetylaspartate content using magnetic resonance spectroscopy and apparent diffusion coefficient using diffusion-weighted imaging (Nakasu *et al.*, 1995; Wang *et al.*, 1996; Tokumitsu *et al.*, 1997), whereas T2 hyperintensity, although present, may be less apparent than the other findings. Magnetic resonance properties of tissue following injury due to limbic seizures in animal models are rapidly changing, dynamic variables. The apparent diffusion constant has been observed to decline within 10 to 20 minutes following the onset of flurothyl-induced generalized seizures in rat brain and, if the seizure is terminated by injection of pentobarbital, the apparent diffusion constant rapidly returns toward normal values (Zhong et al., 1995). T2 hyperintensity may be later and longer lasting than reductions of apparent diffusion constant. In the rat model of intraperitoneally administered kainic acid-induced limbic status, T2 signal intensity peaked at 24 to 48 hours and resolved after 72 hours, whereas apparent diffusion constants reached a nadir at 24 hours and were not significantly different than normal by 48 hours (Righini et al., 1994). Following injection of kainic acid into the posterior hippocampus to provoke focal seizures, N-acetylaspartate in the posterior hippocampus fell significantly by 1 day and reached a nadir at 14 days and was still significantly reduced at 84 days (Tokumitsu et al., 1997). Concomitantly, there was a nonsignificant initial decline in the apparent diffusion constant and then a significant increase by 28 days and very little change in the T2 intensity. In a different study, 72 hours following systemic kainic acid-induced limbic status epilepticus in eleven rats, all animals had significant reductions in N-acetylaspartate in pyriform cortex, amygdala, and hippocampus. However, on T2-weighted MRI imaging, although the amygdala and pyriform cortex were consistently abnormal, only 20% of the hippocampi were abnormal (Ebisu et al., 1994). MRI evidence of T2 hyperintensity has been documented in a primate model of limbic status epilepticus, although the time course of the MRI abnormalities is not yet known (Gunderson et al., 1999).

There are no detailed time course data on diffusion-weighted imaging, magnetic resonance spectroscopy, and MRI changes in humans following status. A decreased apparent diffusion constant has been reported during seizure activity in neocortex both with (Lansberg et al., 1999; Wieshmann et al., 1997) and without (Kassem-Moussa et al., 2000) accompanying T2 hyperintensity. In addition, an increased apparent diffusion constant has been reported interictally in the sclerotic hippocampi of patients with TLE (Hugg et al., 1999), but we are not aware of any data on hippocampal apparent diffusion constant changes soon after status epilepticus in humans. Based on TLE studies, magnetic resonance spectroscopy may be slightly more sensitive to chronic hippocampal injury compared to T2 intensity (Cendes et al., 1997), but it is unclear whether this applies to acute hippocampal injury in humans. Therefore, based on the limited data, early imaging between 24 and 72 hours following the seizures would seem advisable and evaluation of the relative sensitivity of diffusion-weighted imaging, T2 weighting, and magnetic resonance spectroscopy is needed. However, incorporating several extra pulse protocols is a real challenge in infants who are sick and must be sedated for MRI studies. Regarding which modality is most sensitive, we are currently comparing the usefulness of T2-weighted MRI and diffusion-weighted imaging in evaluating postictal injury in infants with complex febrile seizures.

B. Problems Associated with Hippocampal Volume Measurements in Infants

The critical determination of whether a particular hippocampal volume measurement is abnormal requires normative pediatric data, and very few are available. The existing data show that MRI-measured hippocampal volume rapidly increases during the first 2 years of life and then increases slowly (Utsunomiya *et al.*, 1999; Pfluger *et al.*, 1999) or is relatively stable (Giedd *et al.*, 1996b) thereafter. There may be gender differences in the velocity of growth (Pfluger *et al.*, 1999), and final volumes in males are slightly larger than in females. As in adults, the right hippocampus tends to be larger. Variability in hippocampal volume across same-aged individuals is quite large. The coefficient of variation of hippocampal volumes, a measure of between-individual variability, averaged 11% in children aged 4 to 20 years (Lange *et al.*, 1997) and may be greater in those under 4 years. The inherent variability and gender differences and a rapidly changing hippocampal volume during this age period suggest that a large number of control hippocampal volumes will be required to construct a growth curve with reliable confidence intervals. We have found repeatedly that al-

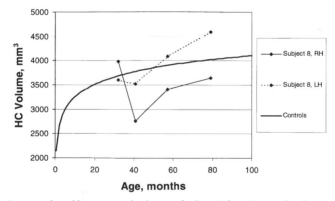

FIGURE 3   Sequential total hippocampal volumes of subject 8 from 32 months, the time of the complex febrile seizure, to 79 months, taken from four sequential MRIs. Note that the right hippocampus (RH) was initially larger than the left (LH) and that the sizes are reversed by the time of the first follow-up MRI. However, there was subsequent growth of both hippocampi on follow-up. In addition, there was a slight initial decline in the volume of the left hippocampus, suggesting that although the predominant insult was on the right, there may have been some injury to the left as well. This pattern of initial marked decline in size with some subsequent growth but not complete recovery argues for an acute insult during the complex febrile seizure at the time of the first MRI. Abnormalities in growth pattern like this may be the best way to detect injury due to acute insults. The solid line is a logarithmic regression fitted to the hippocampi of 31 control infants. Adapted from MRI evidence of hippocampal injury after prolonged, focal febrile convulsions. K. E. VanLandingham, E. R. Heinz, J. E. Cavazos, and D. V. Lewis; *Ann. Neurol.* Copyright © 1998, John Wiley & Sons, Inc.

though hippocampal volume may appear increased on visual inspection following a complex febrile seizure, the change in measured volume is not statistically significant due to a limited number of age-matched controls with large variance. However, with the acquisition of serial scans for an individual patient, one may assess volumetric change over time. Inspection of the hippocampal growth curve for an individual may provide the most sensitive measure of damage if the expected developmental trajectory is not achieved (Figure 3). This method would be particularly useful in cases of predominantly unilateral damage, where the growth of the relatively intact hippocampus can be compared to the growth of the damaged hippocampus (VanLandingham et al., 1998).

C. MRI Acquisition

The determination of hippocampal damage requires high-quality, high-resolution MRI images. The extant studies on hippocampal volumetry employ a variety of MRI protocols. Because the goal in these volumetric studies is to calculate accurately the number of voxels specifically within the hippocampus, good contrast is important for delineating the structure. This is particularly important when imaging patients between the ages of about 6 and 14 months, when contrast between gray and white matter is poor in both T2- and T1-weighted protocols, presumably because of immature myelination. The optimal protocol for this age range has not been determined and ultimately may require the acquisition of multiple contrasts to achieve accurate identification of the hippocampus.

Finally, because the change in hippocampal volume and T2 signal over time intervals of 6 to 12 months may be very critical in determining whether hippocampal injury has occurred, the stability of the MRI scanner(s) with which the data are acquired is a critical issue. Because the initial scan is often performed on a sick infant who is postictal or in intensive care, the luxury of using the same dedicated research scanner for all subjects is not an option. To detect and correct for differences between scanners or instability with time, we have begun to use phantom standards for both T2 relaxation time and geometry; these are scanned with each patient. A geometry phantom can be scanned just following the clinical scan using the same patient protocol. These phantoms contain calibrated markers in all three image axes, and errors in field homogeneity or geometry measured from a phantom scan could be used to correct the hippocampal volume measurements on a given patient.

T2 signal intensity standards with known relaxation times are placed on the infant's head within the head coil during a multiecho spin echo sequence. We are using these standards with known relaxation times in combination with dual-echo spin echo sequences to estimate the T2 relaxation time constants of each subject's hippocampi and neocortex as described by Duncan *et al.* (1996).

VI. SUMMARY

MRI has provided convincing evidence that hippocampal injury can occasionally occur during very prolonged febrile seizures. The MRI results combined with the clinical data suggest that duration and focality of seizure activity may be major risk factors predictive of hippocampal injury and, in addition, have given some support to the concept that preexisting hippocampal and other brain pathologies act as cofactors in the mechanism of injury.

However, much work remains to be done. The incidence of injury and the mechanisms at work in the clinical setting of hippocampal injury remain to be clearly determined. In addition, the clinical correlates and evolution of the hippocampal sclerosis in infants who have not yet manifested TLE must be determined.

By pursuing these imaging studies, we may uncover other new risk factors and mechanisms of injury and also be able ultimately to consider therapeutic intervention in infants who present with MRI evidence of acute hippocampal injury.

REFERENCES

Abou-Khalil, B., Andermann, E., Andermann, F., Olivier, A., and Quesney, L. F. (1993). Temporal lobe epilepsy after prolonged febrile convulsions: Excellent outcome after surgical treatment. *Epilepsia* 34, 878–883.

Annegers, J. F., Hauser, W. A., Shirts, S. B., and Kurland, L. T. (1987). Factors prognostic of unprovoked seizures after febrile convulsions. *N. Engl. J. Med.* 316, 493–498.

Babb, T. L., and Brown, W. J. (1987). Pathological findings in epilepsy. *In* "Surgical Treatment of the Epilepsies" (J. Engel, Jr., ed.), p. 511. Raven Press, New York.

Baram, T. Z., and Ribak, C. E. (1995). Peptide induced infant status epilepticus causes neuronal death and synaptic reorganization. *NeuroReport* 6, 277–280.

Baram, T. Z., Gerth, A., and Schultz, L. (1997). Febrile seizures: An appropriate-aged model suitable for long term studies. *Dev. Brain Res.* 98, 265–270.

Berg, A. T., and Shinnar, S. (1996). Complex febrile seizures. *Epilepsia* 37, 126–133.

Caserta, M. T., Hall, C. B., Schnabel, K., McIntyre, K., Long, C., Costanzo, M., Dewhurst, S., Insel, R., and Epstein, L. G. (1994). Neuroinvasion and persistence of human herpesvirus 6 in children. *J. Infect. Dis.* 170, 1586–1589.

Cavalheiro, E. A., Silva, D. F., Turski, W. A., Calderazzo-Filho, L. S., Bortolotto, Z. A., and Turski, L. (1987). The susceptibility of rats to pilocarpine induced seizures is age dependent. *Dev. Brain Res.* 37, 43–58.

Cendes, F., Andermann, F., Dubeau, F., Gloor, P., Evans, A., Jones-Gotman, M., Olivier, A., Andermann, E., Robitaille, Y., Lopes-Cendes, I., Peters, T., and Melanson, D. (1993). Early childhood prolonged febrile convulsions, atrophy and sclerosis of mesial structures, and temporal lobe epilepsy: An MRI volumetric study. *Neurology* **43**, 1083–1087.

Cendes, F., Caramanos, Z., Andermann, F., Dubeau, F., and Arnold, D. L. (1997). Proton magnetic resonance spectroscopic imaging and magnetic resonance imaging volumetry in the lateralization of temporal lobe epilepsy: A series of 100 patients. *Ann. Neurol.* **42**, 737–746.

Chan, S., Chin, S. S. M., Kartha, K., Nordi, D. R., Goodman, R. R., Pedley, T. A., and Hilal, S. K. (1996). Reversible signal abnormalities in the hippocampus and neocortex after prolonged seizure. *Am. J. Neuroradiol.* **17**, 1725–1731.

Commission on Epidemiology and Prognosis of the International League Against Epilepsy (1993). Guidelines for epidemiologic studies on epilepsy. *Epilepsia* **34**, 592–596.

Corey, L. A., Pellock, J. M., Boggs, J. G., Miller, L. L., and DeLorenzo, R. J. (1998). Evidence for a genetic predisposition for status epilepticus. *Neurology* **50**, 558–560.

Cross, J. H., Jackson, G. D., Neville, B. G. R., Connelly, A., Kirkham, F. J., Boyd, S. G., Pitt, M. C., and Gadian, D. G. (1993). Early detection of abnormalities in partial epilepsy using magnetic resonance. *Arch. Dis. Child.* **69**, 104–109.

Davidson, S., and Falconer, M. A. (1975). Outcome of surgery in 40 children with temporal-lobe epilepsy. *Lancet,* 1260–1263.

DeCarolis, P., Crisci, M., Laudadio, S., Baldrati, A., and Sacquegna, T. (1991). Transient abnormalities on magnetic resonance imaging after partial status epilepticus. *Ital. J. Neurol. Sci.* **13**, 267–269.

DeLong, G. R., and Heinz, E. R. (1997). The clinical syndrome of early-life bilateral hippocampal sclerosis. *Ann. Neurol.* **42**, 11–17.

Duncan, J. S., Bartlett, P., and Barker, G. J. (1996). Technique for measuring hippocampal T2 relaxation time. *Am. J. Neuroradiol.* **17**, 1805–1810.

Ebisu, T., Rooney, W. D., Graham;, S. H., Weiner, M. W., and Maudsley, A. A. (1994). N-Acetylaspartate as an *in vivo* marker of neuronal viability in kainate-induced status epilepticus: ^1H magnetic resonance spectroscopic imaging. *J. Cereb. Blood Flow Metab.* **14**, 373–382.

Fernandez, G., Effenberger, O., Vinz, B., Steinlein, O., Elger, C. E., Dohring, W., and Heinze, H. H. (1998). Hippocampal malformation as a cause of familial febrile convulsions and subsequent hippocampal sclerosis. *Neurology* **50**, 909–917.

French, J. A., Williamson, P. D., Thadani, V. M., Darcey, T. M., Mattson, R. H., Spencer, S. S., and Spencer, D. D. (1993). Characteristics of medial temporal lobe epilepsy: I. Results of history and physical examination. *Ann. Neurol.* **34**, 774–780.

Germano, I. M., Zhang, Y. F., Sperber, E., and Moshe, S. (1996). Neuronal migration disorders increase susceptibility to hyperthermia induced seizures in developing rats. *Epilepsia* **37**, 902–910.

Giedd, J. N., Snell, J. W., Lange, N., Rajapakse, J. C., Casey, B. J., Kozuch, P. L., Vaituzis, A. C., Vauss, Y. C., Hamburger, S. D., Kaysen, D., and Rapoport, J. L. (1996a). Quantitative magnetic resonance imaging of human brain development: Ages 4–18. *Cereb. Cortex* **6**, 551–560.

Giedd, J. N., Vaituzis, A. C., Hamburger, S. D., Lange, N.,Rajapakse, J. C., Kaysen, D., Vauss, Y. C., and Rapoport, J. L. (1996b). Quantitative MRI of the temporal lobe, amygdala, and hippocampus in normal human development: Ages 4–18 years. *J. Comp. Neurol.* **366**, 223–230.

Gratten-Smith, J. D., Harvey, A. S., Desmond, P. M., and Chow, C. W. (1993). Hippocampal sclerosis in children with intractable temporal lobe epilepsy: Detection with MR imaging. *Am. J. Roentgenol.* **161**, 1045–1048.

Gross, D. W., and Andermann, F. (1998). Catastrophic deterioration and hippocampal atrophy after childhood status epilepticus. *Ann. Neurol.* **43**, 687.

Gruenthal, M. (1998). Electroencephalographic and histological characteristics of a model of limbic status epilepticus permitting direct control over seizure duration. *Epilepsy Res.* **29**, 221–232.

Gunderson, V. M., Dubach, M., Szot, P., Born, D. E., Wenzel, H. J., Maravilla, K. R., Zierath, D. K.,

Robbins, C. A., and Schwartzkroin, P. A. (1999). Development of a model of status epilepticus in pigtailed macaque infant monkeys. *Dev. Neurosci.* 21, 352–364.

Hall, C. B., Long, C. E., Schnabel, K. C., Caserta, M. T., McIntyre, K. M., Costanzo, M. A., Knott, A., Dewhurst, S., Insel, R. A., and Epstein, L. G. (1994). Human herpesvirus-6 infection in children. *N. Engl. J. Med.* 331, 432–438.

Hardiman, O., Burke, T., Phillips, J., Murphy, S., O'Moore, B., Staunton, H., and Farrell, M. A. (1988). Microdysgenesis in resected temporal neocortex: Incidence and clinical significance in focal epilepsy. *Neurology* 38, 1041–1047.

Harvey, A. S., Gratten-Smith, J. D., Desmond, P. M., Chow, C. W., and Berkovic, S. F. (1995). Febrile seizures and hippocampal sclerosis: Frequent and related findings in intractable temporal lobe epilepsy of childhood. *Pediatr. Neurol.* 12, 201–206.

Harvey, A. S., Berkovic, S. F., Wrennall, J. A., and Hopkins, I. J. (1997). Temporal lobe epilepsy in childhood: Clinical, EEG and neuroimaging findings and syndrome classification in a cohort with new onset seizures. *Neurology* 49, 960–968.

Ho, S. S., Kuzniecky, R., Gilliam, F., Faught, E., and Morawetz, R. B. (1998). Temporal lobe developmental malformations and epilepsy. *Neurology* 50, 748–754.

Holopainen, I. E., Valtonen, M. E., Komu, M. E., Sonninen, P. H., Manner, T. E., Lundbom, N. M. I., and Sillanpää, M. L. (1998). Proton spectroscopy in children with epilepsy and febrile convulsions. *Pediatr. Neurol.* 19, 93–99.

Hosoya, M., Honzumi, K., and Suzuki, H. (1997). Detection of enterovirus by polymerase chain reaction and culture in cerebrospinal fluid of children with transient neurologic complications associated with acute febrile illness. *J. Infect. Dis.* 175, 700–703.

Hugg, J. W., Butterworth, E. J., and Kuzniecky, R. I. (1999). Diffusion mapping applied to mesial temporal lobe epilepsy: Preliminary observations. *Neurology* 53, 173–176.

Jack, Jr., C. R., Bentley, M. D., Twomey, C. K., and Zinsmeister, A. R. (1990). MR imagining-based volume measurements of the hippocampal formation and anterior temporal lobe: Validation studies. *Radiology* 176, 205–209.

Jack, Jr., C. R., Sharbrough, F. W., Cascino, G. D., Hirschorn, K. A., O'Brien, P. C., and Marsh, W. R. (1992). Magnetic resonance image-based hippocampal volumetry: Correlation with outcome after temporal lobectomy. *Ann. Neurol.* 31, 138–146.

Jackson, G. D., Berkovic, S. F., Tress, B. M., Kalnins, R. M., Fabinyi, G. C. A., and Bladin, P. F. (1990). Hippocampal sclerosis can be reliably detected by magnetic resonance imaging. *Neurology* 40, 1869–1875.

Jackson, G. D., McIntosh, A. M., Briellmann, R. S., and Berkovic, S. F. (1998). Hippocampal sclerosis studied in identical twins. *Neurology* 51, 78–84.

Kanemoto, K., Kawasaki, J., Miyamoto, T., Obayashi, H., and Nishimura, M. (2000). Interleukin (IL)-1β, IL-1α, and IL-1 receptor antagonist gene polymorphisms in patients with temporal lobe epilepsy. *Ann. Neurol.* 47, 571–574.

Kassem-Moussa, H., Provenzale, J. M., Petrella, J. R., and Lewis, D. V. (2000). Early diffusion weighted MR abnormalities in status epilepticus. *Am. J. Roentgenol.* 174, 1304–1306.

Kuks, J. B. M., Cook, M. J., Fish, D. R., Stevens, J. M., and Shorvon, S. D. (1993). Hippocampal sclerosis in epilepsy and childhood febrile seizures. *Lancet* 342, 1391–1394.

Lange, N., Giedd, J. N., Castellonos, F. X., Vaituzis, A. C., and Rapoport, J. L. (1997). Variability of human brain structure size: Ages 4–20 years. *Psychiatry Res.* 74, 1–12.

Lansberg, M. G., O'Brien, M. W., Norbash, A. M., Moseley, M. E., Morrell, M., and Albers, G. W. (1999). MRI abnormalities associated with partial status epilepticus. *Neurology* 52, 1021–1027.

Lencz, T., McCarthy, G., Bronen, R. A., Scott, T. M., Inserni, J. A., Sass, K. J., Novelly, R. A., Kim, J. H., and Spencer, D. D. (1992). Quantitative magnetic resonance imaging in temporal lobe epilepsy: Relationship to neuropathology and neuropsychological function. *Ann. Neurol.* 31, 629–637.

Maher, J., and McLachlan, R. S. (1995). Febrile convulsions: Is seizure duration the most important predictor of temporal lobe epilepsy? *Brain* 118, 1521–1528.

Mathern, G. W., Babb, T. L., Vickrey, B. G., Melendez, M., and Pretorius, J. (1995a). The clinical
pathogenic mechanisms of hippocampal neuron loss and surgical outcome in temporal lobe
epilepsy. *Brain* 118, 105–118.

Mathern, G. W., Pretorius, J., and Babb, T. L. (1995b). Influence of the type of initial precipitating
injury and at what age it occurs on the course and outcome in patients with temporal lobe
seizures. *J. Neurosurg.* 82, 220–227.

Maytal, J., and Shinnar, S. (1990). Febrile status epilepticus. *Pediatrics* 86, 611–616.

Meencke, H. J., and Veith, G. (1991). Hippocampal sclerosis in epilepsy. *In* "Epilepsy Surgery" (H.
Lüders, ed.), pp. 705–718. Raven Press, New York.

Meldrum, B., and Brierley, J. B. (1973). Prolonged epileptic seizures in primates. *Arch. Neurol.* 28,
10–17.

Nakasu, Y., Nakasu, S., Morikawa, S., Uemura, S., Inubushi, T., and Handa, J. (1995). Diffusion
weighted MR in experimental sustained seizures elicited with kainic acid. *AJNR Am. J. Neuroradiol.* 16, 1185–1192.

Nelson, K. B., and Ellenberg, J. H. (1976). Predictors of epilepsy in children who have experienced
febrile seizures. *N. Engl. J. Med.* 295, 1029–1033.

Nishimura, S., Ushijima, H., Shiraishi, H., Kanazawa, C., Abe, T., Kaneko, K., and Fukuyama, Y.
(1993). Detection of rotavirus in cerebrospinal fluid and blood of patients with convulsions and
gastroenteritis by means of the reverse transcription polymerase chain reaction. *Brain Dev.* 15,
457–459.

Nitecka, L., Tremblay, E., Charton, G., Bouillot, J. P., Berger, M. L., and Ben-Ari, Y. (1984). Maturation of kainic acid seizure brain damage syndrome in the rat: II. Histopathological sequelae.
Neuroscience 13, 1073–1094.

Nohria, V., Tien, R. D., Lee, N., Heinz, E. R., Smith, J. S., DeLong, G. R., Skeen, M. B., and Lewis,
D. V. (1994). MRI evidence of hippocampal sclerosis in progression: A case report. *Epilepsia* 35,
1332–1336.

Perez, E. R., Maeder, P., Villemure, K. M., Vischer, V. C., Villemure, J. G., and Deonna, T. (2000).
Acquired hippocampal damage after temporal lobe seizures in 2 infants. *Ann. Neurol.* 48, 384–
387.

Pfluger, T., Weil, S., Weis, S., Vollmar, C., Heiss, D., Egger, J., Scheck, R., and Hahn, K. (1999). Normative volumetric data of the developing hippocampus in children based on magnetic resonance
imaging. *Epilepsia* 40, 414–423.

Racacho, L. J., McLachlan, R. S., Ebers, G. C., Maher, J., and Bulman, D. E. (2000). Evidence favoring genetic heterogeneity for febrile convulsions. *Epilepsia* 41, 132–139.

Righini, A., Pierpaoli, C., Alger, J. R., and DiChiro, G. (1994). Brain parenchyma apparent diffusion coefficient alterations associated with experimental complex partial status epilepticus.
Magn. Reson. Imaging 12, 865–871.

Sagar, H. J., and Oxbury, J. M. (1987). Hippocampal neuron loss in temporal lobe epilepsy: Correlation with early childhood convulsions. *Ann. Neurol.* 22, 334–340.

Seress, L. (1992). Morphological variability and developmental aspects of monkey and human granule cells: Differences between the rodent and primate dentate gyrus. *In* "The Dentate Gyrus and
Its Role in Seizures" (C. E. Ribak, C. M. Gall, and I. Mody, eds.), p. 3. Elsevier, Amsterdam.

Spencer, S. S., McCarthy, G., and Spencer, D. D. (1993). Diagnosis of temporal lobe seizure onset:
Relative specificity and sensitivity of quantitative MRI. *Neurology* 43, 2117–2124.

Sperber, E. F., Haas, K. Z., Stanton, P. K., and Moshe, S. L. (1991). Resistance of the immature hippocampus to seizure-induced synaptic reorganization. *Dev. Brain Res.* 60, 88–93.

Stafstrom, C. E., Tien, R. D., Montine, T. J., and Boustany, R. M. (1996). Refractory status epilepticus associated with progressive magnetic resonance imaging signal change and hippocampal
neuronal loss. *J. Epilepsy* 9, 253–258.

Suga, S., Suzuki, K., Ihira, M., Yoshikawa, T., Kajita, Y., Ozaki, T., Iida, K., Saito, Y., and Asano, Y. (2000). Clinical characteristics of febrile convulsions during primary HHV-6 infection. *Arch. Dis. Child.* 82, 62–66.

Szabó, C. Á., Wyllie, E., Siavalas, E. L., Najm, I., Ruggieri, P., Kotogal, P., and Luders, H. (1999). Hippocampal volumetry in children 6 years or younger: Assessment of children with and without complex febrile seizures. *Epilepsy Res.* 33, 1–9.

Thompson, K., and Wasterlain, C. (1997). Lithium–pilocarpine status epilepticus in the immature rabbit. *Dev. Brain Res.* 100, 1–4.

Thompson, K., Holm, A. M., Schousboe, A., Popper, P., Micevych, P., and Wasterlain, C. (1998). Hippocampal stimulation produces neuronal death in the immature brain. *Neuroscience* 82, 337–348.

Tien, R. D., Felsberg, G. J., Campi de Castro, C., Osumi, A. K., Lewis, D. V., Friedman, A. H., Crain, B., and Radtke, R. A. (1993). Complex partial seizures and mesial temporal sclerosis: Evaluation with fast spin echo MR imaging. *Radiology* 189, 835–842.

Tokumitsu, T., Mancuso, A., Weinstein, P. R., Weiner, M. W., Naruse, S., and Maudsley, A. A. (1997). Metabolic and pathological effects of temporal lobe epilepsy in rat brain detected by proton spectroscopy and imaging. *Brain Res.* 744, 57–67.

Trenerry, M. R., Jack, Jr., C.R., Sharbrough, F. W., Cascino, G. D., Hirschorn, K. A., Marsh, W. R., Kelly, P. J., and Meyer, F. B. (1993). Quantitative MRI hippocampal volumes: Association with onset and duration of epilepsy, and febrile convulsions in temporal lobectomy patients. *Epilepsy Res.* 15, 247–252.

Tsujimura, H., Iseki, T., Date, Y., Watanabe, J., Kumagai, K., Kikuno, K., Yonemitsu, H., and Saisho, H. (1998). Human herpesvirus-6 encephalitis after bone marrow transplantation: Magnetic resonance imaging could identify the involved sites of encephalitis. *Eur. J. Haematol.* 61, 284–285.

Utsunomiya, H., Takano, K., Okazaki, M., and Mitsudome, A. (1999). Development of the temporal lobe in infants and children: Analysis by MR based volumetry. *Am. J. Neuroradiol.* 20, 717–723.

van den Berg, J. S. P., van Zeijl, J. H., Rotteveel, J. J., Melchers, W. J. G., Gabreels, F. J. M., and Galema, J. (1999). Neuroinvasion by human herpesvirus type 7 in a case of exanthum subitum with severe neurologic manifestations. *Neurology* 52, 1077–1079.

VanLandingham, K. E., Heinz, E. R., Cavazos, J. E., and Lewis, D. V. (1998). MRI evidence of hippocampal injury after prolonged, focal febrile convulsions. *Ann. Neurol.* 43, 413–426.

Verity, C. M., Ross, E. M., and Golding, J. (1993). Outcome of childhood status epilepticus and lengthy febrile convulsions: Findings of a national cohort study. *Br. Med. J.* 307, 225–228.

Vicedomini, J. P., and Nadler, J. V. (1987). A model of status epilepticus based on electrical stimulation of hippocampal afferent pathways. *Exp. Neurol.* 96, 681–691.

Wallace, S. J. (1982). Prognosis after prolonged unilateral febrile convulsions. In "Advances in Epileptology: XIIIth Epilepsy International Symposium" (H. Akimoto, H. Kazamatsuri, M. Seino, and A. Ward, eds.), p. 97. Raven Press, New York.

Wang, Y., Majors, A., Najm, I., Xue, M., Comair, Y., Modic, M., and Ng, T. C. (1996). Postictal alteration of sodium content and apparent diffusion coefficient in epileptic rat brain induced by kainic acid. *Epilepsia* 37, 1000–1006.

Wieshmann, U. C., Symms, M. R., and Shorvon, S. D. (1997). Diffusion changes in status epilepticus. *Lancet* 350, 493–494.

Williamson, P. D., French, J. A., Thadani, V. M., Kim, J. H., Novelly, R. A., Spencer, S. S., Spencer, D. D., and Mattson, R. H. (1993). Characteristics of medial temporal lobe epilepsy: II. Interictal and ictal scalp electroencephalography, neuropsychological testing, neuroimaging, surgical results and pathology. *Ann. Neurol.* 34, 781–787.

Zhong, J., Petroff, O. A. C., Prichard, J. W., and Gore, J. C. (1995). Barbiturate-reversible reduction of water diffusion coefficient in flurothyl-induced status epilepticus. *Magn. Reson. Med.* 33, 253–256.

CHAPTER 9

Do Prolonged Febrile Seizures Injure Hippocampal Neurons? Insights from Animal Models

ROLAND A. BENDER AND TALLIE Z. BARAM

Departments of Pediatrics and Anatomy/Neurobiology, University of California at Irvine, Irvine, California 92697

Whether febrile seizures, the most common seizure type in young children, induce death of hippocampal neurons and consequent limbic epilepsy has remained controversial, with conflicting data from prospective and retrospective studies. This chapter describes the use of an immature rat model of prolonged febrile seizures to evaluate the acute and chronic effects of hyperthermic seizures on hippocampal cell survival, proliferation, and integrity. Using DNA fragmentation analysis, we demonstrated that these experimental prolonged febrile seizures did not result in acute death of hippocampal neurons. No evidence of loss of specific, often seizure-vulnerable populations of hippocampal cells was found, nor was the rate of granule cell neurogenesis altered. However, prolonged hyperthermic seizures—but not hyperthermia alone—led to neuronal injury, manifested as avidity to silver staining (argyrophilia) in hippocampal regions commonly affected by excitotoxic processes. This "febrile seizure"-induced injury was evident within 24 hours and persisted for at least 2 weeks. The involved cells were not lost, but—as shown in accompanying studies—were profoundly altered, in a manner sufficient to result in significant changes of the functional properties of the hippocampal network. In summary, in an immature rat model, prolonged hyperthermic seizures lead to striking, transient alterations in neuronal structure that are sufficient to induce long-term alterations of neuronal function. © 2002 Academic Press.

I. INTRODUCTION

Febrile seizures affect 2–5% of all children between the ages of 6 months and 5 years, with peak incidence at about 18 months (see Chapters 1 and 2). The impact of these seizures on the immature brain has not been fully resolved. In particular, whether these seizures constitute a risk factor for the development of epilepsy later in life has been a focus of intense research, as discussed in Chapters 5, 6, and 7. Results obtained from an animal model developed to study the effects of febrile seizures (Baram *et al.*, 1997) indicate that these seizures can indeed have long-lasting consequences. Dube *et al.* (2000) demonstrated that rats that had experienced prolonged febrile seizures early in life had, as adults, a lower threshold for developing limbic seizures than did age-matched controls. The mechanisms that cause this increased susceptibility to seizures later in life have remained elusive.

A common mechanism, and an underlying theme in seizure-induced alteration of brain excitability and the consequent evolution of epilepsy (epileptogenesis), involves death of specific types of hippocampal neurons. Thus, prolonged seizures induced by pilocarpine (Clifford *et al.*, 1987; Mello *et al.*, 1993; Obenaus *et al.*, 1993; Liu *et al.*, 1994; Rossart *et al.*, 2001), kainic acid (Nadler *et al.*, 1978; Sperk *et al.*, 1983; Ben-Ari, 1985; Pollard *et al.*, 1994; Buckmaster and Dudek, 1997), or electrical stimulation (Sloviter, 1987, 1991; Wasterlain *et al.*, 1999) lead to death of seizure-sensitive neurons in the vulnerable hippocampal subfields CA1, CA3, and the hilus of the dentate gyrus. The loss of these cells and the resulting, partially compensatory, changes in hippocampal circuitry (for review, see Houser, 1999) are considered the principal neuroanatomical basis of epileptogenesis. This view is strongly supported by neuroanatomical studies of human tissue from patients with temporal lobe epilepsy (Margerison and Corsellis, 1966; Bruton, 1988; deLanerolle *et al.*, 1989; Sutula *et al.*, 1989; Babb *et al.*, 1991). Human hippocampus from these patients demonstrates a pattern of neuronal loss in vulnerable regions and layers of the hippocampal formation, with associated gliosis, comprising the typical "mesial temporal sclerosis" (MTS) (Falconer *et al.*, 1964). Because seizures in animal models can lead to both epilepsy and to neuroanatomical changes highly reminiscent of the human ones, it has been widely hypothesized that (1) the lesion (MTS) in the human is a consequence of previous seizure-induced injury, and (2) that this seizure-induced injury plays a key role in the development of epilepsy. These hypotheses have been particularly prominent in considering the relationship of prolonged febrile seizures and subsequent temporal lobe epilepsy (Cendes *et al.*, 1993; French *et al.*, 1993; Davies *et al.*, 1996).

In this chapter, we describe experiments that address these notions, using animal models for febrile seizures. This chapter does not discuss neuronal injury in models of a brain with preexisting abnormality or lesion; these are discussed in Chapter 10. This chapter focuses on findings derived from an experimental model for prolonged febrile seizures (which is described in detail in Chapter 15), and compares them to other data (e.g., Jiang *et al.*, 1999), when available. Specific questions that are addressed here include examining whether experimental prolonged febrile seizures caused acute death or long-term loss of specific populations of hippocampal neurons, whether the seizures influenced neuronal birth rate, and whether neuronal injury, short of actual death, was responsible for the functional changes observed after these seizures in this experimental animal model (Chapters 14 and 15).

II. DO PROLONGED EXPERIMENTAL FEBRILE SEIZURES CAUSE ACUTE HIPPOCAMPAL CELL DEATH?

For all of the experiments from the authors' laboratory, an immature rat model of prolonged febrile seizures, described in more detail in Chapter 15 and the papers cited there, was used. Briefly, on postnatal days (P)10–11, brain and core temperatures were elevated, using a constant, calibrated stream of warm air. This led to seizures when brain and core temperatures reach 40.9°C. Seizure duration was regulated to approximate the condition of prolonged (complex) febrile seizures in the human, i.e., those associated in retrospective studies with temporal lobe epilepsy. The electrophysiological correlates of the behavioral seizures, and their involvement of the hippocampal formation, have been verified (see Chapter 15).

For all analyses, the effects of the hyperthermic seizures were distinguished from potential effects of hyperthermia alone, by using a control group that experienced the same duration and degree of hyperthermia, but in whom the seizures were prevented using a short-acting barbiturate (hyperthermic controls). An additional, normothermic control group was also evaluated.

Because no gross injury or tissue loss was observed on routine histochemistry after the seizures, death of individual neurons, expected to proceed via the apoptotic (programmed cell death) cascade, was examined, using methods visualizing DNA fragmentation. Because these methods, *in situ* end labeling (ISEL) or terminal end labeling (TUNEL), label neurons only during a very short window in the process of apoptotic death, ISEL was performed on sections obtained from rats sacrificed 1, 4, 8.5, 20, or 48 hours after the seizures, to provide the complete time course of potential apoptotic cell death (Toth *et al.*, 1998). An additional group of animals was subjected to hyperthermia twice, leading to total seizure duration of 60 ± 2 minutes, and was sacrificed 20 hours following the second seizure episode. As a "positive control," sections from adult rats subjected to kainic acid-induced status epilepticus and allowed a 20-hour survival time were run in parallel. These sections revealed numerous dying limbic neurons, confirming the validity of the ISEL method.

The results of these experiments were quite unequivocal: whereas an occasional dying neuron was visualized, as expected in the P10–P11 rat, no excess of cell death was found at any of the time points analyzed. Therefore, it can be concluded that acute, apoptotic cell death is not induced by prolonged (20 or 60 minutes) experimental febrile seizures. These findings are in line with other triggered seizures early in life (Sperber *et al.*, 1992; Baram and Hatalski, 1998; Jensen and Baram, 2000). They also emphasize that cell death is not a prerequisite for fundamental alteration of excitability in the hippocampal network.

III. DO EXPERIMENTAL FEBRILE SEIZURES INDUCE LOSS OF SPECIFIC, VULNERABLE POPULATIONS OF HIPPOCAMPAL NEURONS?

Neuronal cell loss in the hilus of the dentate gyrus and in regions of the pyramidal cell layer considered "vulnerable" (CA1, CA3) is one of the pathological alterations most frequently observed among patients with temporal lobe epilepsy, and could contribute significantly to the hyperexcitability of the neuronal network in these patients. As discussed above, experimental prolonged febrile seizures did not induce *acute* cell death in the hippocampus, but they still could lead to slow or delayed death and to neuronal loss long term. We therefore tested the hypothesis that a delayed death of neurons in the seizure-sensitive hippocampal subfields CA1 and hilus (Sankar *et al.*, 1998) contributed to the increased excitability of the hippocampal network observed in rats that had sustained prolonged febrile seizures during development (see Chapter 15).

The overall approach was to evaluate specific neuronal populations in hippocampal sections from adult (3-month-old) rats that had either experienced prolonged febrile seizures on P10 or served as age-matched controls. Coronal sections (50 μm) from perfused brains were processed for *in situ* hybridization (ISH) for glutamate decarboxylase 67 (GAD67) mRNA, immunocytochemistry (ICC) for glutamate receptor subunits 2/3 (GluR2/3), or parvalbumin, as well as for cresyl violet staining. In CA1 and hilus, numbers of total neurons (cresyl violet), of GABAergic interneurons (GAD67-ISH), of hilar mossy cells (GluR2/3-ICC), and of parvalbumin-expressing neurons were determined in anatomically matched series of sections by investigators who were unaware of the treatment.

Again, the results were unequivocal: no differences in the number of cells be-

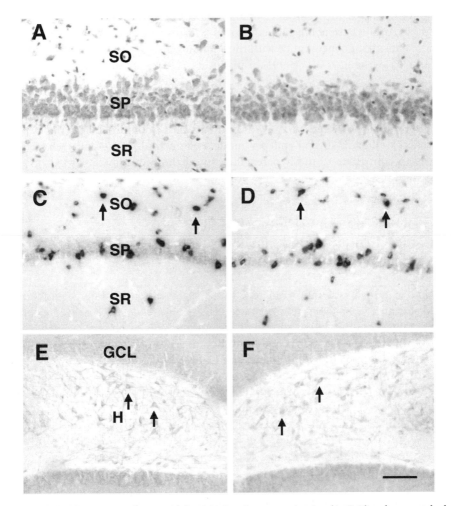

FIGURE 1 Comparison of neuronal densities in seizure-experiencing (A, C, E) and age-matched control rats (B, D, F) 3 months after hyperthermic seizures. Coronal sections stained with cresyl violet (A, B) or processed for GAD67 mRNA-ISH (C, D) show CA1 pyramidal layer (SP), stratum oriens (SO), and stratum radiatum (SR) of a seizure-experiencing (A, C) and a control rat (B, D). No sign of neuronal cell loss is evident in seizure-experiencing rats. Densities of either pyramidal cells (A, B) or GAD67 mRNA-expressing GABAergic interneurons (C, D) do not differ between the two groups. Note that GABAergic interneurons in stratum oriens (arrows in C, D), found to be particularly vulnerable in several models of experimental epilepsy (Rossart et al., 2001), are not affected by hyperthermic seizures. (E, F) Sections show GluR2/3-immunoreactive mossy cells (arrows) in the hilus (H) of a seizure-experiencing (E) and a control rat (F). Numbers of these neurons, found to be sensitive to seizure-induced death (Houser, 1999), were not altered after hyperthermic seizures. GCL, Granule cell layer. Scale bar, 50 μm.

longing to any of the neuronal populations counted were evident in sections from seizure-experiencing rats compared to those from controls (Figure 1). These data are in concordance with those obtained in the febrile seizure model employed by Jiang *et al.* (1999), in juvenile (22-day-old) rats on elevation of core temperatures to 44°C. Exposure of these juvenile rats to a single seizure did not lead to neuronal degeneration (Jiang *et al.*, 1999). Thus, these data indicate that prolonged "febrile" seizures in immature rat models do not cause neuronal cell loss. Neuronal loss—as found in many temporal lobe epilepsy patients as well as in several epilepsy models using adult rats—is therefore not likely to contribute to the hyperexcitability of the hippocampal network observed in these models.

IV. DO PROLONGED "FEBRILE SEIZURES" ALTER NEUROGENESIS OF THE DENTATE GYRUS GRANULE CELLS?

A change in the proliferation rate of granule cell layer neuronal stem cells could lead to a surplus or shortage of dentate gyrus granule cells. Because of the complex excitatory innervation pattern of the granule cells, such changes may perturb the balance of excitation and inhibition in the hippocampus (Parent *et al.*, 1997). In addition, altered proliferation rate of granule cells has been described after seizures in adult experimental animals. Therefore, the question of whether prolonged hyperthermic seizures influenced the proliferation rate of neuronal stem cells in the dentate gyrus was addressed.

As described above, rat pups were subjected to approximately 20-minute hyperthermic seizures on P10 and, together with age-matched controls, were injected with bromodeoxyuridine (BrdU, 50 mg/kg) at several time points later (3, 7, or 25 days after the seizures). Rats were perfused 48 hours after the injections, and coronal sections (50 μm) were processed for BrdU detection. Labeled cells were counted in the dentate gyrus of six anatomically matched sections per brain, by investigators without knowledge of treatment.

The results of these experiments indicated that the rate of proliferation of neurons in the hilus or at the base of the granule cell layer, typical locations of new granule cell formation, was not altered at any of the time points investigated. This is in contrast to enhanced proliferation of granule cells after prolonged seizures in the adult, or to reduced rate of proliferation in immature rats subjected to numerous recurrent seizures (McCabe *et al.*, 2001). Importantly, these findings indicate that prolonged experimental febrile seizures did not lead to long-term enhanced hippocampal excitability by increasing or decreasing the number of granule cells that provide excitatory innervation of CA3 pyramidal cells and hilar mossy cells.

V. DO PROLONGED "FEBRILE" SEIZURES INJURE SPECIFIC POPULATIONS OF HIPPOCAMPAL NEURONS?

The experiments described above demonstrated a dichotomy in the functional and neuroanatomical changes induced by hyperthermic seizures. Namely, enhanced susceptibility to further seizures was observed long term, but this was achieved without any evidence for acute or chronic cell death (or altered numbers of excitatory afferents of pyramidal and mossy cells). Therefore, we evaluated the possibility that experimental prolonged febrile seizures induced neuronal injury that was sufficient to alter permanently the properties of these neurons, without leading to their death. A method considered sensitive to changes in cytoskeletal elements of neurons was chosen (Gallyas et al, 1990; Toth et al., 1998), to visualize potential effects of hyperthermic seizures on neuronal structure. The overall approach involved a comparison of three experimental groups: normothermic and hyperthermic controls and animals subjected to prolonged experimental febrile seizures. For analysis of neuronal injury using the Gallyas "dark"-neuron silver stain, animals were sacrificed 24 hours, 1 week, or 2 weeks after seizure induction. For cell counting, animals ($n = 12$, 4 per experimental group) were sacrificed 4 weeks following the hyperthermic seizures.

As shown in Figure 2, significant and prolonged alterations in the physicochemical properties of neurons in the pyramidal layer of the hippocampal CA1 and all the CA3 subfields were found. Specifically, starting within 24 hours of seizures and persisting for at least 2 weeks, numerous pyramidal cells as well as less abundant hilar neurons exhibited pronounced avidity to silver stain (argyrophilia). The distribution of these argyrophilic neurons indicated the pattern of neuronal vulnerability to febrile seizures in this model, and shared significant similarities with the pattern of injury found with other limbic seizure types (and in human temporal lobe epilepsy). In the hippocampus, major involvement of CA3 and CA1 pyramidal cell layers and relative sparing of the granule cell layer and subiculum were consistent with vulnerability patterns in adult models of kainic acid-induced (Nadler et al., 1978; Sperk et al., 1983; Ben-Ari, 1985; Pollard et al., 1994) and pilocarpine-induced (Clifford et al., 1987; Mello et al., 1993; Liu et al., 1994) status epilepticus.

However, unlike the chronic outcome of these seizures in adult rats, no evidence of neuronal cell loss was found at any time after the hyperthermic seizures, and cell counts revealed no evidence of loss in specific vulnerable hippocampal cell populations (see above). Thus, these data, revealing profound but transient alterations of neuronal integrity in regions known to be affected by other limbic seizure paradigms, may provide a mechanism to reconcile conflicting reports regarding the effects of developmental limbic seizures on neu-

Bender and Baram

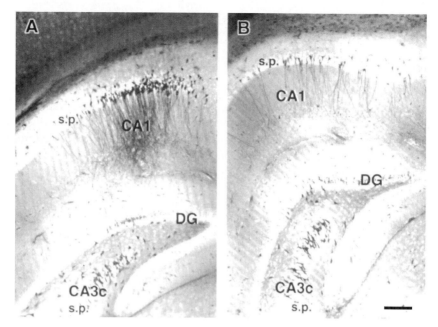

FIGURE 2   Persistent injury to hippocampal neurons after hyperthermic seizures. Sections obtained from immature rats killed 1 week (A) or 2 weeks (B) after hyperthermic seizures are shown.
Silver-stained neurons are evident in the pyramidal cell layer and in the hilus at both time points.
Decreased numbers of affected neurons are apparent at the 2-week time point. DG, Dentate gyrus;
s.p., stratum pyramidale. Scale bar, 50 μm. Modified with permission from Toth *et al.* (1998). Copyright 1998 by the Society for Neuroscience.

ronal survival. Specifically, our findings suggest that similar neuronal populations share vulnerability to limbic seizures in both the immature and mature
hippocampus, but immature neurons may undergo injury followed by recovery,
whereas mature neurons progress from injury to death (Chang and Baram,
1994; Owens *et al.*, 1997).

VI. CONCLUSION

In conclusion, the experiments described in this chapter indicate that experimental febrile seizures, though shown to alter excitability in the hippocampal
network, do not produce this long-lasting effect by acute or chronic alteration
of cell numbers. Thus, no death of typically vulnerable neuronal populations
was found, nor changes in proliferation rates of granule cells. These findings
are important, because they lead away from the straightforward notion that cell
death is required for the process of epileptogenesis. In addition, this finding may

have an important implication for clinical studies of the outcome of febrile seizures: recent and ongoing imaging studies target acute injury (swelling) of hippocampal structures, as well as volume reduction (presumably due to hippocampal cell loss) as a chronic consequence of these seizures. Data from our animal model suggest that the latter measure may not be a sensitive or required marker for alteration of the underlying limbic circuit.

ACKNOWLEDGMENTS

Studies in the authors' laboratory were supported in part by NIH Grant NS 35439 (TZB) and an Epilepsy Foundation of America Postdoctoral Research Award (RAB).

REFERENCES

Babb, T. L., Kupfer, W. R., Pretorius, J. K., Crandall, P. H., and Levesque, M. F. (1991). Synaptic reorganization by mossy fibers in human epileptic fascia dentata. *Neuroscience* 42, 351–363.

Baram, T. Z., and Hatalski, C. G. (1998). Neuropeptide-mediated excitability: A key triggering mechanism for seizure generation in the developing brain. *Trends Neurosci.* 21, 471–476.

Baram, T. Z., Gerth, A., and Schultz, L. (1997). Febrile seizures: An appropriate-aged model suitable for long-term studies. *Brain Res. Dev. Brain Res.* 98, 265–270.

Ben-Ari, Y. (1985). Limbic seizure and brain damage produced by kainic acid: Mechanisms and relevance to human temporal lobe epilepsy. *Neuroscience* 14, 375–403.

Bruton, C. J. (1988). "The Neuropathology of Temporal Lobe Epilepsy" (Maudsley Monographs, no. 31). Oxford University Press, New York.

Buckmaster, P. S., and Dudek, F. E. (1997). Neuron loss, granule cell axon reorganization and functional changes in the dentate gyrus of epileptic kainate-treated rats. *J. Comp. Neurol.* 385, 385–404.

Cendes, F., Andermann, F., Dubeau, F., Gloor, P., Evans, A., Jones-Gotman, M., *et al.* (1993). Early childhood prolonged febrile convulsions, atrophy and sclerosis of mesial structures, and temporal lobe epilepsy: An MRI volumetric study. *Neurology* 43, 1083–1087.

Chang, D., and Baram, T. Z. (1994). Status epilepticus results in reversible neuronal injury in infant rat hippocampus: Novel use of a marker. *Brain Res. Dev. Brain Res.* 77, 133–136.

Clifford, D. B., Olney, J. W., Maniotis, A., Collins, R. C., and Zorumski, C. F. (1987). The functional anatomy and pathology of lithium-pilocarpine and high-dose pilocarpine seizures. *Neuroscience* 23, 953–968.

Davies, K. G., Hermann, B. P., Dohan, F. C. Jr., Foley, K. T., Bush, A. J., and Wyler, A. R. (1996). Relationship of hippocampal sclerosis to duration and age of onset of epilepsy, and childhood febrile seizures in temporal lobectomy patients. *Epilepsy Res.* 24, 119–126.

deLanerolle, N. C., Kim, J. H., Robbins, R. J., and Spencer, D. D. (1989). Hippocampal interneuron loss and plasticity in human temporal lobe epilepsy. *Brain Res.* 495, 387–395.

Dube, C., Chen, K., Eghbal-Ahmadi, M., Brunson, K., Soltesz, I., and Baram, T. Z. (2000). Prolonged febrile seizures in immature rat model enhance hippocampal excitability long-term. *Ann. Neurol.* 47, 336–344.

Falconer, M. A., Serafetinides, E. A., and Corsellis, J. A. N. (1964). Etiology and pathogenesis of temporal lobe epilepsy. *Arch. Neurol.* 10, 233–248.

French, J. A., Williamson, P. D., Thadani, V. M., Darcey, T. M., Mattson, R. H., Spencer, S. S., and Spencer, D. D. (1993). Characteristics of medial temporal lobe epilepsy: I. Results of history and physical examination. *Ann. Neurol.* **34**, 774–780.

Gallyas, F., Guldner, F. H., Zoltay, G., and Wolff, J. R. (1990). Golgi-like demonstration of "dark" neurons with an argyrophil III method for experimental neuropathology. *Acta Neuropathol. (Berl.)* **79**, 620–628.

Houser, C. R. (1999). Neuronal loss and synaptic reorganization in temporal lobe epilepsy. *In* "Jasper's Basic Mechanisms of the Epilepsies" (A. V. Delgado-Escueta, W. A. Wilson, R. W. Olsen, and R. J. Porter, eds.), Vol. 79, pp. 743–761. Lippincott Williams & Wilkins, Philadelphia.

Jensen, F. E., and Baram, T. Z. (2000). Developmental seizures induced by common early-life insults: Short- and long-term effects on seizure suseptibility. *Mental Retardations Dev. Disabil. Res. Rev.* **6**, 253–257.

Jiang, W., Duong, T. M., and deLanerolle, N. C. (1999). The neuropathology of hyperthermic seizures in the rat. *Epilepsia* **40**, 5–19.

Liu, Z., Nagao, T., Desjardins, G. C., Gloor, P., and Avoli, M. (1994). Quantitative evaluation of neuronal loss in the dorsal hippocampus in rats with long-term pilocarpine seizures. *Epilepsy Res.* **17**, 237–247.

Margerison, J. H., and Corsellis, J. A. (1966). Epilepsy and temporal lobes. A clinical, electroencephalographic and neuropathological study of the brain in epilepsy, with particular reference to the temporal lobes. *Brain* **89**, 499–530.

McCabe, B. K., Silveira, D. C., Cilio, M. R., Cha, B. H., Liu, X., Sogawa, Y., and Holmes, G. L. (2001). Reduced neurogenesis following neonatal seizures. *J. Neurosci.* **21**, 2094–2103.

Mello, L. E., Cavalheiro, E. A., Tan, A. M., Kupfer, W. R., Pretorius, J. K., Babb, T. L., and Finch, D. M. (1993). Circuit mechanisms of seizures in the pilocarpine model of chronic epilepsy: Cell loss and mossy fiber sprouting. *Epilepsia* **34**, 985–995.

Nadler, J. V., Perry, B. W., and Cotman, C. W. (1978). Intraventricular kainic acid preferentially destroys hippocampal pyramidal cells. *Nature* **271**, 676–677.

Obenaus, A., Esclapez, M., and Houser, C. R. (1993). Loss of glutamate decarboxylase mRNA-containing neurons in the rat dentate gyrus following pilocarpine-induced seizures. J. Neurosci. **13**, 4470–4485.

Owens, J. Jr., Robbins, C. A., Wenzel, H. J., and Schwartzkroin, P. A. (1997). Acute and chronic effects of hypoxia on the developing hippocampus. *Ann. Neurol.* **41**, 187–199.

Parent, J. M., Yu, T. W., Leibowitz, R. T., Geschwind, D. H., Sloviter, R. S., and Lowenstein, D. H. (1997). Dentate granule cell neurogenesis is increased by seizures and contributes to aberrant network reorganization in the adult rat hippocampus. *J. Neurosci.* **17**, 3727–3738.

Pollard, H., Charriaut-Marlangue, C., Cantagrel, S., Represa, A., Robain, Q., Moreau, J., and Ben-Ari, Y. (1994). Kainate-induced apoptotic cell death in hippocampal neurons. *Neuroscience* **63**, 7–18.

Rossart, R., Dinocourt, C., Hirsch, J. C., Merchan-Perez, A., De Felipe, J., Ben-Ari, Y., Esclapez, M., and Bernard, C. (2001). Dendritic but not somatic GABAergic inhibition is decreased in experimental epilepsy. *Nat. Neurosci.* **4**, 63–71.

Sankar, R., Shin, D. H., Liu, H., Mazarati, A., Pereira de Vasconcelos, A., and Wasterlain, C. (1998). Patterns of status epilepticus-induced neuronal injury during development and long-term consequences. *J. Neurosci.* **18**, 8382–8393.

Sloviter, R. S. (1987). Decreased hippocampal inhibition and a selective loss of interneurons in experimental epilepsy. *Science* **235**, 73–76.

Sloviter, R. S. (1991). Permanently altered hippocampal structure, excitability, and inhibition after experimental status epilepticus in the rat: The 'dormant basket cell' hypothesis and its possible relevance to temporal lobe epilepsy. *Hippocampus* **1**, 41–66.

Sperber, E. F., Stanton, P. K., Haas, K., Ackerman, R. F., and Moshe, S. L. (1992). Developmental differences in the neurobiology of epileptic brain damage. *In* "Molecular Neurobiolgy of Epilepsy" pp. 67–81. Elsevier, Amsterdam.

Sperk, G., Lassmann, H., Baran, H., Kish, S. J., Seitelberger, F., and Hornykiewicz, O. (1983). Kainic acid induced seizures: Neurochemical and histopathological changes. *Neuroscience* 10, 1301–1315.

Sutula, T., Cascino, G., Cavazos, J., Parada, I., and Ramirez, L. (1989). Mossy fiber synaptic reorganization in the epileptic human temporal lobe. *Ann. Neurol.* 26, 321–330.

Toth, Z., Yan, X. X., Haftoglou, S., Ribak, C .E., and Baram, T. Z. (1998). Seizure-induced neuronal injury: Vulnerability to febrile seizures in an immature rat model. *J. Neurosci.* 18, 4285–4294.

Wasterlain, C. G., Mazarati, A. M., Shirasaka, Y., Thompson, K. W., Peniz, L., Liu, H., and Katsumori, H. (1999). Seizure-induced hippocampal damage and chronic epilepsy: A Hebbian Theory of epileptogenesis. *In* "Jasper's Basic Mechanisms of the Epilepsies" (A. V. Delgado-Escueta, W. A. Wilson, R. W. Olsen, and R. J. Porter, eds.), Vol. 79, pp. 829–843. Lippincott Williams & Wilkins, Philadelphia.

CHAPTER 10

Do Effects of Febrile Seizures Differ in Normal and Abnormal Brain?

Ellen F. Sperber,*,†,§ Solomon L. Moshé,*,†,‡
and Isabelle M. Germano‖

*Departments of *Neurology, †Neuroscience, and ‡Pediatrics, Albert Einstein
College of Medicine, Bronx, New York 10461, §Department of Psychology,
Mercy College, Dobbs Ferry, New York 10522, and ‖Department of Neurosurgery,
Mt. Sinai School of Medicine, New York, New York 10029*

Febrile seizures are the most common form of convulsions in infants and young children. The presence of these seizures early in life is frequently correlated with hippocampal sclerosis and temporal lobe epilepsy in adulthood. Although several studies have addressed this issue, a causal relationship has not been established. The important question is whether febrile seizures result in neuronal damage and epilepsy later in life or whether some preexisting damage predisposed the child to febrile seizures and subsequently to neuronal loss and epilepsy. Hyperthermia has been used as a model of febrile seizures and has several advantages to clinical studies. In general, our studies indicate that single, short hyperthermic seizures in young rats do not have any long-term effect on seizure susceptibility or produce any obvious brain injury. In contrast, rats with a preexisting pathology demonstrate a lowered seizure threshold and neuronal loss. © 2002 Academic Press.

I. INTRODUCTION

High fever is a common occurrence in childhood. However, periodically, the fever may be accompanied by convulsions. Approximately 3–5% of infants and young children experience febrile seizures before the age of 5 years (Hauser and Kurland, 1975; Woodbury, 1977). Studies suggest that a large number of adults (30–50%) with temporal lobe epilepsy and mesial temporal sclerosis report a history of febrile seizures (Cendes *et al.*, 1993; Gloor, 1991). Thus, it has been suggested that neuronal loss, as a consequence of febrile seizures, results in temporal lobe epilepsy in adulthood (Falconer, 1970).

On the other hand, it has been argued that relatively few children with high fevers develop febrile convulsions. And furthermore, only a small percentage of those children with febrile seizures later develop epilepsy. In fact, it has been demonstrated that seizure recurrence in children with symptomatic seizures can be predicted by the presence of prior febrile seizures (Shinnar *et al.*, 1990). These latter studies argue that some underlying abnormality was present and increased the likelihood of febrile seizures in childhood and temporal lobe epilepsy in adulthood. In this regard, a few epidemiological studies suggest that children with preexisting brain damage have an increased incidence of febrile seizures. In particular, children with static encephalopathy, previous neurological insult (Shinnar *et al.*, 1990; Ellenberg *et al.*, 1984), or perinatal ischemic brain injury (Aicardi and Chevrie, 1970; Hill and Volpe, 1981) have an increased incidence of seizures of all types, including febrile seizures.

In humans, it is difficult to study the effects of febrile seizures and neuronal loss on the development of temporal lobe epilepsy later in life. Longitudinal studies are generally expensive and time consuming. Therefore, most of our knowledge has been obtained from retrospective reports of patients with temporal lobe epilepsy. Unfortunately, such reports start off with people who have epilepsy, and may thus suffer from recall bias. In addition, neither longitudinal nor retrospective studies can be used to establish a causal relationship between febrile seizures early in life and the development of temporal lobe epilepsy in adulthood. In this regard, basic research has proved to be a great asset. Such studies have addressed the following issues: (1) whether febrile seizures produce neuronal loss ("brain damage") that may be responsible for the development of seizures later in life and (2) whether there is an increased likelihood of febrile seizures in an immature brain with a preexisting pathology.

Several different techniques have been devised to induce hyperthermic convulsions in young rats as a model of febrile seizures. For instance, circulation of warm air either with a hair dryer (Baram *et al.*, 1997; Toth *et al.*, 1998; Dube *et al.*, 2000) or fan (Morimoto *et al.*, 1990; Gilbert and Cain, 1985) has been found effective in producing hyperthermic seizures in rat pups. Other studies have incorporated a microwave (Hjeresen and Diaz, 1988) or heated metal chamber with an infrared light source (Holtzman *et al.*, 1981; Zhao *et al.*, 1985a,b; Chilsolm *et al.*, 1985) to produce seizures. And still other laboratories have found that merely placing young rats either directly onto a heated surface (Sarkisian *et al.*, 1999), into a tank of warm water (Jiang *et al.*, 1999; Klauenberg and Sparber, 1984), or in a container floating in warm water (Germano *et al.*, 1996) will produce seizures. For detailed discussions of these models, the reader is referred to Chapter 13.

II. EFFECTS OF FEBRILE SEIZURES
IN THE NORMAL DEVELOPING RAT

Clinical studies frequently cite the association between the presence of febrile seizures in childhood and the development of temporal lobe epilepsy in adulthood. The initial basic research studies in this field addressed this issue by examining the effects of exposure to a single febrile seizure early in life on seizure susceptibility in adulthood. Typically, seizures were produced during development and seizure threshold was determined at maturity. For instance, rat pups experienced hyperthermic seizures and as adults their seizure susceptibility was determined by either pentylenetetrazol (PTZ) or kindled seizures. Rats having a hyperthermic seizure at 5–20 days of age were exposed to PTZ as adults and were found to have more severe seizures. As adults, these rats displayed a shorter seizure latency to seizure onset and an increased probability of developing status (McCaughran and Schecter, 1982). Similarly, rat pups that had a hyperthermic seizure at 1 day of age required fewer stimulations to develop kindled seizures in adulthood. However, 5- or 10-day-old rats that had either single or multiple hyperthermic seizures had no change in their kindling rates in adulthood (Gilbert and Cain, 1985). It appears that there may be a small window of increased sensitivity to the effects of hyperthermic seizures. It is also possible that febrile seizures may alter the immature brain subtly (Chen et al., 1999), without inducing neuronal death (Toth et al., 1998). Along these lines, a study by Dube and colleagues (Dube et al., 2000) demonstrates that febrile seizures do not produce behavioral or electrographic seizure in adulthood. However, adult rats had a heightened sensitivity to seizures induced in vivo with kainic acid or in vitro by electrical stimulation. This suggests that febrile seizures may at times produce subtle, yet persistent changes in neuronal excitability, which may lower seizure threshold later in life.

If, indeed, early exposure to febrile seizures results in an increased seizure vulnerability in adulthood, the early seizure must result in some neuropathological alterations. Several reports have attempted to determine if hyperthermic seizures may compromise neuronal integrity either structurally or functionally. Adult rats exposed to hyperthermic seizures prior to 10 days of age did not show signs of neuronal loss, morphological changes, or gross damage in areas of the brain typically affected by limbic seizures, such as the hippocampus, particularly CA1 and CA3, piriform cortex, or neocortex (Gilbert and Cain, 1985). These results are confirmed by a study of Sarkisian et al. (1999) in which stereological cell counts were performed in immature rats 10 days after seizures induced by hyperthermia and continuous hippocampal stimulation. In this study, no neuronal loss or abnormalities were observed in the hippocampal CA1, CA3, dentate gyrus, or hilus. Similarly, Germano et al. (1996) observed no difference

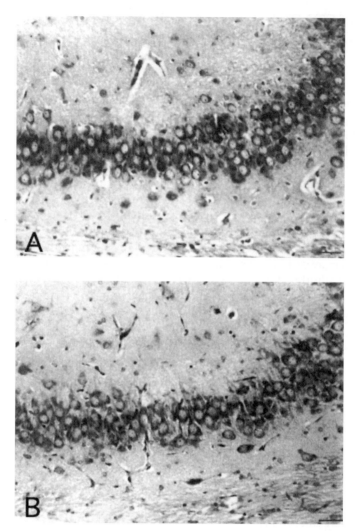

FIGURE 1 Hippocampal section of normal developing rat after exposure to hyperthermic seizure at 14 days of age. Photomicrographs of coronal section of the CA3 pyramidal cell layer of a normal control rat (A) and normal rat 4 weeks following a single exposure to hyperthermia (B). Histological examination reveals no significant morphological changes and cell counts indicate that no neuronal loss occurred following hyperthermia. Cresyl violet stain; bar, 200 mm. Reprinted with permission from I. M. Germano, Y. F. Zhang, E. F. Sperber, and S. L. Moshé (1996). Neuronal migration disorders increase seizure susceptibility to febrile seizures. *Epilepsia* 37, 902–910.

4 weeks after hyperthermia in the appearance of the CA3 pyramidal cells of 2-week-old rats with or without exposure to hyperthermia (Figure 1).

Several other histological techniques have been used to determine if hyperthermic seizures alter neuronal integrity and produce neuronal degeneration. Jiang *et al.* (1999) reported that single and multiple hyperthermic seizures in rats beginning at 22 days of age did not result in degeneration of hippocampal cells. Interestingly, a small percentage of the rats exposed to hyperthermic seizures went into status epilepticus as adults (2–6 months later). In these rats, as expected in adult rats following status epilepticus, extensive neuronal damage was present throughout the temporal lobe (hippocampus, amygdala, piriform cortex and entorhinal cortex). The observed damage appeared to be a consequence of the occurrence of status epilepticus in adulthood and not the initial hyperthermic seizure(s) during development. Therefore, these studies indicate that hyperthermic seizures at an early age do not result in neuronal alterations in adulthood.

A study by Baram and colleagues (Toth *et al.*, 1998) demonstrated extensive changes following hyperthermic seizures in young rats; however, these changes appeared to be transient. The brains of 11-day-old rats were examined 24 hours after a hyperthermic seizure. Extensive argyrophylic cells indicating neuronal injury were present in the hippocampal CA1 and CA3 pyramidal cells in addition to a large number of cells throughout the amygdala. However, DNA fragmentation beyond that observed in control animals was not apparent. The argyrophylic changes persisted for at least 2 weeks. However, 4 weeks after the seizure, these changes were no longer observable and neuronal loss had not occurred.

There is one report of hyperthermic seizures in young rats in which seizure induced neuropathological changes were not apparent until adulthood (Chilsolm *et al.*, 1985). It was found that adult rats that had previously been exposed to hyperthermic seizures at 15 days of age had extensive morphological changes in hippocampal neurons. The pyramidal cells appeared basophilic and shrunken with pyknotic nuclei or nucleoli. In addition, increased extraneuronal space was also apparent. However, despite extensive neuronal injury in the hippocampus, no degenerating debris or lesion was present indicating that cell loss had not occurred. In addition, these changes were only transient and were not apparent at 30 days of age.

Taken together, these studies suggest that febrile seizures do not result in neuronal loss or mesial temporal epilepsy in the normal developing rat. This is further demonstrated in several other seizure models. For instance, immature rats do not show hippocampal cell loss following seizures induced by kainic acid (Nitecka *et al.*, 1984; Holmes and Thompson, 1988; Sperber *et al.*, 1991), pilocarpine (Cavalheiro *et al.*, 1987; Hirsch *et al.*, 1992), kindling (Haas *et al.*, 2001), or flurothyl (Sperber *et al.*, 1999). One exception is Sankar *et al.* (1999). Along these lines, neurophysiological changes using paired pulse inhibition in dentate granule cells of 2-week-old rats have also not been observed 2–4 weeks following kainic acid (Sperber *et al.*, 1991), flurothyl (Sperber *et al.*, 1999), or kindled seizures (Haas *et al.*, 2001).

In summary, in the normal developing rat, seizures early in life do not result in permanent neuronal loss indicative of mesial temporal epilepsy. Thus, if there is a link between febrile seizures and adult epilepsy, it is unlikely that the link is mesial temporal neuronal loss. Nonetheless, it is possible that the presence of extensive neuronal injury, even if only transient, may result in altered functional and electrophysiological circuitry. This seems possible because seizures early in life may subsequently produce some behavioral or learning deficits in adulthood (Stafstrom *et al.*, 1993; Koh *et al.*, 1999). In fact a study by Chen *et al.* (1999) suggests that febrile seizures may produce effects more subtle than neuronal degeneration, such as changes in hippocampal neuronal excitability. Hippocampal slice recordings were obtained following hyperthermic seizures in 10-day-old rats. At 1 week and again 10 weeks after hyperthermic seizures, an increase in inhibitory synaptic signaling was present. These results indicate that seizures, or at least limbic seizures, at any early age may produce permanent neurophysiological changes in the absence of neuropathological changes. Whether this is true of other hyperthermic seizure models or nonlimbic seizures has not yet been determined.

III. EFFECTS OF FEBRILE SEIZURES IN THE ABNORMAL DEVELOPING RAT

Several clinical studies contend that the presence of febrile seizures is not the determining factor for adult epilepsy (see Chapters 5–7). First, only a small percentage of children with febrile seizures develop recurrent seizures (Maytal and Shinnar, 1990; Berg *et al.*, 1998). Second, there is an increased likelihood of febrile seizures in children with prior brain damage (Lennox-Buchthal, 1973; Nelson and Ellenberg, 1976). It has been suggested that the link between febrile seizures and temporal lobe epilepsy is the presence of an underlying abnormality that renders the brain vulnerable both to febrile seizures in childhood and subsequently to temporal lobe epilepsy in adulthood.

Early studies such as that by Zhao *et al.* (1985b) suggested that rats with a genetic predisposition may have an increased vulnerability to febrile seizures. Subsequently, these rats were more susceptible to other seizure models in adulthood. Rats that were genetically prone to audiogenic seizures were found to have shorter latencies to the onset of hyperthermic seizures. Furthermore, when later exposed to either kainic acid (Zhao *et al.*, 1985a) or kindled seizures (Zhao *et al.*, 1985b) they demonstrated an increased seizure susceptibility. Along these lines, a study by Kanemoto and co-workers (Kanemoto *et al.*, 2000) suggests that a subpopulation of patients with temporal lobe epilepsy may also have a genetic predisposition for the development of hippocampal sclerosis following febrile seizures. These studies should not be taken to indicate that all genetic anomalies increase susceptibility to febrile seizure or that a genetic anomaly is the only means to increase vulnerability to febrile seizures. Lowered seizure thresholds also occur in the presence of a variety of malformations, some of which may or may not be genetic in origin.

Along these lines, Olson *et al.* (1985) was one of the first to address directly the question of whether the presence of prior brain damage increases vulnerability to febrile seizures. The study examined the effects of ischemic injury on sensitivity to hyperthermic seizures in the developing rat. Ischemia was produced by ligation of the carotid artery and anoxia at 1–2 days of age. At 5–20 days of age, rats were exposed to hyperthermia until they convulsed. At 5 days of age, the presence of prior ischemic damage had no effect on susceptibility to hyperthermic seizure. However, in 10-, 15-, and 20-day-old rats with ischemic injury, there was a significant decrease in temperature thresholds and decrease in survivability with age. These findings indicate that in the presence of prior brain damage, there is an increased vulnerability to febrile seizures throughout the developmental period. This supports clinical reports of increased seizures in children with perinatal brain injury (Chevrie and Aicardi, 1977; Hill and Volpe, 1981).

In another study, Germano and collegues (1996) examined the effects of disordered neuronal migration on susceptibility to febrile seizures. Neuronal migration disorder (NMD) in humans may range from a few ectopic cells to severe disruption of the cortical and hippocampal cytoarchitecture. Histological abnormalities can be experimentally induced by *in utero* treatment with a potent alkylating agent, methylazoxymethanol (MAM). Treatment on embryonic day 15 results in histological features that closely parallel the human pathological state. These include cortical and hippocampal laminar disorganization, ectopic neurons in the subcortical white matter and hippocampus, persistent granular layer, and marginal glioneuronal heterotopia (Germano and Sperber, 1998). Germano and associates (1996) treated rats with MAM *in utero* and on postnatal day 15 the rats were exposed to a febrile seizure. Results of the study indicate that rats pups with NMD were significantly more vulnerable to the effects of elevated core body temperatures. These rats had a greater incidence of both single and multiple seizures, more severe seizures, and a higher mortality rate, irrespective of seizure occurrence. These effects increased as the exposure time to hyperthermia increased.

Several additional studies further indicate that the presence of an underlying brain pathology may increase susceptibility to other types of seizures, as well. For instance, it has been demonstrated that 14-day-old rats with NMD have a shorter latency to seizure and higher mortality rate following kainic acid (Germano *et al.*, 1993). Similarly, studies demonstrate that 15-day-old rats with NMD have an increased vulnerability to kainic acid and bicuculline-induced seizures (de Feo *et al.*, 1995). de Feo and colleagues (1995) observed that the increased sensitivity to seizures in NMD rats was not permanent because the increased susceptibility was present at 15 days of age but not at 30. However, others report that the effects of an early brain injury on seizure susceptibility are permanent.

Baraban and Schwartzkroin (1996) demonstrated that adult rats with NMD had lowered seizure threshold as indicated by a shorter latency to the onset of flurothyl seizures. The discrepency between these two studies may be due to differences in either the seizure model or the extent of cortical dysplasia.

Evidence from *in vitro* studies further indicate that prior neuronal brain injury in developing rats may result in lowered seizure thresholds. Baraban and Schwartzkroin (1996) obtained differences in electrophysiological recordings from hippocampal slices derived from NMD and normal rats (25–35 days of age). Their results demonstrate significantly more stimulus evoked and spontaneous epileptiform discharge activity from CA1 pyramidal cells from NMD slices. This suggests that dysplastic cells are in a sense "primed" for seizure activity.

The results of these studies indicate that the presence of an underlying brain pathology may lower the threshold to seizures, in particular, febrile seizures. Clinical findings further indicate increased vulnerability to seizures when a neurological abnormality has been determined. Shinnar and associates (1990 and 1992) demonstrated that a prior neurologic abnormality has a high probability of being associated with development of an epileptic syndrome. Children with febrile seizures who later developed epilepsy were more likely to have been diagnosed with remote symptomatic etiology at the time of the initial unprovoked seizure. In addition, neuroimaging studies (Fernandez *et al.*, 1998; VanLandingham *et al.*, 1998; Jackson *et al.*, 1998), reviewed in detail in Chapter 8, suggest that a previous pathological condition may leave the brain vulnerable to febrile seizures and possibly the development of hippocampal sclerosis.

It appears that the occurrence of a febrile seizure may sometimes be a marker of an underlying disease. Furthermore, it is possible that in these circumstances, when the brain is already in a compromised state, the febrile seizure may produce hippocampal injury. In fact, recent studies indicate that prior brain damage increases the vulnerability to seizure-induced damage, in contrast to normal developing rats, which have been repeatedly shown to have a greater resistance than adult rats to seizure-induced damage.

The studies discussed thus far have examined the relationship between prior brain injury and the increased vulnerability to seizures. Few studies, however, have determined the effects of prior injury on the vulnerability to seizure-induced damage. Germano *et al.* (1996, 1998) addressed this question in rats with neuronal migration disorders. Their results demonstrate that that immature rats with NMD show evidence of brain injury following a single exposure to hyperthermia at 2 weeks of age (Germano *et al.*, 1996). Neuronal counts 4 weeks later revealed pyramidal cell loss in the hippocampal CA1 and CA 3 areas in all rats with NMD (Figure 2). Furthermore, the extent of the loss correlated with the duration of exposure to hyperthermia. Neuronal injury was characterized by loss of pyramidal cells or damaged cytoplasm. In addition, astrocyte proliferation, another marker of neuronal injury, was increased in le-

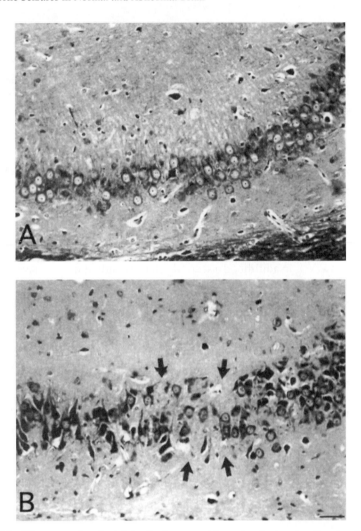

FIGURE 2   Hippocampal region of developing rats with neuronal migration disorders following exposure to hyperthermia at 14 days of age. Photomicrographs of coronal section of the CA3 pyramidal cell layer of a control rat with neuronal migration disorder (A) and rat with neuronal migration disorder 4 weeks after exposure to hyperthermia (B). Arrows indicate the extensive neuronal degeneration and cell loss present in the neuronal migration disorder rat following hyperthermia (B). Cresyl violet stain; bar, 200 mm. Reprinted with permission from I. M. Germano, Y. F. Zhang, E. F. Sperber, and S. L. Moshé (1996). Neuronal migration disorders increase seizure susceptibility to febrile seizures. *Epilepsia* **37**, 902–910.

sioned areas. In the rats with NMD, hyperthermia with or without convulsions resulted in a similar pattern of damage.

Further studies with NMD in young rats demonstrate that these rats are more vulnerable to acute kindling (Germano *et al.,* 1998) or kainic acid (Germano and Sperber, 1998) seizure-induced damage: 24 hours after kainic acid seizure, numerous darkened and shrunken pyramidal cells were observed only in treated rats. These studies with NMD and hyperthermia, in particular, suggest that that the initial dysplasia or pathology may be the relevant factor in determining whether hippocampal damage is likely to be present, and not necessarily seizure occurrence alone. Nonetheless, these studies suggest that a "dual pathology" may be necessary for the development of seizure-induced hippocampal injury and subsequently epilepsy (Levesque *et al.,* 1991).

Thus, the studies by Germano *et al.* (1996, 1998) suggest a "two-hit" hypothesis—that is, in the presence of a brain anomaly (such as NMD) there is an increased susceptibility to seizure-induced hippocampal damage. The idea of a two-hit hypothesis is further supported by others. Koh and colleagues (1999) have demonstrated that when 2-week-old rats experienced kainic acid seizures no hippocampal injury was detected by DNA fragmentation or histological staining. However, in adulthood a second seizure resulted in extensive neuronal injury that was significantly greater than in adult rats exposed only to kainic acid during adulthood. In preliminary studies, Sperber and colleagues have demonstrated that hippocampal lesions at 2 weeks of age increased the amount of granule cell mossy fiber sprouting in adulthood following kainic acid or kindled seizures. Taken together, these studies suggest that the two-hit hypothesis does not necessitate that the initial trauma be a specific brain anomaly such as NMD. Rather, any trauma to the brain may compromise the developing brain so that it is more vulnerable to seizure-induced damage. This may be relevant to the clinical situation: Mathern and co-workers (1997) demonstrated that the hippocampi of patients with intractable epilepsy who had an initial precipitating injury early in life had more severe sclerosis than did those without a precipitating injury.

ACKNOWLEDGMENTS

This work was supported by NIH grants NS-30387 (EFS) and NS-20253 (SLM). Dr. Moshé is the recepient of a Martin A. and Emily L. Fisher Fellowship in Neurology and Pediatrics. With thanks to Dr. J. Veliskova for manuscript preparation and Dr. A. Galanopoulou for photographic assistance.

REFERENCES

Aicardi, J., and Chevrie, J. J. (1970). Convulsive status epilepticus in infants and children. *Epilepsia* 11, 187–197.
Baraban, S. C., and Schwartzkroin, P. A. (1996). Flurothyl seizure susceptibility in rats following prenatal methylazoxymethanol treatment. *Epilepsy Res.* 23, 189–194.

Baram, T. Z., Gerth, A., and Schultz, L. (1997). Febrile seizures: An appropriate-aged model suitable for long-term studies. *Brain Res. Dev. Brain Res.* **246**, 134–143.

Berg, A. T., Darefsky, A. S., and Holford, T. R. (1998). Seizures with fever after unprovoked seizures: An analysis on children followed from the time of a first febrile seizure. *Epilepsia* **39**, 77–80.

Cavalheiro, E. A., Silva, D. F., Turski, W. A., Calderazzo-Filho, L. S., Bartolotto, Z., and Turski, L. (1987). The susceptibility of rats to pilocarpine-induced seizures is age dependent. *Dev. Brain Res.* **37**, 43–58.

Cendes, F., Andermann, F., Gloor, P., Lopes-Cendes, I., Andermann, E., Melanson, D., Jones-Gotman, M., Robitaille, Y., Evans, A., and Peters, T. (1993). Atrophy of mesial structures in patients with temporal lobe epilepsy: Cause or consequence of repeated seizures? *Ann. Neurol.* **34(6)**, 795–801.

Chen, K., Baram, T. Z., and Soltesz, I. (1999). Febrile seizures in the immature brain result in persistent modification of neuronal excitability in limbic circuits. *Nat. Med.* **5**, 888–894.

Chevrie, J. J., and Aicardi, J. (1977). Convulsive disorders in the first year of life: Etiologic factors. *Epilepsia* **18**, 489–498.

Chilsolm, J., Kellogg, C., and Frank, J. E. (1985). Developmental hyperthermic seizures alter adult hippocampal benzdiazepine binding and morphology. *Epilepsia* **26**, 151–157.

de Feo, M. R., Mecarelli, O., and Ricci, G. F. (1995). Seizure susceptibility in immature rats with microenecphaly induced by prenatal exposure to methylazoxymethanol acetate. *Pharm. Res.* **31**, 109–114.

Dube, C., Chen, K., Eghbal-Ahmadi, M., Brunson, K. L., Soltesz, I., and Baram, T. Z. (2000). Prolonged febrile seizures in the immature rat model enhance hippocampal excitability long term. *Ann. Neurol.* **47**, 336–344.

Ellenberg, J. H., Hirtz, D. H., and Nelson, K. B. (1984). Age at onset of seizures in young children. *Ann. Neurol.* **15**, 127–134.

Falconer, M. A. (1970). The pathological substrate of temporal lobe epilepsy. *Guy's Hosp. Rep.* **119**, 47–60.

Fernandez, G., Effenberger, O., Vinz, B., Steinlein, O., Elger, C. E., Döhring, W., and Heinze, H. J. (1998). Hippocampal malformation as a cause of familial febrile convulsions and subsequent hippocampal sclerosis. *Neurology* **50**, 909–916.

Germano, I. M., and Sperber, E. F. (1998). Transplacentally induced neuronal migration disorders: An animal model for the study of the epilepsies. *J. Neurosci. Res.* **51**, 473–488.

Germano, I. M., Zhang, Y. F., Sperber, E. F., and Moshé, S. L. (1993). Expression of GABA and glutamate in a rat model of epilepsy. *Soc. Neurosci. Abstr.* **21**, 1467.

Germano, I. M., Zhang, Y. F., Sperber, E. F., and Moshé, S. L. (1996). Neuronal migration disorders increase seizure susceptibility to febrile seizures. *Epilepsia* **37**, 902–910.

Germano, I. M., Sperber, E. F., Ahuja, S., and Moshé, S. L. (1998). Evidence of enhanced kindling and hippocampal neuronal injury in immature rats with neuronal migration disorders. *Epilepsia* **39(12)**, 1253–1260.

Gilbert, M. E., and Cain, D. P. (1985). A single neonatal pentylenetetrazol or hyperthermia convulsion increases kindling susceptibility in the adult rat. *Brain Res,* **354**, 169–180.

Gloor, P. (1991). Mesial temporal sclerosis: Historical background and overview from a modern perspective. *In* "Epilepsy Surgery" (H. O. Luders, ed.), pp. 689–703. Raven Press, New York.

Haas, K. Z., Sperber, E. F., Opanashuka, L. A., Stanton, P. K., and Moshé, S. L. (2001). Resistance of the immature hippocampus to morphologic and physiologic alterations following status epilepticus or kindling. *Hippocampus* (in press).

Hauser, W. A., and Kurland, L. T. (1975). The epidemiology of epilepsy in Rochester, Minnesota, 1935–1967. *Epilepsia* **16**, 1–66.

Hill, A., and Volpe, J. (1981). Seizures, hypoxic-ischemia, and intraventricular hemorrhage in the newborn. *Ann. Neurol.* **10**, 109–122.

Hirsch, E., Baram, T. Z., and Snead III, O. C. (1992). Ontogenic study of lithium–pilocarpine-induced status epilepticus in rats. *Brain Res.* 583, 120–126.

Hjeresen, D. L., and Diaz, J. (1988). Ontogeny of susceptibility to experimental febrile seizures in rats. *Dev. Psychobiol.* 21, 261–275.

Holmes, G. L., and Thompson, J. L. (1988). Effects of kainic acid on seizure susceptibility in the developing brain. *Dev. Brain Res.* 39, 51–59.

Holtzman, D., Obana, K., and Olson, J. (1981). Hyperthemia-induced seizures in the rat pup: A model for febrile convulsions. *Science* 213, 1034–1036.

Jackson, G. D., McIntosh, A. M., Briellman, R. S., and Berkovic, S. F. (1998). Hippocampal sclerosis studied in identical twins. *Neurology* 51, 78–84.

Jiang, W., Duong, T. M., and Lanerolle, D. (1999). The neuropathology of hyperthermic seizures in the rat. *Epilepsia* 40, 5–19.

Kanemoto, K., Kawasaki, J., Miyamoto, T., Obayashi, H., and Nishimura, M. (2000). Interleukin (IL)-1β, IL-1α, and IL-1 receptor antagonist gene polymorhisms in patients with temporal lobe epilepsy. *Ann. Neurol.* 47, 571–574.

Klauenberg, B. J., and Sparber, S. B. (1984). A kindling-like effect induced by repeated exposure to heated water in rats. *Epilepsia* 25, 292–301.

Koh, S., Storey, T. W., Santos, T. C., Mian, A. Y., and Cole, A. J. (1999). Early-life seizures in rats increases susceptibility to seizure-induced brain injury in adulthood. *Neurology* 53, 915–921.

Lennox-Buchthal, M. (1973). Febrile convulsions: A reappraisal. *Electroencephalogr. Clin. Neurophysiol.* 32, 1–132.

Levesque, M. F., Nakast, N., Vinters, H., and Babb, T. L. (1991). Surgical treatment of limbic epilepsy associated with intrahippocamapl lesions: The problem of dual pathology. *J. Neurosurg.* 75, 364–370.

Mathern, G. W., Babb, T. L., and Armstrong, D. L. (1997). Hippocampal sclerosis. *In* "Epilepsy: A Comprehensive Textbook" (J. J Engel and T. A. Pedley, eds.), pp. 133–155. Lippincott-Raven, Philadelphia.

Maytal, J., and Shinnar, S. (1990). Febrile status epilepticus. *Pediatrics* 86, 611–616.

McCaughran, J. A. J., and Schecter, N. (1982). Experimental febrile convulsions: Long-term effects of hyperthermia-induced convulsions in the developing rat. *Epilepsia* 23, 173–183.

Morimoto, T., Nagao, H., Sano, N., Takahashi, M., and Matsuda, H. (1990). Hyperthermia-induced seizures with a servo system: Neurophysiological roles of age, temperature elevation rate and regional GABA content in the rat. *Brain Dev.* 12, 279–283.

Nelson, K. B., and Ellenberg, J. H. (1976). Predictors of epilepsy in children who have experienced febrile seizures. *N. Engl. J. Med.* 295, 1029–1033.

Nitecka, L., Tremblay, E., Charton, G., Bouillot, J. P., Berger, M. L., and Ben-Ari, Y. (1984). Maturation of kainic acid seizure-brain damage syndrome in the rat. II. Histopathological sequelae. *Neuroscience* 13, 1073–1094.

Olson, J. E., Horne, D. S., Holtzman, D., and Miller, M. (1985). Hyperthermia-induced seizures in rat pups with preexisting ischemic brain injury. *Epilepsia* 26, 360–364.

Sankar, R., Shin, D., Mazarati, A. M., Liu, H., and Wasterlain, C. G. (1999). Ontogeny of self-sustaining status epilepticus. *Dev. Neurosci.* 21, 345–351.

Sarkisian, M. R., Holmes, G. L., Carmant, L., Liu, Z., Yang, Y., and Stafstrom, C. E. (1999). Effects of hyperthermia and continuous hippocampal stimulation on the immature and adult brain. *Brain Dev.* 21, 318–325.

Shinnar, S., Berg, A. T., Moshé, S. L., Petix, M., Maytal, J., Kang, H., Goldensohn, E. S., and Hauser, W. A. (1990). Risk if seizure recurrence following a first unprovoked seizure in childhood. *Pediatrics* 85, 1076–1085.

Shinnar, S., Maytal, J., Krasnoff, L., and Moshé, S. L. (1992). Recurrent status epilepticus in children. *Ann. Neurol.* 31, 598–604.

Sperber, E. F., Haas, K. Z., Stanton, P. K., and Moshé, S. L. (1991). Resistance to damage of the immature hippocampus to flurothyl induced status epilepticus. *Ann. Neurol.* **30**, 495.

Sperber, E. F., Haas, K. Z., Romero, M. T., Stanton, P. K., and Moshé, S. L. (1999). Flurothyl status epilepticus in developing rats: Behavioral, electrographic, histological and electrophysiological studies. *Dev. Brain Res.* **116**, 59–68.

Stafstrom, C. E., Chronopoulos, A., Thurber, S., Thompson, J. L., and Holmes, G. L. (1993). Age-dependent cognitive and behavioral deficits after kainic acid seizures. *Epilepsia* **34**, 420–432.

Toth, Z., Yan, X. X., Heftoglu, S., Ribak, C. E., and Baram, T. Z. (1998). Seizure-induced neuronal injury: Vulnerability to febrile seizures in an immature rat model. *J. Neurosci.* **18**, 4285–4294.

VanLandingham, K. E., Heinz, E. R., Cavazos, J. E., and Lewis, D. V. (1998). Magnetic resonance imaging evidence of hippocampal injury after prolonged focal febrile convulsions. *Ann. Neurol.* **43**, 413–426.

Woodbury, L. A. (1977). Incidence and prevalence of seizure disorders including the epilepsies in the USA. A review and analysis of the literature. *In* "Plan for the Nationwide Action of Epilepsy," Vol. IV, pp. 24–77. DHEW Publication. GPO, Washington, D.C.

Zhao, D., Wu, X., Pei, Y., and Zuo, Q. (1985a). Long-term effects of febrile convulsions on seizure susceptibility in P77PMC rat—Resistant to accoustic stimuli but susceptible to kainiate-indued seizures. *Exp Neurol* **88**, 688–695.

Zhao, D., Wu, X., and Zuo, Q. (1985b). Kindling phenomenon of hyperthermic seizures in the epilepsy-prone versus the epilepsy-resistant rat. *Brain Res* **358**, 390–393.

CHAPTER 11

Why Does the Developing Brain Demonstrate Heightened Susceptibility to Febrile and Other Provoked Seizures?

FRANCES E. JENSEN AND RUSSELL M. SANCHEZ

Department of Neurology, Children's Hospital and Program in Neuroscience,
Harvard Medical School, Boston, Massachusetts 02115

The majority of human seizures occur early in life, and many developmental seizures occur only during discrete windows of development. Understanding the mechanisms and consequences of these early-life seizures, including the features that distinguish them from seizures in the fully mature brain, is a requisite for delineating the consequences of these seizures on structural and functional integrity of the developing central nervous system. This chapter reviews experimental evidence from studies of the maturational changes in neurotransmitter and other effector systems that modulate the balance of excitation and inhibition early in postnatal life, influencing the susceptibility of the immature brain to seizures. These maturational changes also govern the mechanisms by which developmental seizures influence the developing brain long-term. © 2002 Academic Press.

I. INTRODUCTION

The immature brain differs from the adult brain in its susceptibility to seizures, seizure characteristics, and responses to antiepileptic drugs (AEDs). Experimental evidence from animal models has revealed factors that may contribute to the age dependence of epileptic syndromes, and further suggests that early-life seizures or treatment with AEDs can alter the normal maturation of brain function (Holmes, 1997). To fully understand the age-dependence of childhood epilepsies and to optimize treatments, it is necessary to consider maturational differences in the cellular and molecular mechanisms of epilepsy and how these may be functionally altered by early-life seizures or AED treatment.

II. THE CLINICAL PROBLEM

Most early-life seizures are not genetically determined, and the majority of seizures occurring during infancy and early childhood are not spontaneous but are triggered (Baram and Hatalski, 1998) by fever (Shinnar, 1998), hypoxia (Jensen et al., 1991; Bellinger, et al., 1995; Nelson and Ellenberg, 1986), or trauma (Dinner, 1993). In general, these triggered seizures demonstrate a high degree of age specificity. Hypoxia-related seizures occur primarily in neonates (Jensen et al., 1991, 1998; Volpe, 1989, 2000), febrile seizures are exclusive to infancy and childhood (see Chapters 1–3), and early traumatic seizures (distinct from posttraumatic epilepsy) are far more common in children (Jennett and Lewin, 1960).

Why does the developing brain demonstrate heightened susceptibility to proconvulsant triggers? Human studies have been unable to resolve this question (French et al., 1993; Cendes et al., 1993). However, recent experimental observations from animal models of epilepsy and development suggest that many factors that enhance neuronal excitability are overexpressed during the normal brain maturation. This relative imbalance of excitation over inhibition is postulated to be important for activity-dependent synaptogenesis and synaptic plasticity during a window of development characterized by enhanced rates of learning and brain growth.

Why do some seizures during development induce long-term susceptibility to seizures and/or epilepsy? A related issue is whether seizures occurring in a growing brain can alter subsequent neuronal development and cognitive outcome. For example, in the case of short seizures provoked by fever (simple febrile seizures), prospective epidemiological studies have demonstrated a benign outcome, without cognitive dysfunction (Verity et al., 1998) (see Chapter 4) or subsequent epilepsy (Shinnar, 1998), (see Chapters 5 and 7). However, the relationship between prolonged febrile seizures and temporal lobe epilepsy (TLE) has been a subject of conflicting data and interpretation (see Chapters 5–8). Patients with intractable TLE, reported in retrospective risk-factor analyses, have a high incidence (30–60%) of a history of prolonged febrile seizures (French et al., 1993; Cendes et al., 1993) (see Chapter 6), compared to the 3–5% incidence of febrile seizures in the general population. It is widely hypothesized that febrile seizures produce temporal lobe injury and this leads to spontaneous seizures (Falconer et al., 1964; Annegers et al., 1987; French et al., 1993) (see Chapters 6 and 15). Alternatively, rather than a causal relationship between early febrile seizures and TLE, others hypothesize that a common predisposing tendency to neuronal excitability in these individuals results in their lowered threshold to febrile seizures as well as later development of epilepsy (Verity and Golding, 1991; Shinnar, 1998; Lewis, 1999) (see Chapters 5–7). This hypothesis is supported by the fact that TLE after prolonged febrile seizures is more frequent in individuals with preexisting brain abnormalities compared to those with normal neurological status and neuroimaging studies (Maytal and Shinnar, 1990).

Similarly, perinatal hypoxia has been variably associated with the development of epilepsy in later life (Bergamasco *et al.*, 1984; Nelson and Ellenberg, 1986). Hypoxic encephalopathy occurs in neonates with multisystem failure, and thus represents a heterogeneous population that confounds clinical outcome studies. Nevertheless, under more controlled conditions of infants undergoing cardiac bypass surgery for repair of congenital heart defects, electroencephalographic (EEG) monitoring revealed a high incidence of postoperative epileptiform events, and EEG abnormalities were the major predictor of subsequent structural abnormalities on magnetic resonance imaging (MRI) (Bellinger *et al.*, 1995).

A. Animal Models of Seizures and Status Epilepticus in the Immature Brain

A number of experimental seizure models have at least in part recapitulated components of the age-specific seizure syndromes (Moshe and Albala 1983; Albala *et al.*, 1984; Stafstrom *et al.*, 1992; Sperber, 1996). Symptomatic early-onset seizures can be modeled in the developing brain by exposure to chemoconvulsants such as kainate, pilocarpine, flurothyl, and tetanus toxin, or by repeated electrical stimulation (kindling). Seizure thresholds to chemoconvulsant and kindling stimuli are much lower in immature animals (Albala *et al.*, 1984; Moshe *et al.*, 1983; Baram *et al.*, 1993). Additionally, certain pathophysiological conditions such as hypoxia or hyperthermia may precipitate seizures in the immature animal, while having no epileptogenic effect in the adult (Dube *et al.*, 2000; Jensen and Wang, 1996).

In general, these models exhibit age dependence not only in their efficacy for inducing seizures, but also in their long-term effects on brain function. Unlike the adult, the immature brain appears to be relatively resistant to seizure-induced neuronal injury (Sperber, 1996; Holmes, 1997; Toth *et al.*, 1998). Kainate injections induce status epilepticus in immature animals with no delayed neuronal loss despite 2 hours or more of continuous seizures (Chang and Baram, 1994; Sperber *et al.*, 1991; Nitecka *et al.*, 1984; Liu *et al.*, 1995). More severe proconvulsant conditions have been found to both induce seizures and cause neuronal injury in the immature brain (Thompson *et al.*, 1998), and pilocarpine status-induced neuronal death in the immature brain has been reported (Sankar *et al.*, 1998). However, the extent of death is significantly less than that seen after status in the adult brain (Wasterlain, 1997). These data suggest that although the resistance of the immature brain to chemoconvulsant-induced neuronal death is not absolute, it is much greater relative to the adult brain.

Despite the lack of significant injury in the immature brain in these experimental models, other evidence suggests that neonatal seizures may adversely alter the function of surviving neurons and neuronal circuitry to chronically lower seizure thresholds or promote epileptogenesis. In rat pups at postnatal age day 10 (P10), global hypoxia induced spontaneous seizures and resulted in chronically decreased thresholds to chemoconvulsant-induced seizures (Jensen *et al.*, 1992) and increased excitability in hippocampal slices (Jensen *et al.*, 1998), despite no apparent neuronal injury (Jensen *et al.*, 1991). These seizures are suppressed by an antagonist specific to a glutamate receptor subtype, indicating that maturational changes in glutamate receptors play a role in the generation of seizures (Jensen *et al.*, 1995). Similarly, hyperthermia-induced convulsions in the P10 rat do not cause acute cell death (Toth *et al.*, 1998), yet result in long-lasting changes in inhibitory synaptic transmission (Chen *et al.*, 1999) and chronically decreased seizure threshold and increased hippocampal excitability (Dube *et al.*, 2000). Intrahippocampal tetanus toxin injections in P10 rats result in the development of acute seizures that lead to spontaneous recurrent seizures later in life and aberrant mossy fiber sprouting in the dentate gyrus (Anderson *et al.*, 1997, 1999).

Recurrent (25–50) seizures induced by repeated flurothyl inhalation or pentylenetetrazol administration beginning on the first day of life or during the second postnatal week can result in long-term increases in seizure susceptibility, with selective mossy fiber sprouting in hippocampal subfields (Huang *et al.*, 1999; Holmes *et al.*, 1998, 1999). Notably, animals that experienced repeated flurothyl-induced seizures also showed modest but significant impairment in learning and memory in adulthood (Huang *et al.*, 1999). The cellular and molecular events that mediate these morphological and functional changes are still under investigation, but these data reiterate the concept that seizures can induce long-lasting, potentially adverse functional changes in the immature brain that may not appear acutely as injury.

B. MATURATIONAL FACTORS THAT MAY ENHANCE SEIZURE SUSCEPTIBILITY IN THE IMMATURE BRAIN

Animal studies indicate that early postnatal development is a critical window during which synaptogenesis and neuronal plasticity are peaking (Swann *et al.*, 1999; Fox *et al.*, 1996; Huttenlocher *et al.*, 1982; Rakic *et al.*, 1989). Excitatory synaptic transmission mediated by glutamate receptors is required for these processes and their expression is enhanced in the immature brain, compared to the adult brain (Fox *et al.*, 1996; Huttenlocher *et al.*, 1982; Rakic *et al.*, 1989; Insel *et al.*, 1990; McDonald *et al.*, 1992). In the rat, glutamate receptor expression is highest in the second postnatal week (McDonald *et al.*, 1992; Insel *et al.*, 1990). Although precise correlations of rat and human neurodevelopmental profiles are problematic, brain growth and myelination evidence suggest that the first 2 weeks of postnatal development in the rat correspond to the transition from infancy to childhood in the human (Gottlieb *et al.*, 1977; Romijn *et al.*, 1991). Additional factors that govern synaptic transmission and neuronal excitability continue to change during this developmental window, including the expression and molecular composition of neurotransmitter receptors and transporters, neuromodulatory peptides and neuropeptide receptors, voltage-gated ion channels, and mechanisms of ionic homeostasis. These factors and their possible relationship to epilepsy in the developing brain are discussed below.

1. Glutamate Receptors

a. Ionotropic Glutamate Receptors

Glutamate is the major excitatory neurotransmitter in the brain, and there are several subtypes of glutamate receptor. These include the N-methyl-D-aspartate (NMDA), α-amino-3-hydroxy-5-methyl-4-isoxazolepropionic acid (AMPA), and kainate (KA) subtypes of ionotropic receptor (Dingledine *et al.*, 1999) as well as different classes of metabotropic glutamate receptor (Conn and Pin, 1997; Wong *et al.*, 1999). AMPA and KA receptors mediate fast excitatory signaling; NMDA receptors play a more modulatory role. NMDA receptor channels are highly permeable to Ca^{2+} (in addition to Na^+ and K^+), and the influx of Ca^{2+} through NMDA receptors can trigger signaling pathways that regulate synaptic function and activity-driven synaptogenesis (Aamodt and Constantine-Paton, 1999; Vallano, 1998). NMDA receptors are critical for pathophysiological processes such as ictal seizure discharges and hypoxic/ischemic neuronal injury (Chapman, 1998; Michaelis, 1998; Meldrum, 1994).

Binding studies in the rat indicate that NMDA receptor density peaks late in the first postnatal week in many forebrain structures, including hippocampus and neocortex (Insel *et al.*, 1990). AMPA receptor density appears to peak later in the second postnatal week around P10 (Insel *et al.*, 1990), whereas kainate receptor development varies with subunit (Miller *et al.*, 1990; Bahn *et al.*, 1994; Kidd and Isaac, 1999). During the first 2–3 postnatal weeks, glutamate-mediated synaptic plasticity is enhanced (Swann *et al.*, 1999) and certain brain regions exhibit heightened susceptibility to the convulsant and excitotoxic effects of glutamate receptor agonists (McDonald *et al.*, 1992; Johnston, 1995; Liu *et al.*, 1996; Young *et al.*, 1991). Thus, the overshoot in expression of functional glutamate receptors is likely to increase excitability of the immature postnatal brain.

The functional properties of glutamate receptors are determined by the particular combination of molecular subunits (Dingledine *et al.*, 1999). In neocortex and hippocampus, expression of the NMDA receptor subunit NR2B relative to the expression of NR2A is much higher during early postnatal development compared to adulthood (Zhong *et al.*, 1995; Monyer *et al.*, 1994). Recombinant NMDA receptors composed predominantly of NR2B exhibit slower decay times compared to those composed predominantly of NR2A (Monyer *et al.*, 1994), and the developmental increase in NR2A expression results in a maturational shortening of NMDA receptor-mediated synaptic currents (Flint *et al.*, 1997). Thus, synaptic excitability and plasticity may be increased in the immature brain by the increased duration of NMDA receptor-mediated excitation and increased Ca^{2+} influx.

In the mature brain, AMPA and kainate receptors are relatively impermeable to Ca^{2+}, but in the immature brain these channels may exhibit Ca^{2+} permeability (Pellegrini-Giampietro *et al.*, 1992). AMPA receptors lacking a GluR2(B) subunit are more permeable to Ca^{2+} than are those that contain a GluR2(B) subunit (Burnashev *et al.*, 1992; Jonas *et al.*, 1994; McBain and Dingledine, 1993; Washburn *et al.*, 1997), and the ratio of expression of GluR2 subunits to that of other AMPA receptor subunits is significantly lower in immature neocortex and hippocampus compared to the adult (Pellegrini-Giampietro *et al.*, 1991). Hence, this suggests that a larger proportion of AMPA receptors are permeable to Ca^{2+} in immature neurons in these brain regions, and may therefore mediate pathophysiological events in early postnatal life, similarly to NMDA receptors (Pellegrini-Giampietro *et al.*, 1992, 1997). This notion is supported by the report that transient knockdown of GluR2 expression in hippocampus of young rats caused spontaneous seizurelike behavior (Friedman and Koudinov, 1999).

b. Metabotropic Glutamate Receptors

There are currently at least eight cloned metabotropic glutamate receptors classified into three groups (Conn and Pin, 1997). Group I receptors are coupled to phosphoinositide (PI) hydrolysis, leading to Ca^{2+} mobilization from intracellular stores, whereas Group II and Group III receptors are negatively coupled to adenylyl cyclase (AC) activity. In general, postsynaptic Group I mGluR activation increases the intrinsic excitability of principal neurons mainly via down-modulation of voltage-gated potassium channels (Gerber and Gahwiler, 1994), and therefore, activation of PI-coupled mGluRs is proconvulsant. Conversely, presynaptic Group II and Group III receptor activation inhibits glutamate release and depresses excitatory synaptic transmission (Glaum and Miller, 1994), and therefore activation of AC-coupled mGluRs is likely to be anticonvulsant.

Developmental regulation of mGluR function also may contribute to the increased seizure susceptibility of the immature brain. mGluR agonist-stimulated PI turnover has been shown to be relatively robust in slices of immature rat brain (Nicoletti et al., 1994). In contrast, the activity of mGluRs negatively coupled to AC is more robust in adult compared to neonatal hippocampus (Casabona et al., 1992; Schoepp and Johnson, 1993). Thus, the developmental pattern of mGluR function may favor a hyperexcitable state, as the activity of postsynaptic mGluRs that promote increased intrinsic neuronal excitability can predominate over mGluRs that presynaptically regulate neurotransmitter release.

c. Glutamate Uptake

The expression of glutamate transporters also is developmentally regulated and may play a role in the enhanced excitability of the immature brain. Glutamate transporters function to eliminate glutamate from the synaptic cleft into neurons or glial cells by active uptake mechanisms. In animal models, decreased expression of glutamate transporters can lead to seizures or lower seizure thresholds (Meldrum et al., 1999; Tanaka et al., 1997; Watanabe et al., 1999). Notably, the expression of both the GLT-1 and GLAST astrocytic glutamate transporters gradually increases during postnatal development in the rat (Furuta et al., 1997). Thus, a relatively lower activity of certain glutamate transporters during development could contribute to enhanced seizure susceptibility in the immature brain.

2. GABA Receptors

γ-Aminobutyric acid (GABA) is the predominant inhibitory neurotransmitter in the brain, and the expression and function of GABA receptors also are developmentally regulated. $GABA_A$ receptors, which mediate postsynaptic responses to GABA in central neurons, are expressed at embryonic stages (Laurie et al., 1992). However, in the first postnatal week, activation of $GABA_A$ receptors causes membrane depolarization rather than the hyperpolarization typical of mature GABAergic synapses (Ben-Ari et al., 1997; Swann et al., 1999). This difference results from maturational changes in the transmembrane chloride ion gradient that governs the equilibrium potential for $GABA_A$ channels (Staley et al., 1995). Inhibitory (hyperpolarizing) $GABA_A$ receptor-mediated potentials gradually appear and are present by the end of the first postnatal week (Ben-Ari et al., 1997; Rivera et al., 1999). Thus, although functional GABA receptors are present very early in development, the delayed onset of functional GABAergic inhibition may contribute to the enhanced excitability of the immature brain.

The molecular composition of $GABA_A$ receptors also is developmentally regulated, with associated changes in functional properties (Paysan and Fritschy, 1998; Hevers and Luddëns, 1998). For example, the expression of $GABA_A$ receptor $\alpha 1$ subunits is low at birth and gradually increases with age (Brooks-Kayal et al., 1998; Dunning et al., 1999; Laurie et al., 1992; Fritschy et al., 1994), and is associated with a gradual shift toward the more rapid kinetics and increased sensitivity to certain benzodiazepines (e.g., diazepam) that are characteristic of most $GABA_A$ receptors in the adult brain (Dunning et al., 1999; Kapur and Macdonald, 1999; Hollrigel and Soltesz, 1997). Such a developmental change in the pharmacological properties of $GABA_A$ receptors suggests that the neonatal brain may respond differently than the adult brain to AEDs that act by enhancing $GABA_A$ receptor function.

Unlike $GABA_A$ receptors, the G protein-coupled $GABA_B$ receptors are activated both pre- and postsynaptically, with opposite effects on synaptic transmission (Gaiarsa et al., 1995). Postsynaptic $GABA_B$ receptors mediate relatively slowly activating and long-lasting membrane hyperpolarization through the activation of a K^+ conductance, while the activation of presynaptic $GABA_B$ receptors decreases neurotransmitter release through the inhibition of Ca^{2+} channels (Gaiarsa et al., 1995). $GABA_B$ receptor binding in rat brain increases during postnatal development and peaks in a regionally specific manner during the first 3 weeks before declining to adult levels. Notably, in hippocampus the presynaptic effects of $GABA_B$ receptor activation are observable earlier in development compared to the postsynaptic effects (Gaiarsa et al., 1995). If the activation of presynaptic $GABA_B$ receptors depresses GABA release, then the earlier appearance of presynaptic $GABA_B$ receptor function would be expected to promote synaptic excitability.

C. OTHER FACTORS MODULATING SYNAPTIC TRANSMISSION AND INTRINSIC NEURONAL EXCITABILITY

The expression of certain neuromodulatory peptides that influence neuronal excitability is developmentally regulated. The excitatory neuropeptide corticotropin-releasing hormone (CRH) is potently proconvulsant (Wasterlain and Mazarati, 1997; Baram and Hatalski, 1998) and may play a critical role in the "triggering" of seizures (by fever, hypoxia, etc.) in the immature brain (Baram and Hatalski, 1998; Jensen and Baram, 2000). CRH expression in immature rat hippocampus is far higher than in the hippocampal formation of the adult rodent (Yan *et al.*, 1998; Chen *et al.*, 2001). In addition, in both immature rat hippocampus and amygdala, the expression of CRH receptors reaches twice that of the adult level in the second postnatal week, a developmental stage during which the immature brain is most susceptible to CRH-induced seizures (Baram *et al.*, 1997; Avishai-Eliner *et al.*, 1996).

Neuropeptide Y and somatostatin also can modulate seizures (Wasterlain and Mazarati, 1997) and their function and expression are developmentally regulated (Lee *et al.*, 1998; Burgunder, 1994). However, the role of these neuropeptides in epileptogenesis in the immature brain is not well understood.

The intrinsic excitability of postsynaptic and axonal membranes is largely determined by the activity of voltage-gated ion channels. In general, the developmental patterns of expression and function of voltage-gated ion channels promote increased intrinsic membrane excitability during embryogenesis and early postnatal development. Spontaneous electrical activity is necessary for cell differentiation, migration, and synaptogenesis (Moody, 1998). Action potentials in immature neurons are of significantly longer duration compared to their adult counterparts, largely due to slower activation rates of delayed rectifier K^+ channels that repolarize the action potential (Moody, 1998; Behrens and Latorre, 1991). The longer action potentials in immature neurons play a key role in activity-driven Ca^{2+}-dependent developmental events. For example, premature shortening of the action potential by overexpression of a delayed rectifier K^+ channel (Kv1.1) in embryonic *Xenopus* spinal neurons decreases neuronal differentiation (Jones and Ribera, 1994). Knockout mice lacking Kv1.1 exhibit spontaneous seizures beginning in the third postnatal week (Smart *et al.*, 1998).

The developmental regulation of voltage-gated channels in axons and at presynaptic terminals may be particularly critical in the generation of seizure activity through their influence on neurotransmitter release. In epileptic DBA/2J mice, a strain genetically prone to audiogenic seizures, binding of a radiolabeled N-type Ca^{2+}-channel toxin (conotoxin GVIA) indicated that the expression of these presynaptic Ca^{2+} channels abnormally increased between postnatal days 2–8 in parallel with seizure susceptibility (Esplin *et al.*, 1994). Wild-type mice showed no change in GVIA binding during the same period, but exhibited a rapid increase in binding between postnatal days 11–14 (Litzinger *et al.*, 1993). This period of N-channel proliferation coincides with the period of heightened susceptibility in rodents to seizures induced by hypoxia or hyperthermia, as discussed below. Thus, the developmental change in presynaptic Ca^{2+} channels may contribute to enhanced seizure susceptibility in the immature brain.

Mechanisms of ion homeostasis are also changing during development. As mentioned earlier, the neuronal expression of chloride transporters has a postnatal onset, and in their absence, the transmembrane Cl^- gradient is such that

Cl^--mediated currents are depolarizing (Staley *et al.*, 1995). The major neuronal Na^+/K^+-ATPase also is less abundant in the immature brain (Haglund and Schwartzkroin, 1990), and thus moderate increases in neuronal activity could regeneratively cause extracellular K^+ to rise to epileptogenic levels. Intracellular Ca^{2+} homeostasis also may be developmentally regulated. For example, the calcium-binding protein calbindin D28K is not expressed in immature hippocampal dentate granule cells, but is expressed by these same cells as they mature (Goodman *et al.*, 1993).

III. CONCLUSION

Developmental changes in factors that regulate neuronal excitability can alter seizure susceptibility, and seizures can alter the normal pattern of brain development. There is likely to be considerable overlap between mechanisms responsible for the exaggerated plasticity and synaptogenesis that characterizes normal brain development and those mechanisms critical to epileptogenesis. An improved understanding of this critical interaction is necessary to devise optimal age-specific therapeutic strategies for the treatment of neonatal and childhood seizures.

REFERENCES

Aamodt, S. M., and Constantine-Paton, M. (1999). The role of neural activity in synaptic development and its implications for adult brain function. *Adv. Neurol.* **79**, 133–144.

Albala, B. J., Moshe, S. L., and Okada, R. (1984). Kainic-acid-induced seizures: A developmental study. *Brain Res.* **315**(1), 139–148.

Anderson, A. E., Hrachovy, R. A., and Swann, J. W. (1997). Increased susceptibility to tetanus toxin-induced seizures in immature rats. *Epilepsy Res.* **26**, 433–442.

Anderson, A. E., Hrachovy, R. A., Antalffy, B. A., Armstrong, D. L., and Swann, J. W. (1999). A chronic focal epilepsy with mossy fiber sprouting follows recurrent seizures induced by intrahippocampal tetanus toxin injection in infant rats. *Neuroscience* **92**(1), 73–82.

Annegers, J. F., Hauser, W. A., Shirts, S. B., *et al.* (1987). Factors prognostic of unprovoked seizures after febrile convulsions. *N. Engl. J. Med.* **316**, 493–498.

Avishai-Eliner, S., Yi, S. J., and Baram, T. Z. (1996). Developmental profile of messenger RNA for the corticotropin-releasing hormone receptor in the rat limbic system. *Brain Res. Dev. Brain Res.* **91**(2), 159–163.

Bahn, S., Volk, B., and Wisden, W. (1994). Kainate receptor gene expression in the developing rat brain. *J. Neurosci.* **14**(9), 5525–5547.

Baram, T. Z., and Hatalski, C. G. (1998). Neuropeptide-mediated excitability: A key triggering mechanism for seizure generation in the developing brain. *Trends Neurosci.* **21**(11), 471–476.

Baram, T. Z., Hirsch, E., and Schultz, L. (1993). Short-interval amygdala kindling in neonatal rats. *Dev. Brain Res.* **73**, 79–83.

Baram, T. Z., Chalmers, D. T., Chen, C., Koutsoukos, Y., and De Souza, E. B. (1997). The CRF1 receptor mediates the excitatory actions of corticotropin releasing factor (CRF) in the developing rat brain: *In vivo* evidence using a novel, selective, non-peptide CRF receptor agonist. *Brain Res.* 770(1–2), 89–95.

Behrens, M. I., and Latorre, R. (1991). Potassium channels in developing excitable cells. *In* "Developmental Biology of Membrane Transport Systems; Current Topics in Membranes." (D. J. Benos, ed.), pp. 327–355. Academic Press, San Diego.

Ben-Ari, Y., Khazipov, R., Leinekugel, X., Caillard, O., and Gaiarsa, J.-L. (1997). GABA-A, NMDA, and AMPA receptors: A developmentally regulated "ménage à trois." *Trends Neurosci.* 20, 523–529.

Bellinger, D. C., Jonas, R. A., Rappaport, L. A., Wypij, D., Wernovsky, G., Kuban, K., Barnes, P. D., Holmes, G. L., Hickey, P. R., Strand, R. D., *et al.* (1995). Developmental and neurologic status of children after heart surgery with hypothermic circulatory arrest or low flow cardiopulmonary bypass. *N. Engl. J. Med.* 332, 549–555.

Bergamasco, B., Penna, P., Ferrero, P., and Gavinelli, R. (1984). Neonatal hypoxia and epileptic risk: A clinical prospective study. *Epilepsia* 25, 131–146.

Brooks-Kayal, A., Jin, H., Price, M., and Dichter, M. A. (1998). Developmental expression of GABA(A) receptor subunit mRNAs in individual hippocampal neurons *in vitro* and *in vivo*. *J. Neurochem.* 70(3), 1017–1028.

Burgunder, J. M. (1994). Ontogeny of somatostatin gene expression in rat forebrain. *Brain Res. Dev. Brain Res.* 78(1), 109–122.

Burnashev, N., Monyer, H., Seeburg, P. H., and Sakmann, B. (1992). Divalent ion permeability of AMPA receptor channels is dominated by the edited form of a single subunit. *Neuron* 8, 189–198.

Casabona, G., Genazzani, A. A., Di Stefano, M., Sortino, M. A., and Nicoletti, F. (1992). Developmental changes in the modulation of cyclic AMP formation by the metabotropic glutamate receptor agonist 1S,3R-aminocyclopentane-1,3-dicarboxylic acid in brain slices. *J. Neurochem.* 59, 1161–1163.

Cendes, F., Andermann, F., Dubeau, F., *et al.* (1993). Early childhood prolonged febrile convulsions, atrophy and sclerosis of mesial structures, and temporal lobe epilepsy: An MRI volumetric study. *Neurology* 43, 1083–1087.

Chang, D., and Baram, T. Z. (1994). Status epilepticus results in reversible neuronal injury in infant rat hippocampus: Novel use of a marker. *Brain Res. Dev. Brain Res.* 77(1), 133–136.

Chapman, A. G. (1998). Glutamate receptors in epilepsy. *Prog. Brain Res.* 116, 371–383.

Chen, K., Baram, T. Z., and Soltesz, I. (1999). Febrile seizures in the developing brain result in persistent modification of neuronal excitability in limbic circuits. *Nat. Med.* 5(8), 888–894.

Chen, Y., Bender, R. A., and Baram, T. Z. (2001). Novel and transient populations of corticotropin-releasing hormone-expressing neurons in developing hippocampus suggest unique functional roles: A quantitative spatiotemporal analysis. *J. Neurosci.* (in press).

Conn, P. J., and Pin, J.-P. (1997). Pharmacology and functions of metabotropic glutamate receptors. *Annu. Rev. Pharmacol. Toxicol.* 37, 205–237.

Dingledine, R., Borges, K., Bowie, D., and Traynelis, S. F. (1999). The glutamate receptor ion channels. *Pharmacol. Rev.* 51(1), 7–61.

Dinner, D. S. (1993). Posttraumatic epilepsy. *In* "The Treatment of Epilepsy: Principles and Practice" (E. Wyllie, ed.), pp. 654–658. Lea & Febiger, Philadelphia.

Dube, C., Chen, K., Eghbal-Ahmadi, M., Brunson, K., Soltesz, I., and Baram, T. Z. (2000). Prolonged febrile seizures in the immature rat model enhance hippocampal excitability long term. *Ann. Neurol.* 47, 336–344.

Dunning, D. D., Hoover, C. L., Soltesz, I., Smith, M. A., and O'Dowd, D. K. (1999). GABAA receptor-mediated miniature postsynaptic currents and α-subunit expression in developing cortical neurons. *J. Neurophysiol.* 82, 3286–3297.

Esplin, M. S., Abbott, J. R., Smart, M. L., Burroughs, A. F., Frandsen, T. C., and Litzinger, M. J. (1994). Voltage-sensitive calcium channel development in epileptic DBA/2J mice suggests altered presynaptic function. *Epilepsia* 35(5), 911–914.

Falconer, M. A., Serafetinides, E. A., and Corsellis, J.A.N. (1964). Etiology and pathogenesis of temporal lobe epilepsy. *Arch. Neurol.* 10, 233–248.

Fishman, M. A. (1979). Febrile seizures: The treatment controversy. *J. Pediatr.* 94, 177–184.

Flint, A. C., Maisch, U. S., Weishaupt, J. H., Kriegstein, A. R., and Monyer, H. (1997). NR2A subunit expression shortens NMDA receptor synaptic currents in developing neocortex. *J. Neurosci.* 17(7), 2469–2476.

Fox, K., Schlaggar, B. L., Glazewski, S., and O'Leary, D.D.M. (1996). Glutamate receptor blockade at cortical synapses disrupts development of thalamocortical and columnar organization in somatosensory cortex. *Proc. Natl. Acad. Sci. U.S.A.* 93, 5584–5589.

French, J. A., Williamson, P. D., Thadani, V. M., *et al.* (1993). Characteristics of medial temporal lobe epilepsy. I. Results of history and physical examination. *Ann. Neurol.* 34, 774–780.

Friedman, L. K., and Koudinov, A. R. (1999). Unilateral GluR2(B) hippocampal knockdown: A novel partial seizure model in the developing rat. *J. Neurosci.* 19(21), 9412–9425.

Fritschy, J. M., Paysan, J., Enna, A., and Mohler, H. (1994). Switch in the expression of rat GABAA-receptor subtypes during postnatal development: An immunohistochemical study. *J. Neurosci.* 14(9), 5302–5324.

Furuta, A., Rothstein, J. D., and Martin, L. J. (1997). Glutamate transporter subtypes are expressed differentially during rat CNS development. *J. Neurosci.* 17, 8363–8375.

Gaiarsa, J.-L., McLean, H., Congar, P., Leinekugel, X., Khazipov, R., Tseeb, V., and Ben-Ari, Y. (1995). Postnatal maturation of gamma-aminobutyric acid A and B-mediated inhibition in the CA3 hippocampal region in the rat. *J. Neurobiol.* 26(3), 339–349.

Gerber, U., and Gahwiler, B. H. (1994). Modulation of ionic currents by metabotropic glutamate receptors. *In* "The Metabotropic Glutamate Receptors" (P. J. Conn and J. Patel, eds.), pp. 125–146. Humana Press, Totowa, NJ.

Glaum, S. R., and Miller, R. J. (1994). Acute regulation of synaptic transmission by metabotropic glutamate receptors. *In* "The Metabotropic Glutamate Receptors" (P. J. Conn and J. Patel, eds.), pp. 147–172. Humana Press, Totowa, NJ.

Goodman, J. H., Wasterlain, C. G., Massarweh, W. F., Dean, E., Sollas, A. L., and Sloviter, R. S. (1993). Calbindin-D28k immunoreactivity and selective vulnerability to ischemia in the dentate gyrus of the developing rat. *Brain Res.* 606(2), 309–314.

Gottlieb, A., Keydar, Y., and Epstein, H. T. (1977). Rodent brain growth stages: An analytical review. *Biol. Neonate* 32, 166–176.

Haglund, M. M., and Schwartzkroin, P. A. (1990). Role of Na-K pump potassium regulation and IPSPs in seizures and spreading depression in immature rabbit hippocampal slices. *J. Neurophysiol.* 63(2), 225–239.

Hevers, W., and Luddëns, H. (1998). The diversity of GABAA receptors. *Mol. Neurobiol.* 18(1), 35–86.

Hollrigel, G. S., and Soltesz, I. (1997). Slow kinetics of miniature IPSCs during early postnatal development in granule cells of the dentate gyrus. *J. Neurosci.* 17(13), 5119–5128.

Holmes, G. L. (1997). Epilepsy in the developing brain: Lessons from the laboratory and clinic. *Epilepsia* 38, 12–30.

Holmes, G. L., Gairsa, J. L., Chevassus-Au-Louis, N., and Ben-Ari, Y. (1998). Consequences of neonatal seizures in the rat: Morphological and behavioral effects. *Ann. Neurol.* 44, 845–857.

Holmes, G. L., Sarkisian, M., Ben-Ari, Y., and Chevassus-Au-Louis, N. (1999). Mossy fiber sprouting after recurrent seizures during early development in rats. *J. Comp. Neurol.* 404(4), 537–553.

Huang, L., Cilio, M. R., Silveira, D. C., McCabe, B. K., Sogawa, Y., Stafstrom, C. E., and Holmes, G. L. (1999). Long-term effects of neonatal seizures: A behavioral, electrophysiological, and histological study. *Brain Res. Dev. Brain Res.* 118(1–2), 99–107.

Huttenlocher, P. R., deCourten, C., Garey, L. J., and Van der Loos, H. (1982). Synaptogenesis in human visual cortex—Evidence for synapse elimination during normal development. *Neurosci. Lett.* **33**, 247–260.

Insel, T. R., Miller, L. P., and Gelhard, R. E. (1990). The ontogeny of excitatory amino acid receptors in the rat forebrain I: *N*-Methyl-D-aspartate and quisqualate receptors. *Neuroscience* **35**, 31–43.

Jennett, W. B., and Lewin, W. (1960). Traumatic epilepsy after closed head injuries. *J. Neurol. Neurosurg. Psychiatry* **23**, 295–301.

Jensen, F. E., and Baram, T. Z. (2000). Developmental seizures induced by common early-life insults. Short and long-term effects on seizure susceptibility. *Ment. Retard. Dev. Disabil. Res. Rev.* **6**, 253–257.

Jensen, F. E., and Wang, C. (1996). Hypoxia-induced hyperexcitability *in vivo* and *in vitro* in the immature hippocampus. *Epilepsy Res.* **26**(1), 131–140.

Jensen, F. E., Applegate, C. D., Holtzman, D., Belin, T., and Burchfiel, J. (1991). Epileptogenic effects of hypoxia in immature rodent brain. *Ann. Neurol.* **29**, 629–637.

Jensen, F. E., Holmes, G. H., Lombroso, C. T., Blume, H., and Firkusny, I. (1992). Age dependent long term changes in seizure susceptibility and neurobehavior following hypoxia in the rat. *Epilepsia* **33**(6), 971–980.

Jensen, F. E., Alvarado, S., Firkusny, I. R., and Geary, C. (1995). NBQX blocks the acute and late epileptogenic effects of perinatal hypoxia. *Epilepsia* **36**(10), 966–972.

Jensen, F. E., Wang, C., Stafstrom, C. E., Liu, Z., Geary, C., and Stevens, M. C. (1998). Acute and chronic increases in excitability in rat hippocampal slices after perinatal hypoxia *in vivo. J. Neurophysiol.* **79**, 73–81.

Johnston, M. V. (1995). Neurotransmitters and vulnerability of the developing brain. *Brain Dev.* **17**(5), 301–306.

Jonas, P., Racca, C., Sakmann, B., Seeburg, P. H., and Monyer, H. (1994). Differences in Ca^{2+} permeability of AMPA-type glutamate receptor channels in neocortical neurons caused by differential expression of the GluR-B subunit. *Neuron* **12**, 1281–1289.

Jones, S. M., and Ribera, A. B. (1994). Overexpression of a potassium channel gene perturbs neuronal differentiation. *J. Neurosci.* **14**, 2789–2799.

Kapur, J., and Macdonald, R. L. (1999). Postnatal development of hippocampal dentate granule cell γ-aminobutyric acidA receptor pharmacological properties. *Mol. Pharmacol.* **55**, 444–452.

Kidd, F. L., and Issac, J. T. (1999). Developmental and activity-dependent regulation of kainate receptors at thalamocortical synapses. *Nature (London)* **400**, 569–573.

Laurie, D. J., Wisden, W., and Seeburg, P. H. (1992). The distribution of thirteen GABAA receptor subunit mRNAs in the rat brain. III. Embryonic and postnatal development. *J. Neurosci.* **12**(11), 4151–4172.

Lee, E. Y., Lee, T. S., Baik, S. H., and Cha, C. I. (1998). Postnatal development of somatostatin- and neuropeptide γ-immunoreactive neurons in rat cerebral cortex: A double-labeling immunohistochemical study. *Int. J. Dev. Neurosci.* **16**(1), 63–72.

Lewis, D. V. (1999). Febrile convulsions and mesial temporal sclerosis. *Curr. Opin. Neurol.* **12**, 197–201.

Litzinger, M. J., Grover, B. B., Saderup, S., and Abbott, J. R. (1993). Voltage sensitive calcium channels mark a critical period in mouse neurodevelopment. *Int. J. Dev. Neurosci.* **11**(1), 17–24.

Liu, Z., Mikati, M., and Holmes, G. L. (1995). Mesial temporal sclerosis: Pathogenesis and significance. *Pediatr. Neurol.* **12**(1), 5–16.

Liu, Z., Stafstrom, C. E., Sarkisian, M., Tandon, P., Yang, Y., Hori, A., and Holmes, G. L. (1996). Age-dependent effects of glutamate toxicity in the hippocampus. *Brain Res. Dev. Brain Res.* **97**(2), 178–184.

Maytal, J., and Shinnar, S. (1990). Febrile status epilepticus. *Pediatrics* **86**, 611–616.

McBain, C. J., and Dingledine, R. (1993). Heterogeneity of synaptic glutamate receptors on CA3 stratum radiatum interneurones of rat hippocampus. *J. Physiol.* **462**, 373–392.

McDonald, J. W., Trescher, W. H., and Johnston, M. V. (1992). Susceptibility of brain to AMPA induced excitotoxicity transiently peaks during early postnatal development. *Brain Res.* **583**(1–2), 54–70.

Meldrum, B. S. (1994). The role of glutamate in epilepsy and other CNS disorders. *Neurology* **44**(Suppl. 8), S14–S23.

Meldrum, B. S., Akbar, M. T., and Chapman, A. G. (1999). Glutamate receptors and transporters in genetic and acquired models of epilepsy. *Epilepsy Res.* **36**(2–3), 189–204.

Michaelis, E. K. (1998). Molecular biology of glutamate receptors in the central nervous system and their role in excitotoxicity, oxidative stress, and aging. *Prog. Neurobiol.* **54**(4), 369–415.

Miller, L. P., Johnson, A. E., Gelhard, R. E., and Insel, T. R. (1990). The ontogeny of excitatory amino acid receptors in the rat forebrain—II. Kainic acid receptors. *Neuroscience* **35**(1), 45–51.

Monyer, H., Burnashev, N., Laurie, D. J., Sakmann, B., and Seeburg, P. H. (1994). Developmental and regional expression in the rat brain and functional properties of four NMDA receptors. *Neuron* **12**, 529–540.

Moody, W. M. (1998). The development of voltage-gated ion channels and its relation to activity-dependent developmental events. *Curr. Top. Dev. Biol.* **39**, 159–185.

Moshe, S. L., and Albala, B. J. (1983). Maturational changes in postictal refractoriness and seizure susceptibility in developing rats. *Ann. Neurol.* **13**, 552–557.

Moshe, S. L., Albala, B. J., Ackermann, R. F., and Engel, Jr. J. (1983). Increased seizure susceptibility of the immature brain. *Brain Res.* **283**(1), 81–85.

Nelson, K. B., and Ellenberg, J. H. (1976). Predictors of epilepsy in children who have experienced febrile seizures. *N. Engl. J. Med.* **295**, 1029–1033.

Nelson, K. B., Ellenberg, J. H. (1986). Antecedents of cerebral palsy. *N. Engl. J. Med.* **315**, 81–86.

Nicoletti, E., Aronica, E., Battaglia, G., Bruno, V., Casabona, G., Catania, M. V., Copani, A., Genazzani, A. A., L'Episcopo, M. R., and Condorelli, D. F. (1994). Plasticity of metabotropic glutamate receptors in physiological and pathological conditions. In "The Metabotropic Glutamate Receptors" (P. J. Conn and J. Patel, eds.), pp. 243–269. Humana Press, Totowa, NJ.

Nitecka, L., Tremblay, E., Charton, G., Bouillot, J. P., Berger, M. L., Ben-Ari, Y. (1984). Maturation of kainic acid seizure-brain damage syndrome in the rat. II. Histopathological sequelae. *Neuroscience* **13**(4), 1073–1094.

Paysan, J., and Fritschy, J. M. (1998). GABAA-receptor subtypes in developing brain. Actors or spectators? *Perspect. Dev. Neurobiol.* **5**(2–3), 179–192.

Pellegrini-Giampietro, D. E., Bennett, M.V.L., and Zukin, R. S. (1991). Differential expression of three glutamate receptor genes in developing rat brain: An *in situ* hybridization study. *Proc. Natl. Acad. Sci. U.S.A.* **88**, 4157–4161.

Pellegrini-Giampietro, D. E., Bennett, M.V.L., and Zukin, R. S. (1992). Are Ca^{2+}-permeable kainate/AMPA receptors more abundant in immature brain? *Neuroscience Lett.* **144**, 65–69.

Pellegrini-Giampietro, D. E., Gorter, J. A., Bennett, M.V.L., and Zukin, R. S. (1997). The GluR2 (GluR-B) hypothesis: $Ca(2+)$-permeable AMPA receptors in neurological disorders. *Trends Neurosci.* **20**, 464–470.

Rakic, P., Bourgeois, J. P., Eckenhoff, M. F., Zecevic, N., and Goldman-Rakic, P. S. (1989). Concurrent overproduction of synapses in diverse regions of primate cortex. *Science* **232**, 232–235.

Rivera, C., Voipio, J., Payne, J. A., Ruusuvuori, E., Lahtinen, H., Lamsa, K., Pirvola, U., Saarma, M., and Kaila, K. (1999). The K^+/Cl^- co-transporter KCC2 renders GABA hyperpolarizing during neuronal maturation. *Nature (London)* **397**, 251–5.

Romijn, H. J., Hofman, M. A., and Gramsbergen, A. (1991). At what age is the developing cerebral cortex of the rat comparable to that of the full term newborn baby? *Early Hum. Dev.* **26**, 61–67.

Sanchez, R. M., and Jensen, F. E. (2001). Maturational aspects of epilepsy mechanisms and consequences for the immature brain. *Epilepsia* **42**, 577–585.

Sankar, R., Shin, D. H., Liu, H., Mazarati, A., Pereira de Vasconcelos, A., and Wasterlain, C. G. (1998). Patterns of status epilepticus-induced neuronal injury during development and long-term consequences. *J. Neurosci.* **18**(20), 8382–8393.

Schoepp, D. D., and Johnson, B. G. (1993). Metabotropic glutamate receptor modulation of cAMP accumulation in the neonatal rat hippocampus. *Neuropharmacol.* **32**(12), 1359–1365.

Shinnar, S. (1998). Prolonged febrile seizures and medial temporal sclerosis. *Ann. Neurol.* **43**, 411–412.

Smart, S. L., Lopantsev, V., Zhang, C. L., Robbins, C. A., Wang, H., Chiu, S. Y., Schwartzkroin, P. A., Messing, A., and Tempel, B. L. (1998). Deletion of the K(V)1.1 potassium channel causes epilepsy in mice. *Neuron* **20**(4), 809–819.

Sperber, E. F. (1996). The relationship between seizures and damage in the maturing brain. *Epilepsy Res.* **S12**, 365–376.

Sperber, E. F., Haas, K. Z., Stanton, P. K., and Moshe, S. L. (1991). Resistance of the immature hippocampus to seizure-induced synaptic reorganization. *Brain Res. Dev. Brain Res.* **60**(1), 88–93.

Stafstrom, C. E., Thompson, J. L., and Holmes, G. L. (1992). Kainic acid seizures in the developing brain: Status epilepticus and spontaneous recurrent seizures. *Brain Res. Dev. Brain Res.* **65**, 227–236.

Staley, K. J., Soldo, B. L., and Proctor, W. R. (1995). Ionic mechanisms of neuronal excitation by inhibitory GABAA receptors. *Science* **269**, 977–981.

Swann, J. W., Pierson, M. G., Smith, K. L., and Lee, C. L. (1999). Developmental neuroplasticity: Roles in early life seizures and chronic epilepsy. *Adv. Neurol.* **79**, 203–216.

Tanaka, K., Watase, K., Manabe, T., Yamada, K., Watanabe, M., Takahashi, K., Iwama, H., Nishikawa, T., Ichihara, N., Kikuchi, T., Okuyama, S., Kawashima, N., Hori, S., Takimoto, M., and Wada, K. (1997). Epilepsy and exacerbation of brain injury in mice lacking the glutamate transporter GLT-1. *Science* **276**, 1699–1702.

Thompson, K., Holm, A. M., Schousboue, A., Popper, P., Micevych, P., and Wasterlain, C. G. (1998). Hippocampal stimulation produces neuronal death in the immature brain. *Neuroscience* **82**, 337–348.

Toth, Z., Yan, X. X., Heftoglu, S., Ribak, C. E., and Baram, T. Z. (1998). Seizure-induced neuronal injury: Vulnerability to febrile seizures in an immature rat model. *J. Neurosci.* **18**, 4285–4294.

Vallano, M. L. (1998). Developmental aspects of NMDA receptor function. *Crit. Rev. Neurobiol.* **12**(3), 177–204.

Verity, C. M., and Golding, J. (1991). Risk of epilepsy after febrile convulsions: A national cohort study. *Br. Med. J.* **303**, 1373–1376.

Verity, C. M., Greenwood, R., and Golding, J. (1998). Long-term intellectual and behavioral outcomes of children with febrile convulsions. *N. Engl. J. Med.* **338**, 1723–1728.

Volpe, J. J. (1989). Neonatal seizures. *Pediatrics* **84**, 422–428.

Volpe, J. J. (2000). "Neurology of the Newborn." Saunders, Philadelphia.

Washburn, M. S., Numberger, M., Zhang, S., and Dingledine, R. (1997). Differential dependence on GluR2 expression of the three characteristic features of AMPA receptors. *J. Neurosci.* **17**, 9393–9406.

Wasterlain, C. G. (1997). Recurrent seizures in the developing brain are harmful. *Epilepsia* **38**, 728–734.

Wasterlain, C. G., and Mazarati, A. M. (1997). Neuromodulators and second messengers. *In* "Epilepsy: A Comprehensive Textbook" (J. Engel, Jr. and T. A. Pedley, eds.), pp. 277–289. Lippincott-Raven, Philadelphia.

Watanabe, T., Morimoto, K., Hirao, T., Suwaki, H., Watase, K., and Tanaka, K. (1999). Amygdala-kindled and pentylenetetrazole-induced seizures in glutamate transporter GLAST-deficient mice. *Brain Res.* **845**(1), 92–96.

Wong, R. K., Bianchi, R., Taylor, G. W., and Merlin, L. R. (1999). Role of metabotropic glutamate receptors in epilepsy. *Adv. Neurol.* **79**, 685–698.

Yan, X. X., Toth, Z., Schultz, L., Ribak, C. E., and Baram, T. Z. (1998). Corticotropin-releasing hormone (CRH)-containing neurons in the immature rat hippocampal formation: Light and electron microscope features and colocalization with glutamate decarboxylase and parvalbumin. *Hippocampus* **8**, 231–243.

Young, R. S., Petroff, O. A., Aquila, W. J., and Yates, J. (1991). Effects of glutamate, quisqualate, and N-methyl-D-aspartate in neonatal brain. *Exp. Neurol.* **111**(3), 362–368.

Zhong, J., Carrozza, D. P., Williams, K., Pritchett, D. B., and Molinoff, P. B. (1995). Expression of mRNAs encoding subunits of the NMDA receptor in developing rat brain. *J. Neurochem.* **64**, 531–539.

CHAPTER 12

Mechanisms of Fever and Febrile Seizures: Putative Role of the Interleukin-1 System

S. Gatti,* A. Vezzani,[†] and T. Bartfai[‡]

*CNS Preclinical Research, Pharmaceutical Division Hoffmann–LaRoche, 4070 Basel, Switzerland; [†]Laboratory of Experimental Neurology, Department of Neuroscience, Mario Negri Institute for Pharmacological Research, 20157 Milan, Italy, and [‡]The Harold L. Dorris Neurological Research Center, Department of Neuropharmacology, The Scripps Research Institute, La Jolla, California 92037

Strategies of antipyretic management are applied in infants during fever crisis mainly to protect them from epileptic seizures. However, it is becoming apparent that the effects of endogenous pyrogens such as interleukin-1 (IL-1) on neuronal excitability can also be direct and not necessarily related to the parallel rise of brain temperature during fever. As presented in this chapter, the IL-1β/IL-1 receptor antagonist ratio seems to affect neuronal excitability in the hippocampus and provides a putative common link between fever and seizure activity. It should be noted that the data presented herein are based on studies in adult animals and thus may have limited relevance in situations arising in infants with febrile seizures.
© 2002 Academic Press.

I. INTRODUCTION

In children, primarily between ages 3 months and 5 years, seizures occur during episodes of fever at a frequency between 2 and 5% in the United States and Western Europe, and as high as 14% in selected other countries. Although many children maintain temperatures of 39°C or lower at the time of their seizure, others, or the same children, may endure higher fevers at later dates without convulsing. Unfortunately, antipyretic therapy has not been shown to protect against recurrences of febrile seizure in the few controlled trials conducted thus far, whereas GABAergic drugs do prevent the seizures. This review covers some essentials on an endogenous pyrogen, IL-1: its action of causing fever by changing the temperature set point and its involvement in changing neuronal excitability and seizure threshold. Unfortunately, most data have been derived from studies of young adult animals rather than of pups. The possibility that the fully developed nervous system might respond differently to a powerful biological agent such as IL-1, compared with the developing nervous system, when human infants manifest febrile seizures, requires an important cautionary note. We believe, however, that it is still worth reviewing the dual role of IL-1 as both pyrogen and convulsant substance.

II. THE FEBRILE RESPONSE

Fever is a stereotyped, systemic response usually defined as a transient shift upward of the core body temperature set point (Gatti and Bartfai, 2000; Sundgren-Andersson *et al.*, 1998b). Fever is triggered by the exposure of immunocompetent cells to a broad variety of viral proteins (Cartmell *et al.*, 1999a,b), bacterial lipopolysaccharides, and peptidoglycans, or occurs during anaphylactic reactions. In all cases, a burst of expression of proinflammatory cytokines, the endogenous pyrogens, mainly in monocytic cell types, and their subsequent release are the common triggering events controlling fever and all the other phases of the innate acute-phase response. Several central nervous system (CNS) cell types, such as microglia and astroglia, can also produce proinflammatory cytokines, and several neuronal cell types, in particular in the hippocampus, carry IL-1, tumor necrosis factor (TNF), and interleukin-6 (IL-6) receptors, from early development.

A. IL-1β IS THE MOST POTENT ENDOGENOUS PYROGEN

IL-1α and IL-1β were among the first cytokines described. In particular, the biological properties of IL-1β as endogenous pyrogen, the "leukocytic pyrogen," were described long before the purification of the protein (see Dinarello, 1996). In general, the concept of a humoral mediator of fever responses is older than the discovery of proinflammatory cytokines and it was initially related to the observation that bacterial debris containing lipopolysaccharide (LPS) could cause fever, with almost 2 hours delay from the time of the injection. LPS effect *in vivo* and on monocytes was also characterized by priming and tolerance, further suggesting the presence of endogenous mediators. The discovery of several pyrogenic cytokines, present in the plasma only during an inflammatory reaction, the study of their production in hypothalamus, and the synergism of their action during a febrile response further clarified the generalizing definition of endogenous pyrogens. All of these (IL-1α and IL-1β, TNFα, and interferons) cause fever when administered into the lateral cerebral ventricles and in the periphery, and they are all released into the circulatory system during a fever response to exogenous pyrogens (Kluger, 1991). IL-1β is the most potent known endogenous pyrogen: 30 ng/kg by intravenous injection is sufficient to cause fever in humans.

Common final mediators of the effect of endogenous pyrogens are prostaglandins, in particular PGE_2, locally produced in the anterior hypothalamus, in the brain nuclei controlling the core body temperature set point and the activation of thermogenesis and vasoconstriction. For this reason, all antipyretic therapies effectively target the production of PGE_2, usually at the level of inhibition of the cyclooxygenase-2 enzyme. Studies have shown that the prostaglandin receptor subtype EP3R is highly expressed in neurons in the anterior hypothalamus and in periventricular organs, and that mice carrying null mutation for EP3R do not develop a febrile response when challenged with proinflammatory cytokines as systemic stimuli (Nakamura et al., 2000; Ek et al., 2000; Dinarello et al., 1999).

B. IL-1 RECEPTORS AND IL-1 RECEPTOR LIGANDS

The family of IL-1 receptor ligands consists of three known members: the agonists IL-1α and IL-1β, and interleukin-1 receptor antagonist (IL-1ra). IL-1α and IL-1β are both agonists acting at the type I IL-1 receptor level and possess overlapping biological activities. IL-1 receptor antagonist is a competitive antagonist at the level of the IL-1 receptors. The endogenous ligands for the IL-1 receptors exert their effect by binding to high-affinity ($K_d < 1$ nM) cell surface receptors, IL-1 receptors type I and type II. Only IL-1 receptor type I transduces the signal into a cellular response. IL-1 receptor type II is a decoy protein present in both a shedded and membrane-bound form (Mantovani et al., 1996).

The secondary and tertiary structures of IL-1α, IL-1β and IL-1ra have been solved using X-ray crystallography and heteronuclear NMR spectroscopy. These studies have demonstrated that, in spite of their low degree of homology at the level of the primary sequence (about 26%) (Simoncsits et al., 1994), all these IL-1 receptor ligands belong to the beta-trefoil fold structural superfamily. The beta-trefoil fold is formed by the arrangement of six pairs of antiparallel beta strands. Using the three-dimensional model of IL-1 structure, other proteins belonging to the same structural group were recently cloned. All of them are proinflammatory cytokines, such as IL-18, and new proteins of unknown function, such as FILδ, FILε and FILη. All of these proteins interact with distinct sets of receptors (Born et al., 2000; Smith et al., 2000) with possibly different roles in the immune network. The possible cross-talk among their cellular effects is mediated by the different receptors via some common accessory proteins, and possibly via common intracellular secondary mechanisms of signal transduction (O'Neill, 2000). Orphan IL-1 receptor-like proteins were also found by homology analysis of genomic sequences (Sana *et al.*, 2000).

The IL-1ra protein represents a unique case in biology: an endogenously occurring antagonist with no other known effect than the blockade of interleukin-1 actions, through competition with the agonists at the level of IL-1 receptor type I. The large increase in the levels of IL-1ra (secreted form, sIL-1ra) in the serum soon after IL-1β injection exerts a complete inhibitory control on all IL-1β effects. Moreover, IL-1 effects can be blocked by a systemic pretreatment with a large excess (100- to 250-fold more) of recombinant IL-1ra. In these studies, animals were injected with IL-1ra 15 minutes before IL-1β, because of the short plasma half-life of the IL-1ra protein (about 6 minutes) (Dinarello, 1996, 2000). At least three isoforms of intracellular IL-1ra and one isoform of secreted sIL-1ra are known. sIL-1ra is secreted by several different cell types via the Golgi apparatus, and keratinocytes and intestinal epithelial cells constitutively express intracellular forms of IL-1ra. These intracellular IL-1ra gene products probably represent a reservoir of IL-1ra, released by endothelial or immunocompetent cells on cell death (Muzio *et al.*, 1999). The gene expression of sIL-1ra and of intracellular IL-1ra is controlled by two different promoters (Jenkins *et al.*, 1997).

In the presence of the agonists, IL-1α and IL-1β, the IL-1 receptor interacts with another membrane-bound protein, the IL-1 receptor accessory protein, leading to the formation of an [IL-1 receptor]–[IL-1 accessory protein] heterodimer that increases the affinity of the agonists for this receptor. The heterodimerization of the intracellular domains of IL-1 receptor type I and the accessory protein is necessary for the intracellular signaling via this receptor.

During inflammation, tissue levels of IL-1 receptor ligands can be rather high because of membrane-bound interleukins produced by activated platelets, macrophages, and microglia. On the other hand, the occupancy of only 5–10% of a cell's receptors is sufficient to trigger the maximal cellular response (at least *in vitro*). For this reason an effective blockade of IL-1α/IL-1β actions can be obtained only by sustaining high circulating levels of IL-1ra. In healthy volunteers, injected intravenously with a low dose of *Escherichia coli* endotoxin (LPS), circulating IL-1ra levels are in a 100-fold molar excess (7000 pg/ml), compared to those of IL-1β (70 pg/ml) (Dinarello, 1996).

Production of IL-1 receptor ligands, agonists and antagonists has been demonstrated both at the mRNA and the protein level in several immunocompetent, tumoral, and endocrine cell types. Particularly relevant for this review are the studies demonstrating production of all three ligands in astrocytes and microglia, in the sympathetic ganglia, and in hypothalamic neurons (IL-1ra)

(Rothwell and Luheshi, 1994; Diana *et al.*, 1999; Bartfai and Schultzberg, 1993; Licinio *et al.*, 1991).

C. Afferent Systems Mediating the Central Effects of IL-1

A concentration of 10 pg/ml of human IL-1β in the serum of a human is sufficient to trigger central events such as fever, anorexia, sleep and sickness behavior, which last for hours after IL-1β injection. Multiple mechanisms of coordination between the peripheral immune response and the signaling to the CNS sustain these effects:

1. The stimulation of circulating immunocompetent cells by IL-1β causes the production of endogenous IL-1 and other pyrogenic cytokines, such as TNFα, amplifying the initial proinflammatory stimulus (Elmquist *et al.*, 1997).

2. Vascular fenestrated endothelium in periventricular organs and in the rostro-ventral hypothalamus express IL-1 receptor type I and can trigger the activation of several hypothalamic nuclei on agonist occupancy (Sundgren-Andersson *et al.*, 1998b);

3. Primary afferent neurons of the vagus nerve are activated after peritoneal administration of either IL-1 or LPS, as demonstrated using immediate-early gene (*c-Fos*) expression as a marker of neuronal activation (Gaykema *et al.*, 1998). This is likely to involve local production of IL-1 in the vagal nerve, as demonstrated by Goehler *et al.* (1998, 1999) using both quantitative assays and immunohistochemistry to show the presence of IL-1β-like immunoreactivity together with the induction of the IL-1 receptor type I.

D. Central and Peripheral Mechanisms Controlling the Change of the Core Body Temperature Set Point

In homeotherms, body temperature is controlled by a neuronal circuit that involves several hypothalamic (preoptic area) and extrahypothalamic regions and defines a set point of the core body temperature, which is integrated with species-specific mechanisms of control dependent on body mass and energy expenditure. The direct control of core body temperature is probably exerted by thermosensitive neurons distributed in several regions of the body (skin, spinal cord, lower brain stem). Thermosensitive neurons are present also in the diencephalon and in the preoptic hypothalamus, where about 40% of neurons are thermosensitive. Thermosensitive neurons are also present in the sensory and motor cortex. The neuronal activity in the preoptic/anterior (POA) hypothalamus is thus sensitive to the local temperature, and also integrates neuronal signals arriving from thermosensitive neurons distributed in the periphery. The firing rate of "warm"- or "cold"-sensitive neurons (neurons that respond to a temperature, respectively, higher and lower than thermoneutrality) can be modified by endogenous pyrogens, thermal stimuli, glucose concentration, osmotic changes, estradiol, and testosterone treatments (Rolfe and Brown, 1997; Gatti *et al.*, 2000).

Extracellularly recorded firing rates of neurons in slices of the preoptic/anterior hypothalamus of the rat have shown that the application of recombinant IL-1β (20 ng/ml) reduced the firing rate and thermosensitivity in linear, warm-sensitive neurons. Moreover, IL-1β shifted the thermal thresholds of activation in threshold warm- and cold-sensitive neurons by 1.1–2.3°C to hyperthermic temperatures. Endogenous pyrogens in general may act on different populations of these thermosensitive neurons to induce fever (Vasilenko *et al.*, 2000). Extrahypothalamic areas are partially involved in the control of fever response, as shown with the injection of 50 μg of IL-1ra in dentate gyrus and hippocampal CA3 region, which delayed the fever response induced by intraperitoneal LPS injection (Cartmell *et al.*, 1999a,b).

The necessary production of heat associated with the shift of the temperature set point is orchestrated mainly by the activation of the sympathetic system. Sympathetic activation can cause an immediate reduction of skin blood flow in thermoregulatory vessels, piloerection, heat production in brown adipose tissue (BAT), muscular shivering, and increased respiratory rate, respectively. In children and in many animal species, the major source of heat is BAT. The mitochondrial uncoupling protein, thermogenin (UCP1), plays the main role in heat production in adipocytes. Heat production in BAT is obtained by dissipation of the protonic gradient across the inner mitochondrial membrane via the activation of thermogenin. Studies indicate that fatty acid-mediated shuttle of protons is responsible for this effect. The system is under the control of β-3 adrenergic receptor activation in several species. The general assumption of a lack of nonshivering thermogenesis in adult humans will have to be re-examined because of the discovery of other uncoupling proteins, UCP2 and UCP3, that are differentially expressed mainly in white adipose tissue and glycolytic muscles of human adults (Garlid *et al.*, 2000; Ricquier *et al.*, 2000).

E. Brain Temperature and Body Temperature during Fever

During fever in rodents, changes in temperature in the hypothalamus and cerebral cortex follow completely changes in temperature observed in the core of the

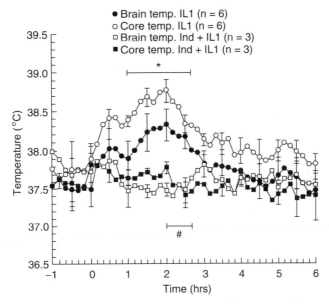

FIGURE 1   Brain (cortex) and core body temperatures during fever. Brain and core temperatures closely follow each other. Fever was induced by intraperitoneal injection of rhIL-1β. Averaged thermal data are from brain and deep core. The febrile response is blocked by indomethacin both in the brain and in the deep core. The difference in amplitude between the brain and core temperatures during the rhIL-1β-induced fever is not statistically significant. [Reproduced from Sundgren-Andersson, A. K., Ostlund, P., and Bartfai, T. (1998a). Simultaneous measurement of brain and core temperature in the rat during fever, hyperthermia, hypothermia, and sleep. Neuroimmunomodulation 5, 241–247, with permission from Karger, Basel.]

body. There has been ample discussion on specific mechanisms of "brain cooling" present in different species, but human adults or infants have not been shown to possess specific brain cooling. Hence, we assume that core body and brain temperature during febrile seizures are the same in infants. Evidence for this notion comes from simultaneous radiotelemetric recording of brain and core temperatures in rats and mice (Sundgren-Andersson *et al.*, 1998a) (Figure 1).

Several studies suggest that hypothalamic temperature plays a key role in the control of core body temperature. The hypothesis of hypothalamic temperature as an independent variable, locally and tightly controlled via integrated peripheral and extrahypothalamic stimuli, is supported by the observation that temperature undergoes smaller fluctuations in the hypothalamus than in other brain and trunk regions in response to several different stimuli. Moreover, small variations of local hypothalamic temperature trigger immediate adjustments on sympathetic activity and thermogenesis (Boulant, 2000; Parmeggiani *et al.*, 2000). In other brain regions, such as the horizontal limb of the diagonal band of Broca, thermosensitive neurons that are responsive to changes in local temperature are hypothesized to participate in sleep–wake control (Parmeggiani, 2000a). γ-Aminobutyric acid (GABA) terminals are abundant in areas containing thermosensitive neurons, and muscimol application causes reductions in both firing rate and thermosensitivity (Hays *et al.*, 1999). A possible link, as yet unknown, between the GABAergic system and thermosensitive neurons is also suggested by the presence of uncoupling proteins (UCP2) in presynaptic mitochondria. The basket cell-like distributions of these presynaptic terminals are strongly suggestive of GABAergic neurons (Horvath *et al.*, 1999).

F. EFFECT OF BRAIN TEMPERATURE ON NEURONAL EXCITABILITY

Much progress has been made in recent years in understanding the molecular basis of warm and cold sensitivity. A large number of ion channels are known to be highly sensitive to temperature changes, at least *in vitro* (Table 1). In many cases, temperature sensitivity is an intrinsic property of the channel, such as for several classes of voltage-dependent K^+ channels (Kv1.1; see also Chapter 16). More recently, attention has been focused on mechanoreceptors such as TREK-1 (Maingret *et al.*, 2000). This protein belongs to the novel family of mammalian two-pore domain K^+ channels with four transmembrane segments, an extended external loop (60–70 residues), and intracellular N and C termini. The gene for TASK-1 encodes a background outward rectifier that is constitutively active at all voltages and is inhibited by mild external acidosis and opened reversibly by heat.

TREK-1 is a mechanosensitive K^+ channel opened by membrane stretch, and mechanical activation is mimicked by polyunsaturated fatty acids such as arachidonic acid, cyclic AMP, and prostaglandin E_2, and by trinitrophenol. The TREK-1 channel is also blockable by chlorpromazine. The high expression levels of TREK-1 in dorsal root ganglia nociceptive neurons, as well as in the CNS in anterior hypothalamus, cortex, and hippocampus, suggest that this ion channel may play a very important physiological role in temperature sensing. TREK-1 may also act as a cold sensor: at physiological temperature, the opening of TREK-1 is hyperpolarizing, whereas at lower temperatures TREK-1 closes and depolarizes neurons, thus possibly signaling "cold information." Dorsal root ganglia neurons are also rich in expression of vanilloid receptor 1, a receptor coupled to a Ca^{2+}/Mg^{2+} ion channel that is acutely activated when temperatures reach 40–43°C (Welch *et al.*, 2000). We know that this receptor is involved in pain transmission, but the central, broad expression of vanilloid receptor 1 mRNA (although low level) seems to suggest other roles for this and

TABLE 1   Effect of Temperature on the Activity/Permeability (Q_{10}) of Different Ion Channels

Name	Q_{10} (T°C range used)	System	References
K$^+$ channels			
Shaker H4			
Activity time constant	+3.14 (20 to 4)	*Xenopus laevis* oocytes	*Exp. Brain Res.* **114**, 138
Decay time constant	+7.2 (20 to 4)	*Xenopus laevis* oocytes	*Exp. Brain Res.* **114**, 138
MinK			
Activity time constant	+4–7	*Xenopus laevis* oocytes	
Na$^+$ channels			
TTX sens non-inactivating			
Na current, curr. amplitude	+4.3–7	Temperature sensitive rat POA neurons	
Ca2$^+$ channels			
HVA calcium channels			
Activity time constant	+ 10	Dorsal raphe neurons	*Neuropharmacol.* **34**(11), 1479
Current amplitude	+1.7	Dorsal raphe neurons	
L-type cardiac CaChs			
Inward currents	+5.8 (15 to 25)	*Xenopus laevis* oocytes	*Pflugers Arch.* **436**(2), 238
HAC	+3–4		
Cl$-$ channels			
From the Torpedo electric organ (slow gate)			
Deactivation potential	+40	*Xenopus laevls* oocytes	*J. Gen. Physiol.* **109**(1), 105
CFTR			
Opening rate	+9.6		*J. Membr. Biol.* **163**(1), 55

possibly other vanilloid receptors of the same class. Currently, it is unclear to what extent the class of receptors/ion channels described here participate in the molecular mechanism sustaining neuronal thermosensitivity; it is also not known if they respond directly or indirectly to endogenous pyrogens.

In other cases, the changes in temperature could affect neuronal excitability in an indirect manner, because of changes in cellular metabolism and possibly intracellular ATP levels. A study by Masino and Dunwiddie (1999) shows that in hippocampal slices, the change of the temperature from 32.5 to 38.5°C degrees is associated with a large and linear inhibition of the amplitude of extracellular field potentials. This effect is mediated by purines, probably adenosine, acting at the level of the A1 adenosine receptor. Interestingly, minute concentrations of IL-1β (10^{-13} M) also cause a depression of extracellular field potentials in hippocampal CA1 and this effect is prevented by pretreatment with IL-1ra or with an A1 receptor antagonist (Luk *et al.*, 1999).

III. IL-1β IN SEIZURES AND EPILEPTOGENESIS

A. IL-1β AND NEURONAL EXCITABILITY

Several lines of evidence point to the functional role of some inflammatory cytokines and related molecules in neuronal network excitability, both under physiological conditions and in pathological neuronal hyperactivity such as that occurring during seizures. Both neurons and glia have been shown to be capable of producing IL-1β, thus indicating a local source of synthesis in the brain (Benveniste, 1992; Bartfai and Schultzberg, 1993; Hopkins and Rothwell, 1995). In particular, receptors for IL-1β have been found at high density in the hippocampus, where they are located on soma and dendrites of granule cells (Takao *et al.*, 1990; Ban *et al.*, 1991; Nishiyori *et al.*, 1997). IL-1 receptors at these sites colocalize with the NMDA receptors that mediate the fast action of glutamate. This places the IL-1 receptor type I, anatomically, at a site crucial for seizure generation, because granule neurons play a pivotal role in gating the excitatory drive through the hippocampus, modulating seizure propagation (McNamara, 1994).

IL-1β and other cytokines have been shown to influence signaling with many neurotransmitters, including norepinephrine, serotonin, GABA, acetylcholine, and adenosine (Rothwell and Hopkins, 1995; Luk *et al.*, 1999), and the expression of various neuropeptides and neurotrophic factors involved in synaptic transmission in several forebrain regions (Scarborough *et al.*, 1989; Spranger *et al.*, 1990; Lapchak *et al.*, 1993). In particular, electrophysiological findings in brain slices have shown that relatively low concentrations of IL-1β (femtomolar to picomolar range) inhibit long-term potentiation (LTP) in CA1, CA3, and dentate gyrus regions of the rodent hippocampus (Katsuki *et al.*, 1990; Bellinger *et al.*, 1993; Cunningham *et al.*, 1996). IL-1β gene expression is substantially increased during LTP, and IL-1 receptor antagonist per se causes a reversible impairment of the maintenance phase of LTP, thus suggesting a functional role of endogenous IL-1β in synaptic plasticity (Schneider *et al.*, 1998). IL-1β has been shown to influence both Ca^{2+} and Cl^- conductances (Miller *et al.*, 1991; Plata-Salaman and French-Mullen, 1992). IL-1β has both inhibitory (Coogan and O'Connor, 1997; D'Arcangelo *et al.*, 1997) and facilitating effects (Zeise *et al.*, 1997; Wang *et al.*, 2000) on glutaminergic transmission. Higher ranges of concentrations of IL-1β (nanomolar to micromolar) are needed to produce excitatory actions in brain, in accordance with previous evidence showing that the effects of IL-1β on neuronal activity and on neuronal viability depend strictly on its concentration (Rothwell and Hopkins, 1995). Several other factors modulate the actions of IL-1β in brain, including the functional state of neurons (healthy or injured), the timing of cytokine release, the duration of tissue exposure, and the brain region examined.

B. IL-1β, GABA, and Glutamate

The functional interactions between IL-1β, GABA, and glutamate are of particular relevance for the convulsant activity of this cytokine. Thus, although the molecular mechanisms underlying the onset, generalization, and recurrence of seizures are mostly unknown, it is well established that these phenomena depend on the imbalance between inhibitory and excitatory neurotransmission in the hippocampus, an area richly endowed with IL-1 receptor type I.

Miller *et al.* (1991) reported that $0.6-6$ nmol/ml of IL-1β inhibited muscimol-induced Cl^- uptake in chick cortical synaptoneurosomes and potentiated GABA-receptor-evoked currents in patch-clamped chick cortical neurons in culture. IL-1ra by itself had no effect in these preparations. The same authors showed that 1 μg of IL-1β given intraperitoneally in mice increased the dose of pentylentetrazol, inducing generalized seizures by 20%. These inhibitory effects of IL-1 were not confirmed in rat cultured hippocampal neurons or hippocampal brain slices (Wang *et al.*, 2000; Zeise *et al.*, 1997). IL-1β ($0.06-0.6$ pmol/ml) was shown to decrease peak magnitude of current elicited by GABA in hippocampal primary cultures as well as inhibitory postsynaptic potentials in CA3 pyramidal cells. It appears, therefore, that IL-1β has multiple actions on neurotransmission, depending on the brain region involved. Thus, inhibitory effects of low doses of IL-1 have been reported in neocortex (D'Arcangelo *et al.*, 1997; Miller *et al.*, 1991; Luk *et al.*, 1999), whereas in the hippocampus both inhibitory and excitatory actions were found depending on the IL-1β concentration (Katsuki *et al.*, 1990; Bellinger *et al.*, 1993; Coogan and O'Connor, 1997; Wang *et al.*, 2000; Zeise *et al.*, 1997).

In vitro and *in vivo* evidence has shown that IL-1β affects Ca^{2+}-dependent glutamate release. In rat hippocampal synaptosomes, IL-1β (0.2 pmol/ml) depressed KCl-stimulated glutamate release (Murray *et al.*, 1998). This effect is likely mediated by the ability of a brief application of low concentrations of IL-1β to increase adenosine release from hippocampal slices, which in turn decreases glutamate release by acting at A_{1A} receptors (Luk *et al.*, 1999). Using *in vivo* microdialysis it was shown that local injection of 0.6 pmol IL-1β enhances extracellular glutamate levels (Kamikawa *et al.*, 1998). This confirms the observation that, in primary cultures of postnatal rat hippocampus, 0.1 pmol/ml IL-1β inhibits astrocytic, high-affinity glutamate uptake and this effect was mediated by nitric oxide production (Ye and Sontheimer, 1996).

Specific interactions between IL-1β and the NMDA subtype of glutamate receptors, which are highly involved in mediating seizure occurrence and, potentially, epileptogenesis (Dingledine *et al.*, 1990), have also been reported. Intracerebral injection of NMDA in perinatal rat brain stimulates the production of IL-1β (Hagan *et al.*, 1996) whereas in adult rat brain IL-1β exacerbates damage induced in the cortex by NMDA application (Loddick and Rothwell, 1996).

In addition, intrahippocampal injection of 1 ng IL-1β induces proconvulsant actions in rats (see below) that are blocked by selective antagonism of NMDA receptors (Vezzani *et al.*, 1999). It is becoming apparent, therefore, that it is important to make a distinction between the effects of pathological (nanomolar or higher) versus physiological (femtomolar–picomolar) levels of IL-1 and to consider the brain areas involved in IL-1β actions.

C. IL-1β AND SEIZURES

Early evidence suggesting an involvement of inflammatory cytokines in epilepsy stems from the findings that various convulsant stimuli induce cytokine mRNA in rodent forebrain areas (Minami *et al.*, 1991; Yabuuchi *et al.*, 1993; Gahring *et al.*, 1997; De Simoni *et al.*, 2000; Plata-Salaman *et al.*, 2000). We have shown by immunocytochemistry that synthesis of IL-1β is, indeed, induced in glial cells in rodent hippocampus and limbic areas after intrahippocampal injection of kainic acid or bicuculline methiodide, producing EEG-detected and/or behavioral seizures (Vezzani *et al.*, 1999, 2000), or after status epilepticus elicited by continuous electrical stimulation of the ventral hippocampus (De Simoni *et al.*, 2000). IL-1β induction was rapid (<2 hours) and reversible within 1 week from seizure onset. In addition, in spontaneously epileptic rats, both the protein and its transcript were still significantly enhanced above their basal levels (De Simoni *et al.*, 2000). IL-1β was enhanced in glia to a larger extent when seizures were associated with neuronal cell loss (i.e., after the kainic acid or electrical stimulation induced status epilepticus) as compared to nonlesional models of seizures (i.e., after bicuculline methiodide) (Vezzani *et al.*, 1999, 2000; De Simoni *et al.*, 2000). Thus, neurodegeneration is likely to contribute to the enhanced IL-1β immunoreactivity, in accordance with previous findings suggesting that degenerating neurons represent a strong signal for IL-1β induction (Rothwell, 1991). In addition, microglia are rapidly activated in response to even minor pathological changes in the CNS (Kreutzberg, 1996) and they represent a source of IL-1 synthesis in the early phases of seizure induction (Vezzani *et al.*, 1999).

Endogenously produced IL-1β may be involved in the pathogenesis of seizures. Thus, limbic seizures are worsened by intracerebral application of picomolar amounts of recombinant IL-1β (Vezzani *et al.*, 1999, 2000). This effect is mediated by the type I IL-1receptor, because it is blocked by coadministration of IL-1 receptor antagonist. Glutamatergic neurotransmission is involved in some way, because a selective competitive antagonist of NMDA receptors prevents the proconvulsant effect of this cytokine (Vezzani *et al.*, 1999). Intrahippocampal administration of 0.1–1 μM IL-1β has been shown to increase body temperature by 2°C above physiological values after 2–4 hours of continuous infusion (Linthorst *et al.*,1994). However, it is unlikely that the increase in body temperature plays a major role in the proconvulsant effect of IL-1β, because values as high as 42°C are needed to provoke seizures, or to enhance EEG activity of seizures induced by kainic acid in rats (Liu *et al.*,1993).

D. Anticonvulsant Action of IL-1ra

The endogenous receptor antagonist of IL-1β (IL-1ra) is markedly induced in glia in the limbic system after status epilepticus following systemic injection of kainic acid or sustained electrical stimulation of the ventral hippocampus in rats (Eriksson *et al.*, 1998; De Simoni *et al.*, 2000) or after intrahippocampal bicuculline methiodide injection in mice (Vezzani *et al.*, 2000). A detailed time course of IL-1ra mRNA changes after electrically induced status epilepticus showed that IL-1ra was enhanced in brain with a significant delay as compared to IL-1β. Thus, IL-1β production peaked between 2 and 4 hours after seizures by IL-1ra was maximally induced between 18 and 24 hours (De Simoni *et al.*, 2000). Moreover, in contrast with septic shock or inflammatory diseases, in which the circulating IL-1ra levels are 100-fold in excess of those of IL-1β (Dinarello, 1997), seizures increase IL-1ra to a similar (De Simoni *et al.*, 2000) or lower extent (Plata-Salaman *et al.*, 2000) compared with IL-1β. Thus, the brain appears less effective in inducing IL-1ra as a mechanism to rapidly block the IL-1receptor (by IL-1ra occupancy) and thus terminate IL-1β actions (Figure 2).

A major finding was that intracerebral application of recombinant IL-1ra dramatically reduced seizure activity in a variety of experimental models (Table 2).

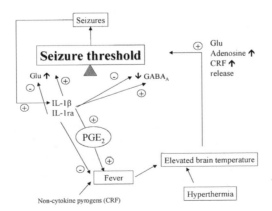

FIGURE 2   Schematic view of the effects of IL-1β/IL-1ra ratios on seizure thresholds in the hippocampus.

TABLE 2   Endogenous (Transgenic) and Exogenous IL-1ra Inhibit Seizure Response
to Bicuculline in Mice

Mediator	Number of mice with seizures		Onset (minutes)		Duration (minutes)	
	Clonic	Tonic	Clonus	Tonus	Clonus	Tonus
Saline	15/15	15/15	2.6	5.8	118	4.3
IL-1ra (icv)	15/15	15/15	5.6	12.1	102	1.1
IL-1ra (transgenic, 15 fold elevated levels)	7/7	4/7	2.5	44.7	22	0.7

Thus, both motor tonic–clonic seizures and EEG ictal activity induced by bicuculline in mice were reduced by 90 and 50%, respectively, by nanomolar
amounts of IL-1ra. Consistent with these findings, mice overexpressing IL-1ra
in astrocytes 15-fold were less susceptible to bicuculline-induced seizures (Vezzani *et al.*, 2000). Analysis of the brain regions affected by seizures using c-*fos*
mRNA as a biochemical marker strongly suggests that IL-1ra reduces bicuculline seizures by inhibiting their generalization from the hippocampus to the
motor cortical areas. The anticonvulsant action of IL-1ra was mediated by IL-1
receptor type I, because IL-1ra was ineffective in mice lacking this receptor subtype (Vezzani *et al.*, 2000). IL-1ra displayed anticonvulsant activity also on
EEG-detected seizures induced by intrahippocampal kainic acid (Vezzani *et al.*,
2000) and reduced generalized motor seizures occurring during electrically induced status epilepticus in rats (De Simoni *et al.*, 2000).

No published studies are available on the involvement of IL-1β and related
molecules in the generation of febrile seizures; in light of the above reported evidence, a detailed investigation in this field is warranted.

IV. HUMAN EPILEPTIC TISSUE

Although the expression of inflammatory cytokines has not yet been investigated in detail in human epileptic brain tissue, an increased production of IL-
1α in glial cells and a functional activation of microglia and astrocytes (the main
source of cytokines in the brain) have been reported in human temporal lobe
epilepsy (Sheng *et al.*, 1994; Barres, 1999). Thus, although constitutive expression of inflammatory cytokines in normal brain is low or barely detectable
(Schobitz *et al.*, 1994), a marked increase can be induced by an acute seizure.

A functional polymorphism in the IL-1β gene promoter, possibly associated with enhanced ability to produce this cytokine, has been found in some temporal lobe epilepsy sufferers (Kanemoto *et al.*, 2000). This suggests that a subtle anomaly in IL-1β/IL-1ra balance or minor developmental events during early life could set up a cascade, leading to hippocampal sclerosis and epilepsy in patients with such genetic predisposition.

V. MECHANISMS OF ACTION AND PHARMACOLOGICAL IMPLICATIONS

It is likely that IL-1β and IL-1ra are released from glia in the extracellular space after their enhanced synthesis. Enhanced release of inflammatory cytokines from hippocampal slices of epileptic tissue has been described (De Bock *et al.*, 1996). The mechanisms by which seizure activity induces these cytokines are unknown. Protein extravasation in the brain parenchyma caused by blood–brain barrier breakdown during seizures (Nitsch *et al.*, 1986), ionic changes induced by seizures in the extracellular environment and in glial cells (Barres, 1999), or glutamate release during seizures may provoke glial cells to synthesize and release higher amount of cytokines. In this scenario, IL-1β will then act on neuronal IL-1 receptor type I (Takao *et al.*, 1990; Ban *et al.*, 1991; Nishiyori *et al.*, 1997) to enhance excitability. This may occur by direct action on ionic currents or indirectly by enhancing extracellular glutamate concentrations or reducing GABA$_A$ receptor function (Zeise *et al.*, 1997; Kamikawa *et al.*, 1998; Wang *et al.*, 2000). IL-1ra will afford protection from seizures by antagonizing the actions of endogenously released IL-1β. Finally, the effect of IL-1β may involve other inflammatory cytokines. Thus, IL-1β induces the synthesis of TNFα and IL-6 in astrocytes and microglia (Bartfai and Schultzberg, 1993; Schobitz *et al.*, 1994) and many actions of IL-1 in the CNS are mediated by these cytokines. IL-6 and TNFα, in turn, have been reported to affect synaptic transmission, and mice overexpressing IL-6 and TNF in glia develop both seizures and neurodegeneration (Campbell *et al.*, 1993; Akassoglou *et al.*, 1997). These hypotheses need to be addressed by *ad hoc* experiments.

In summary, these findings suggest that the balance between IL-1β and IL-1ra during seizures plays a significant role in altering neuronal network excitability, thus affecting the maintenance and spread of seizures, and this may be of pharmacological relevance (cf. Figure 2). Because IL-1ra seems to be a well-tolerated endogenous protein that is highly inducible (Dinarello, 1996), pharmacological means that increase the IL-1ra/IL-1β ratio may be useful for altering seizure threshold and preventing seizures even when brain temperature is elevated and other factors act to increase hippocampal excitability.

ACKNOWLEDGMENTS

We thank Ms. Jennifer Newmann for assistance with manuscript preparation. This manuscript was supported by the Harold L. Dorris Neurological Research Center at The Scripps Research Institute, by the Telethon Onlus Foundation (E.1094), and by Intas (97-2037). This is manuscript #13858-NP from The Scripps Research Institute.

REFERENCES

Akassoglou, K., Probert, L., Kontogeorgos, G., and Kollias, G. (1997). Astrocyte-specific but not neuron-specific transmembrane TNF triggers inflammation and degeneration in the central nervous system of transgenic mice. *J. Immunol.* **158**, 438–445.

Ban, E., Milon, G., Prudhomme, N., Fillion, G., and Haour, F. (1991). Receptors for interleukin-1 (alpha and beta) in mouse brain: Mapping and neuronal localization in hippocampus. *Neuroscience* **43**, 21–30.

Barres, B. A. (1999). New roles for glia. *J. Neurosci.* **11**, 21–30.

Bartfai, T., and Schultzberg, M. (1993). Cytokines in neuronal cell types. *Neurochem. Int.* **22**, 435–444.

Bellinger, F. P., Madamba, S., and Siggins, G. R. (1993). Interleukin 1γ inhibits synaptic strength and long-term potentiation in the rat CA1 hippocampus. *Brain Res.* **628**, 227–234.

Benveniste, E. N. (1992). Inflammatory cytokines within the central nervous system: Sources, function and mechanism of action. *Am. J. Physiol.* **263**, C1–C16.

Born, T.L., Smith, D.E., Garka, K.E., Renshaw, B.R., Bertles, J.S., and Sims, J.E. (2000). Identification and characterization of two members of a novel class of the interleukin-1 receptor (IL-1R) family. *J. Biol. Chem.* **275**, 29946–29954.

Boulant, J. A. (2000). Role of the preoptic-anterior hypothalamus in thermoregulation and fever. *Clin. Infect. Dis.* **31** (Suppl. 5), S157–S166.

Campbell, I. L., Abraham, C. R., Masliah, E., Kemper, P., Inglis, J. D., Oldstone, M. B. A., and Mucke, L. (1993). Neurological disease induced in transgenic mice by cerebral overexpression of interleukin 6. *Proc. Natl. Acad. Sci. U.S.A.* **90**, 10061–10065.

Cartmell, T., Southgate, T., Rees, G. S., Castro, M. G., Lowenstein, P. R., and Luheshi, G. N. (1999a). Interleukin-1 mediates a rapid inflammatory response after injection of adenoviral vectors into the brain. *J. Neurosci.* **19**, 1517–1523.

Cartmell, T., Luheshi, G. N., and Rothwell, N. J. (1999b). Brain sites of action of endogenous interleukin-1 in the febrile response to localized inflammation in the rat. *J. Physiol.* **518**, 585–594.

Coogan, A. and O'Connor, J. J. (1997). Inhibition of NMDA receptor-mediated synaptic transmission in the rat dentate gyrus *in vitro* by IL-1beta. *NeuroReport* **8**, 2107–2110.

Cunningham, A. J., Murray, C. A., O'Neill, L. A., Lynch, M. A., and O'Connor, J. J. (1996). Interleukin-1 beta (IL-1 beta) and tumour necrosis factor (TNF) inhibit long-term potentiation in the rat dentate gyrus *in vitro*. *Neurosci. Lett.* **203**, 17–20.

D'Arcangelo G., Dodt, H., and Zieglgansberger, W. (1997). Reduction of excitation by interleukin-1beta in rat neocortical slices visualized using infrared-darkfield video microscopy. *NeuroReport* **8**, 2079–2083.

De Bock, F., Dornand, J., and Rondouin, G. (1996). Release of TNF alpha in the rat hippocampus following epileptic seizures and excitotoxic neuronal damage. *NeuroReport* **7**, 1125–1129.

De Simoni, M.G., Perego, C., Ravizza, T., Moneta, D., Conti, M., Marchesi, F., De Luigi, A, Garattini, S., and Vezzani, A. (2000). Inflammatory cytokines and related genes are induced in the rat hippocampus by limbic status epilepticus. *Eur. J. Neurosci.* 12, 2623–2633.

Diana, A., Van Dam, A.M., Winblad, B., and Schultzberg, M. (1999). Colocalization of interleukin-1 receptor type I and interleukin-1 receptor antagonist with vasopressin in magnocellular neurons of the paraventricular and supraoptic nuclei of the rat hypothalamus. *Neuroscience* 89, 137–147.

Dinarello, C. A. (1996). Biologic basis for interleukin-1 in disease. *Blood* 87, 2095–2147.

Dinarello, C. A. (1997). Role of pro- and anti-inflammatory cytokines during inflammation: experimental and clinical findings. *J. Biol. Regul. Homeost. Agents* 11, 91–103.

Dinarello, C. A. (2000). The role of the interleukin-1-receptor antagonist in blocking inflammation mediated by interleukin-1. *N. Engl. J. Med.* 343, 732–734.

Dinarello, C. A., Gatti, S., and Bartfai, T. (1999). Fever: Links with an ancient receptor. *Curr. Biol.* 9, R147–R150.

Dingledine, R., McBain, C. J., and McNamara, J. O. (1990). Excitatory amino acid receptors in epilepsy. *Trends Pharmacol. Sci.* 11, 334–338.

Ek, M., Arias, C., Sawchenko, P., and Ericsson-Dahlstrand, A. (2000). Distribution of the EP3 prostaglandin E(2) receptor subtype in the rat brain: Relationship to sites of interleukin-1-induced cellular responsiveness. *J. Comp. Neurol.* 428, 5–20.

Elmquist, J. K., Scammell, T. E., and Saper, C. B. (1997). Mechanisms of CNS response to systemic immune challenge: The febrile response. *Trends Neurosci.* 20, 565–570.

Eriksson, G., Zetterstrom, M., Corets Toro, V., Bartfai, T., and Iverfeldt, K. (1998). Hypersensitive cytokine response to beta-amyloid 25-35 in astroglial cells from IL-1 receptor type 1-deficient mice. *Intl. J. Mol. Med.* 1, 201–206.

Gahring, L. C., White, H. S., Skradski, S. L., Carlson, N. G., and Rogers, S. W. (1997). Interleukin-1alpha in the brain is induced by audiogenic seizure. *Neurobiol Dis.* 3, 263–269.

Garlid, K. D., Jaburek, M., Jezek, P., and Varecha, M. (2000). How do uncoupling proteins uncouple? *Biochim. Biophys. Acta* 1459, 383–389.

Gatti, S., and Bartfai, T. (2000). Febrile response. In "Encyclopedia of Stress" (G. Fink, ed.), Vol.2, pp. 116–120. Academic Press, San Diego.

Gatti, S., Alberati, D., and Bartfai, T. (2000). Thermotolerance, thermoresistance and thermosensitivity. In "Encyclopedia of Stress" (G. Fink, ed.) Vol. 3, pp. 585–560. Academic Press, San Diego.

Gaykema, R. P., Goehler, L. E., Tilders, F. J., Bol, J. G., McGorry, M., Fleshner, M., Maier, S. F., and Watkins, L. R. (1998). Bacterial endotoxin induces fos immunoreactivity in primary afferent neurons of the vagus nerve. *Neuroimmunomodulation* 5, 234–240.

Goehler, L. E., Gaykema, R. P., Hammack, S. E., Maier, S. F., and Watkins, L. R. (1998). Interleukin-1 induces c-Fos immunoreactivity in primary afferent neurons of the vagus nerve. *Brain Res.* 804, 306–310.

Goehler, L. E., Gaykema, R. P., Nguyen, K. T., Lee, J. E., Tilders, F. J., Maier, S. F., and Watkins, L. R. (1999). Interleukin-1beta in immune cells of the abdominal vagus nerve: A link between the immune and nervous systems? *J. Neurosci.* 19, 2799–2806.

Hagan, P., Poole, S., Bristow, A. F., Tilders, F., and Silverstein, F. S. (1996). Intracerebral NMDA injection stimulates production of interleukin-1 beta in perinatal rat brain. *J. Neurochem.* 67, 2215–2218.

Hays, T. C., Szymusiak, R., and McGinty, D. (1999). GABAA receptor modulation of temperature sensitive neurons in the diagonal band of Broca in vitro. *Brain Res.* 845, 215–223.

Hopkins, S. J., and Rothwell, N. J. (1995). Cytokine and the nervous system I: Expression and recognition. *Trends Neurosci.* 18, 83–88.

Horvath, T. L., Warden, C. H., Hajos, M., Lombardi, A., Goglia, F., and Diano, S. (1999). Brain uncoupling protein 2: Uncoupled neuronal mitochondria predict thermal synapses in homeostatic centers. *J. Neurosci.* 19, 10417–10427.

Jenkins, J. K., Drong, R. F., Shuck, M. E., Bienkowski, M. J., Slightom, J. L., Arend, W. P., and Smith, M. F., Jr. (1997). Intracellular IL-1 receptor antagonist promoter: Cell type-specific and inducible regulatory regions. *J. Immunol.* **158,** 748–755.

Kamikawa, H., Hori, T., Nakane, H., Aou, S., and Tashiro, N. (1998). IL-1β increases noreprinephrine level in rat frontal cortex: Involvement of prostanoids, NO, and glutamate. *Am. J. Physiol.* **275,** R806–R810.

Kanemoto, K., Kawasaki, J., Miyamoto, T., Obayashi, H., and Nishimura, M. (2000). Interleukin (IL)-1β, IL-1α, and IL-1 receptor antagonist gene polymorphisms in patients with temporal lobe epilepsy. *Ann. Neurol.* **47,** 571–574.

Katsuki, H., Nakai, S., Hirai, Y., Akaji, K., Kiso, Y., and Satoh, M. (1990). Interleukin-1γ inhibits long-term potentiation in the CA3 region of mouse hippocampal slices. *Eur. J. Pharmacol.* **181,** 323–326.

Kluger, M. J. (1991). *Pharmacol. Rev.* **71,** 93–127.

Kreutzberg, G. W. (1996). Microglia: A sensor for pathological events in the CNS. *Trends Neurosci.* **19,** 312–318.

Lapchak, P. A., Araujo, D. M., and Hefti, F. (1993). Systemic interleukin-1 beta decreases brain-derived neurotrophic factor messenger RNA expression in the rat hippocampal formation. *Neuroscience* **53,** 297–301.

Licinio, J., Wong, M. L., and Gold, P. W. (1991). Localization of interleukin-1 receptor antagonist mRNA in rat brain. *Endocrinology* **129,** 562–564.

Linthorst, A. C. E., Flachskam, C., Holsboer, F., and Reul, J. M. H. M. (1994). Local administration of recombinant human interleukin-1γ in the rat hippocampus increases serotonergic neurotrasmission, hypothalamic-pituitary-adrenocortical axis activity, and body temperature. *Endocrinology* **135,** 520–532.

Liu, Z., Gatt, A., Mikati, M., and Holmes, G. L. (1993). Effect of temperature on kainic acid-induced seizures. *Brain Res.* **631,** 51–58.

Loddick, S. A., and Rothwell, N. J. (1996). Neuroprotective effects of human recombinant interleukin-1 receptor antagonist in focal cerebral ischaemia in the rat. *J. Cerebr. Blood Flow Metab.* **16,** 932–940.

Luk, W. P., Zhang, Y., White, T. D., Lue, F. A., Wu, C., Jiang, C. G., Zhang, L., and Moldofsky, H. (1999). Adenosine: A mediator of interleukin-1β-induced hippocampal synaptic inhibition. *J. Neurosci.* **19,** 4238–4244.

Maingret, F., Lauritzen, I., Patel, A. J., Heurteaux, C., Reyes, R., Lesage, F., Lazdunski, M., and Honore, E. (2000). TREK-1 is a heat-activated background K(+) channel. *EMBO J.* **19,** 2483–2491.

Mantovani, A., Muzio, M., Ghezzi, P., Colotta, F., and Introna, M. (1996). Negative regulators of the interleukin-1 system: Receptor antagonists and a decoy receptor. *Int. J. Clin. Lab. Res.* **26,** 7–14.

Masino, S. A., and Dunwiddie, T. V. (1999). Temperature-dependent modulation of excitatory transmission in hippocampal slices is mediated by extracellular adenosine. *J. Neurosci.* **19,** 1932–1939.

McNamara, J. O. (1994). Cellular and molecular basis of epilepsy. *J. Neurosci.* **14,** 3413–3425.

Miller, L. G., Galpern, W. R., Dunlap, K., Dinarello, C. A., and Turner, T. J. (1991). Interleukin-1 augments gamma-aminobutyric acidA receptor function in brain. *Mol. Pharmacol.* **39,** 105–108.

Minami, M., Kuraishi, Y., and Satoh, M. (1991). Effects of kainic acid on messenger RNA levels of IL-1 beta, IL-6, TNF alpha and LIF in the rat brain. *Biochem. Biophys. Res. Commun.* **176,** 593–598.

Murray, B., Alessandrini, A., Cole, A. J., Yee, A. G., and Furshpan, E. J. (1998). Inhibition of the p44/42 MAP kinase pathway protects hippocampal neurons in a cell-culture model of seizure activity. *Proc. Natl. Acad. Sci. U.S.A.* **95,** 11975–11980.

Muzio, M., Polentarutti, N., Facchetti, F., Peri, G., Doni, A., Sironi, M., Transidico, P., Salmona, M., Introna, M., and Mantovani, A. (1999). Characterization of type II intracellular IL-1 receptor antagonist (IL-1ra3): A depot IL-1ra. *Eur. J. Immunol.* **29,** 781–788.

Nakamura, K., Kaneko, T., Yamashita, Y., Hasegawa, H., Katoh, H., and Negishi, M. (2000). Immunohistochemical localization of prostaglandin EP3 receptor in the rat nervous system. *J. Comp. Neurol.* **421**, 543–569.

Nishiyori, A., Minami, M., Takami, S., and Satoh, M. (1997). Type 2 interleukin-1 receptor mRNA is induced by kainic acid in the rat brain. *Mol. Brain Res.* **50**, 237–245.

Nitsch, C., Goping, G., and Klatzo, I. (1986). Pathophysiological aspects of blood–brain barrier permeability in epileptic seizures. *Adv. Exp. Med. Biol.* **203**, 175–189.

O'Neill, L. (2000). The Toll/interleukin-1 receptor domain: A molecular switch for inflammation and host defence. *Biochem. Soc. Trans.* **28**, 557–563.

Parmeggiani, P. L. (2000). Influence of the temperature signal on sleep in mammals. *Biol. Signals Recept.* **9**, 279–282.

Parmeggiani, P. L., Azzaroni, A., and Calasso, M. (2000). Behavioral state-dependent thermal feedback influencing the hypothalamic thermostat. *Arch. Ital. Biol.* **138**, 277–283.

Plata-Salaman, C. R., and French-Mullen, J. M. (1992). Interleukin-1 beta depresses calcium currents in CA1 hippocampal neurons at pathophysiological concentrations. *Brain Res. Bull.* **29**, 221–223.

Plata-Salaman, C. R., Ilyin, S. E., Turrin, N. P., Gayle, D., Flynn, M. C., Romanovitch, A. E., Kelly, M. E., Bureau, Y., Anisman, H., and McIntyre, D. C. (2000). Kindling modulates the IL-1beta system, TNF-alpha, TGF-beta1, and neuropeptide mRNAs in specific brain regions. *Brain Res. Mol. Brain Res.* **75**, 248–258.

Ricquier, D., Miroux, B., Larose, M., Cassard-Doulcier, A. M., and Bouillaud, F. (2000). Endocrine regulation of uncoupling proteins and energy expenditure. *Int. J. Obes. Relat. Metab. Disord.* **24** (Suppl 2), S86–S88.

Rolfe, D. F., and Brown, G. C. (1997). Cellular energy utilization and molecular origin of standard metabolic rate in mammals. *Physiol Rev.* **77**, 731–758.

Rothwell, N. J. (1991). Functions and mechanisms of interleukin 1 in the brain. *Trends Pharmacol. Sci.* **12**, 430–436.

Rothwell, N. J., and Hopkins, S. J. (1995). Cytokines and the nervous system II: Actions and mechanisms of action. *Trends Neurosci.* **18**, 130–136.

Rothwell, N. J., and Luheshi, G. (1994). Pharmacology of interleukin-1 actions in the brain. *Adv. Pharmacol.* **25**, 1–20.

Sana, T. R., Debets, R., Timans, J. C., Bazan, J. F., and Kastelein, R. A. (2000). Computational identification, cloning, and characterization of IL-1R9, a novel interleukin-1 receptor-like gene encoded over an unusually large interval of human chromosome Xq22.2–q22.3. *Genomics* **69**, 252–262.

Scarborough, D. E., Lee, S. L., Dinarello, C. A., and Reichlin, S. (1989). Interleukin-1 beta stimulates somatostatin biosynthesis in primary cultures of fetal rat brain. *Endocrinology* **124**, 549–51.

Schneider, H., Pitossi, F., Balschun, D., Wagner, A., Del Rey, A., and Besedovsky, H. O. (1998). A neuromodulatory role of interleukin-1b in the hippocampus. *Proc. Natl. Acad. Sci. U.S.A.* **95**, 7778–7783.

Schobitz, B., De Kloet, E. R., and Holsboer, F. (1994). Gene expression and function of interleukin 1, interleukin 6 and tumor necrosis factor in the brain. *Prog. in Neurobiol.* **44**, 397–432.

Sheng, J. G., Boop, F. A., Mrak, R. E., and Griffin, W. S. (1994). Increased neuronal beta-amyloid precursor protein expression in human temporal lobe epilepsy: Association with interleukin-1alpha immunoreactivity. *J. Neurochem.* **63**, 1872–1879.

Simoncsits, A., Bristulf, J., Tjornhammar, M. L., Cserzo, M., Pongor, S., Rybakina, E., Gatti, S., and Bartfai, T. (1994). Deletion mutants of human interleukin 1 beta with significantly reduced agonist properties: Search for the agonist/antagonist switch in ligands to the interleukin 1 receptors. *Cytokine* **6**, 206–214.

Smith, D. E., Renshaw, B. R., Ketchem, R. R., Kubin, M., Garka, K. E., and Sims, J. E. (2000). Four new members expand the interleukin-1 superfamily. *J. Biol. Chem.* **275**, 1169–1175.

Spranger, M., Lindholm, D., Bandtlow, C., Heumann, R., Gnahn, H., Naher-Noÿ, M., and Thoenen, H. (1990). Regulation of nerve growth factor (NGF) synthesis in the rat central nervous system: Comparison between the effects of interleukin-1 and various growth factors in astrocyte cultures and *in vivo*. *Eur. J. Neurosci.* **2**, 69–76.

Sundgren-Andersson, A. K., Ostlund, P., and Bartfai, T. (1998a). Simultaneous measurement of brain and core temperature in the rat during fever, hyperthermia, hypothermia and sleep. *Neuroimmunomodulation* **5**, 241–247.

Sundgren-Andersson, A. K., Gatti, S., and Bartfai, T. (1998b). Neurobiological mechanisms of fever. *Neuroscientist* **4**, 113–121.

Takao, T., Tracey, D. E., Mitchell, W. M., and De Souza, E. B. (1990). Interleukin-1 receptors in mouse brain: Characterization and neuronal localization. *Endocrinology* **127**, 3070–3078.

Vasilenko, V. Y., Petruchuk, T. A., Gourine, V. N., and Pierau, F. (2000). Interleukin-1beta reduces temperature sensitivity but elevates thermal thresholds in different populations of warm-sensitive hypothalamic neurons in rat brain slices. *Neurosci. Lett.* **292**, 207–210.

Vezzani, A., Conti, M., De Luigi, A., Ravizza, T., Moneta, D., Marchesi, F., and De Simoni, M. G. (1999). Interleukin-1beta immunoreactivity and microglia are enhanced in the rat hippocampus by focal kainate application: Functional evidence for enhancement of electrographic seizures. *J. Neurosci.* **19**, 5054–5065.

Vezzani, A., Moneta, D., Conti, M., Richichi, C., Ravizza, T., De Luigi, A., De Simoni, M. G., Sperk, G., Andell-Jonsson, S., Lundkvist, J., Iverfeldt, K., and Bartfai, T. (2000). Powerful anticonvulsant action of IL-1 receptor antagonist on intracerebral injection and astrocytic overexpression in mice. *Proc. Natl. Acad. Sci. U.S.A.* **97**, 11534–11539.

Wang, S., Cheng, Q., Malik, S., and Yang, J. (2000). Interleukin-1β inhibits gamma-aminobutyric acid type A (GABAA) receptor current in cultured hippocampal neurons. *J. Pharmacol. Exp. Ther.* **292**, 497–504.

Welch, J. M., Simon, S. A., and Reinhart, P. H. (2000). The activation mechanism of rat vanilloid receptor 1 by capsaicin involves the pore domain and differs from the activation by either acid or heat. *Proc. Natl. Acad. Sci. U.S.A.* **97**, 13889–13894.

Yabuuchi, K., Minami, M., Katsumata, S., and Satoh, M. (1993). *In situ* hybridization study of interleukin-1 beta mRNA induced by kainic acid in the rat brain. *Brain Res. Mol. Brain Res.* **20**, 153–156.

Ye, Z. C., and Sontheimer, H. (1996). Cytokine modulation of glial glutamate uptake: A possible involvement of nitric oxide. *NeuroReport* **7**, 2181–2185.

Zeise, M. L., Espinoza, J., Morales, P., and Nalli, A. (1997). Interleukin-1β does not increase synaptic inhibition in hippocampal CA3 pyramidal and dentate gyrus granule cells of the rat *in vitro*. *Brain Res.* **768**, 341–344.

CHAPTER 13

Animal Models for Febrile Seizures

TALLIE Z. BARAM

Departments of Pediatrics and Anatomy/Neurobiology,
University of California at Irvine, Irvine, California 92697

Human studies have provided conflicting information regarding the causal relationship between febrile seizures (particularly prolonged ones) and the subsequent development of temporal lobe epilepsy. In addition, it is not possible to study the mechanisms of the development and of the consequences of these seizures in human subjects. Animal models offer the opportunity to induce febrile seizures of controlled duration, and to conduct prospective studies for dissecting out the nature of these seizures and their consequences. This chapter considers the prerequisites of an optimal animal model for febrile seizures, including age specificity, electroencephalographic confirmation, temperature range and validation, pharmacological profile, low morbidity/mortality, and appropriate controls. Models published in the literature are reviewed in this context, and their strength and limitations are discussed. © 2002 Academic Press.

I. INTRODUCTION: WHY USE ANIMAL MODELS TO STUDY FEBRILE SEIZURES?

Although a growing body of epidemiological, genetic, and imaging studies (see chapters in Parts I, II, and V of this book) has focused on febrile seizures, some of the key questions relating to the mechanisms for their generation, and to their acute and chronic effects on the developing brain, cannot be resolved in the human. The reasons are obvious: febrile seizures are typically sudden and unexpected, they occur in circumstances that do not permit monitoring, and are mostly short and often frightening, further interfering even with behavioral observations. Febrile seizures rarely occur in settings where electroencephalographic (EEG) monitoring is possible—indeed, information about the EEG correlates of these seizures is strikingly rare (Morimoto *et al.,* 1991). Importantly, ethical considerations prevent induction of febrile seizures, thus eliminating the possibility of using imaging or electrophysiological methods to study them. Finally, studying specific mechanisms that cause febrile seizures in human infants and children, and testing specific hypotheses about these mechanisms or about prevention of the consequences of these seizures, are not feasible in the clinical situation.

In view of the difficulties of studying both the mechanisms of febrile seizures and the potential direct effects of these seizures on the immature brain, the search for an appropriate animal model has been an ongoing endeavor. Here this issue is discussed from several perspectives. First, the prerequisites of an optimal animal model are addressed; next, several animal models described in the literature are reviewed (this chapter does not deal with the *in vitro* models, which are discussed in Chapter 16).

II. CHARACTERISTICS OF THE OPTIMAL ANIMAL MODEL FOR FEBRILE SEIZURES

Models, by their nature, are only an approximation of the "real" situation. Inherent in a model is a simplification of the condition studied, with elimination of certain complexities. Different models of the same condition may highlight certain features as critical, and omit others. For febrile seizures, parameters that may be considered essential include specific characteristics of the brain that is undergoing the seizures, as well as the features of the seizures. For example, a genetic predisposition of the brain may potentially be required, and is excluded from most models. It should be noted, however, that genetic predisposition to either having febrile seizures or to developing consequences after the seizures is not likely to be a predominant requirement: studies of monozygotic twins with identical genetic makeup demonstrated discordance for both the presence of febrile seizures and the development of mesial temporal sclerosis (Jackson *et al.*, 1998).

By definition, a certain developmental age of the central nervous system (CNS) is required. Temperatures that lead to the seizures should be in the physiological range. The importance of whether these temperatures are generated by induction of fever or by hyperthermia has not been resolved. Whereas the mechanisms of fever involve cytokine activation and other, potentially important, molecular cascades (see Chapter 12 for review), hyperthermia per se has clearly been shown to induce seizures in children, and may be the common denominator of the multitude of fever etiologies in infants and children with febrile convulsions.

Among the characteristics of the provoked seizures, duration should be considered. Is the model designed to reproduce simple febrile seizures (nonfocal, shorter than 15 minutes)? Complex or prolonged febrile seizures (longer than

15 minutes)? Or febrile status epilepticus? Because of potential differences in the outcomes of these entities in the human, careful consideration should be given to the type of febrile seizure that is actually being modeled. Several important criteria for an optimal model for febrile seizures are discussed below.

A. AGE SPECIFICITY

Febrile seizures are seen almost exclusively in infants and young children (Verity *et al.*, 1985; Berg, *et al.*, 1992), specifically between 6 months and 5 years of age (see Chapter 1). Thus, the susceptibility to the convulsant effects of hyperthermia decreases dramatically with age in the human (Fishman, 1979). In the rat, a significant decline in the susceptibility to hyperthermic seizures is evident between the 11th and the 17th day of life (Hjeresen and Diaz, 1988). Though precise correlation of the rat and human neurodevelopmental profile is problematic, brain growth and myelination evidence suggest that the 5- to 7-day-old rat may be "equivalent" to the human neonate (Dobbing and Sands, 1973; Gottlieb *et al.*, 1977). Rat brain development during the period of 10–17 postnatal days best corresponds to the stage of brain development at which human infants and young children are most susceptible to febrile seizures (Dobbing and Sands, 1973; Gottlieb *et al.*, 1977). Therefore, an appropriate rat model for febrile seizures should employ rats during the second and early third week of life.

Using animals at a specific age of brain development is important also to permit proper interpretation of the experimental findings, because maturational processes are very active during the first several postnatal weeks in the rat. These lead to significant differences in the connectivity, excitability, and vulnerability of neurons, which are highly age dependent. Therefore, extrapolating data obtained using older experimental animals to questions of mechanisms and consequences of seizures that occur during younger ages may not be justified. For example, studying the propagation and consequences of experimental hyperthermic seizures in the hippocampus is reasonable, because pronounced cell loss is found in the hippocampal formation (e.g., CA1 and CA3) from human adults with temporal lobe epilepsy and a history of febrile seizures. However, hippocampal circuitry during early postnatal life in the rat is not fully mature, and both inhibitory and excitatory neurotransmissions are in flux (Ben Ari *et al.*, 1997). Thus, Swann *et al.* (1992) demonstrated both anatomical and electrophysiological evidence of immaturity of CA3 neuronal projections during the second and third postnatal weeks, and immaturity of granule cell axon (mossy fiber) synapses in the hilus of the dentate gyrus was demonstrated by Ribak and Navetta (1994). These findings suggest that the mechanisms of hippocampal propagation of age-specific seizures, such as those induced by fever or hyperthermia, may be age dependent. In addition, the consequences of these seizures may also differ from those of similar seizures in older animals. Thus, Sperber *et al.* (1992) and other groups have established the relative resistance of hippocampal neurons to seizure-induced excitotoxicity during this developmental age, whereas seizures of similar severity induced by the same convulsant agents lead to marked cell death in the mature hippocampus (Pollard *et al.*, 1994). Therefore, the age of the animals employed in models of febrile seizures is critical, and should be determined carefully.

B. Electroencephalographic Confirmation of the Seizures

It should be considered whether movements and other behaviors observed under experimental conditions represent seizures. The behaviors induced by hyperthermia in a given animal model are often similar to those seen during seizures. However, automatisms, stiffening, and other motor phenomena may result from nonconvulsive discharges in the brain stem, basal ganglia, etc. Therefore, EEG correlation of these observed behaviors should be obtained.

In infant rats during the second and early third postnatal weeks, hyperthermia induces stereotyped "seizurelike behaviors" (stage 4 in Hjeresen and Diaz, 1988; Baram *et al.*, 1997). These consist of unilateral tonic body posture accompanied by biting and chewing (facial myoclonus), typical markers of limbic origin (Ikonomidou-Turski *et al.*, 1987). EEG correlates should therefore be sought also in limbic regions, particularly in the amygdala and hippocampus. In addition to pinpointing the likely source of the seizures, EEG recording also from limbic rather than only from cortical regions is justified by the normal sequence of maturation in these regions: cortical maturation is incomplete during the second postnatal week in the rat, resulting typically in poorly organized and low-voltage cortical EEG activity (Schickerova *et al.*, 1984; Baram *et al.*, 1992). It should be noted that because EEG correlations of genuine febrile seizures in humans are exceedingly rare (Morimoto *et al.*, 1991), they are not helpful in guiding placement of electrodes in experimental animals.

C. Validation of Temperature Measurement and of Brain Temperatures

The methods for measuring core temperature at baseline and at seizure threshold should be accurate. In addition, the relationship of brain and core temperatures should be considered. Specifically, during fever or hyperthermia (Sundgren-Andersson *et al.*, 1998; Eshel and Safar, 1999) as well as during pathological conditions such as infarction, trauma, or brain death, dissociation of brain temperatures and those measured elsewhere may occur (Mellegard and Nordstroem, 1991; Schwab *et al.*, 1997; Henker *et al.*, 1998; Rumana *et al.*, 1998; Sundgren-Andersson *et al.*, 1998; Eshel and Safar, 1999; Miller *et al.*, 1999). This may be due to malfunction of central regulatory mechanisms of temperature control located in several CNS regions (Cartwell *et al.*, 1999; Bhatnagar and Dallman, 1999) or to inadequate capacity for rapid temperature equilibration under rapidly changing conditions (Sundgren-Andersson *et al.*, 1998; Eshel and Safar, 1999). Indeed, in the immature rat, brain and core temperatures may diverge during normothermia (M. Eghbal-Ahmadi *et al.*, unpublished observations). In addition, the relationship of brain and core temperatures may not be consistent throughout the range of temperatures induced to provoke a hyperthermic seizure. This may result in core temperatures that do not reflect actual brain temperatures. Therefore, calibration and standardization of parameters that influence the relationship of core and brain temperatures—the rate of heating, and volume, direction, and diffusion of heat source—should carefully be standardized for each model. Ideally, chronic measurement of brain temperature should be employed, but this is not feasible in the immature rat.

Of course, this consideration pertains also to the human situation, wherein brain temperature measurement during febrile seizures is not possible. Indeed, a divergence between core and brain temperatures in children, which depends in magnitude on the rate of temperature increase, may underlie the apparent relationship between threshold core temperature and the rapid onset of fever, as reported by some observers.

D. PHARMACOLOGICAL PROFILE

In children, febrile seizures are prevented by certain anticonvulsants (barbiturates, benzodiazepines, and valproate) but not by others (phenytoin and carbamazepine; see also Chapter 19). Optimal animal models should possess a similar pharmacological profile. In the neonatal (5 days old) experimental model (Olson *et al.*, 1984), the appropriate profile of anticonvulsant efficacy has been demonstrated. In models using rats during the third postnatal week or later, a number of pharmacological agents have been shown to increase the threshold temperature for the onset of hyperthermic seizures. These agents include naloxone and calcium channel blockers (Carrillo *et al.*, 1990; Laorden *et al.*, 1988, 1990). It should be noted that the fact that a given agent increases the threshold temperature required for the induction of febrile seizures does not prove that mechanisms blocked by the drug are involved *directly* in the generation of these seizures. The drug may interfere, for example, with the motor aspects of the animal's behavior. The optimal experimental model should permit the use of a variety of pharmaceutical agents to dissect out potential mechanisms underlying the seizures, as well as their potential consequences.

E. BENIGN NATURE

Febrile seizures, whether single, short, and nonfocal (simple) or recurrent, more prolonged, and focal (complex) are by and large benign. Although the role of these seizures in potentiating a long-term propensity to the development of temporal lobe epilepsy remains controversial, adverse short-term outcomes in terms of mortality and morbidity are virtually nil. Therefore, an appropriate animal model of febrile seizures should demonstrate similar low morbidity and mortality. In addition, a fundamental question related to hyperthermic seizures in the young is whether they result in long-term effects, i.e., loss of hippocampal neurons and/or alteration of hippocampal circuitry, leading to epilepsy. Therefore, an optimal model should be suitable for long-term survival without the confounding effects of the major stress (and ethical issues) of burns, infection, or moribund states. Early reported paradigms utilized a heated copper sheet as a heat source, resulting in burns (D. Holtzman, personal communication). Microwave heating has been used for increasing core temperature (e.g., Hjeresen and Diaz, 1988) but unrelated short- and long-term effects of microwaves on neuronal function cannot be excluded. An optimal model should use a defined, benign heating mechanism without unexpected side effects, which is suitable for repeated exposures and long-term studies (see below); models that involve high mortality or significant morbidity (Holtzman et al., 1981; Germano et al., 1996) may thus be less desirable. In summary, benign outcome not only reproduces the human situation, but permits meaningful prospective long-term studies of cognitive outcome and epileptogenicity.

F. HYPERTHERMIC CONTROLS

The goals of setting up models of febrile seizures are to study the mechanisms or the outcomes of these seizures. However, by definition, each model involves subjecting the brain to hyperthermia, to simulate fever. Therefore, the effects of the hyperthermia per se must be distinguished from those of the associated seizures. The potential effects of hyperthermia may not be inconsequential, involving induction of numerous genes (e.g., heat-shock protein) and both deleterious and protective effects on neuronal function and integrity. For example, hyperthermia was shown to enhance seizure severity and neuronal loss induced by kainic acid (Liu et al., 1993) and to cause, by itself, neuronal injury (Germano et al., 1996). Therefore, experiments using febrile seizure models should compare three sets of animals: normothermic controls, hyperthermic controls (in which hyperthermia was induced, but seizures were prevented) (Toth *et al.*, 1998; Chen *et al.*, 1999; see Chapter 15), and the experimental group that has experienced both hyperthermia and seizures.

III. PUBLISHED MODELS OF FEBRILE SEIZURES

One of the first groups to propose an animal model of febrile seizures was Holtzman *et al.* (1981) (see also Olson *et al.*, 1984, 1985). These authors studied rats 5–6 days old (true "neonates") and induced hyperthermia using a copper sheet heated by an infrared source. Their paradigm was lethal to 10-day and older rats, and unsuitable for long-term studies. Cortical EEG data were presented, but no further localization of the seizures was obtained. The model did reproduce the pharmacological profile seen in the human: phenobarbital, diazepam, and valproate increased threshold temperature for hyperthermic seizures, whereas phenytoin did not (Olson *et al.*, 1984).

Subsequently, several additional techniques have been devised to induce hyperthermic convulsions in young rats as a model of febrile seizures. For instance, circulation of warm air using a commercial fan (Morimoto *et al.*, 1990; Gilbert and Cain, 1985) or a hair dryer (Baram *et al.*, 1997; see Chapter 15) was employed. Other groups have utilized microwaves (Hjeresen and Diaz, 1988) or, as mentioned, a heated metal chamber with an infrared light source (Zhao *et al.*, 1985; Chilsolm *et al.*, 1985). Placing immature rats in a tank of heated water (45°C) (Klauenberg and Sparber, 1984; Palmer *et al.*, 1998; Jiang *et al.*, 1999) or in a container floating in warm water (Germano *et al.*, 1996) was used by other groups to provoke hyperthermic seizures; others have placed the subjects directly on a heated surface (Sarkisian *et al.*, 1999).

A critical aspect of the induction of hyperthermic seizure is the ability to measure and regulate accurately both core body temperature and brain temperature (see above). The published models in the literature used highly variable methods of temperature measurements. All those involving infant rats could not utilize permanently implanted sensors (see above), and the differences in measurement devices may account, at least partially, for the somewhat dissimilar threshold temperatures reported. In general, hyperthermic seizures could be induced in younger rats at lower temperatures, such as 40–42°C in rats 7–12 days old (Holtzman *et al.*, 1981; Dube *et al.*, 2000), compared with 42–44°C for older animals (postnatal days 14 or 22–29) (Morimoto *et al.*, 1990; Germano *et al.*, 1996; Jiang *et al.*, 1999). The strikingly lower threshold temperatures reported by Hjeresen and Diaz (1988) (37–39°C) may derive from their use of microwaves. Those may either have unknown effects on neuronal activation that may lead to seizures via mechanisms that are independent from temperature elevation, or may result in a more pronounced divergence of core and brain temperatures. An additional parameter that may be of concern here is the rate of temperature rise. This may be highly different with the use of microwaves, leading to a more rapid temperature increase in the microwave-sensitive, fat- and water-rich brain tissue, compared with core body temperature (see above). Indeed, the rate of temperature rise has been considered by some to be important both in the generation of febrile seizures and in their consequences (Morimoto *et al.,* 1990).

Regardless of variability in absolute values, most groups noted that the propensity to develop hyperthermia-induced seizures was highly age dependent and occurred during a clearly demarcated developmental window. This is an important validation of these models, as discussed above. Several groups also described discrete assessments of this issue. Thus, Hjeresen and Diaz (1988) showed a developmental trend in susceptibility to hyperthermic seizures. Seizure threshold was lowest (i.e., susceptibility was maximal) on postnatal days 11 and 13, and susceptibility then declined rapidly by days P15 and P17. Data from the author's group also demonstrated a maximal propensity for the development of hyperthermic seizures during postnatal days 10–12 (Baram *et al.,* 1997). Though Holtzman *et al.* (1981), evaluating rats in the age range of 2–20 postnatal days, found maximal seizure susceptibility on days P5–7, it is likely that the specific procedure used by these authors and the high mortality may have accounted for this difference.

Interestingly, Morimoto *et al.* (1990) reported that 50% of rats on day P15 and 100% on day P20 developed generalized seizures following hyperthermia, compared to younger (P10) or older (P30 and P40) rats. These data resulted in the use of much older rats by this group. Thus, Morimoto *et al.* (1991, 1993, 1995) reported on a model with EEG-confirmed seizures that used rats on days P24–29 and later. These rats are almost pubertal, and thus are significantly older than the age corresponding to human infants and young children. Further, these older animals were much more resistant to hyperthermic seizures than were younger rats (Hjeresen and Diaz, 1988). Behavioral seizures occurred at 44°C. Morimoto (1991) recorded cortical EEGs only, and suggested that hyperthermic seizures originated from the occipital cortex. This is surprising, because the behavioral seizures reported are typical of limbic origin (Goddard *et al.,* 1969; Haas *et al.,* 1990; Baram *et al.,* 1992).

In subsequent studies, these authors speculated about a role for glutamate in the generation of hyperthermic seizures (Morimoto *et al.,* 1993, 1995). This was based on the release of glutamate into a microdialysis perfusate of brain, and on increase of seizure threshold temperature by a noncompetitive antagonist of N-methyl-D-aspartate (NMDA) (MK-801). However, glutamate was released from brain with hyperthermia alone (air was heated to 50–60°C), and correlated best with the rate of heating (up to a body temperature of 45°C). It should be noted that aside from MK-801, the administration of calcium channel blockers (Carrillo *et al.*, 1990), phenobarbital, diazepam, valproate (Olson *et al.*, 1984), naloxone (Laorden *et al.*, 1988), and competitive blockers of corticotropin-releasing hormone (Baram and Schultz, 1994) has also resulted in elevation of seizure-threshold temperature. Therefore, the effect of MK-801 in juvenile and adult rats cannot be interpreted as proving a specific, mechanistic role for glutamate in the generation of hyperthermic seizures.

Other authors have relied on microwave heating to generate hyperthermic seizures (Hjeresen and Diaz, 1988). These authors demonstrated the rapid decrease in susceptibility to hyperthermia-induced seizures between postnatal days 10 and 17, but, unfortunately, did not provide EEG data.

Several models of febrile seizures have been set up to address the consequences of these seizures, and their potential relationship to temporal lobe epilepsy and mesial temporal sclerosis (see also Chapters 9, 14, and 15). Jiang *et al.* (1999) induced single and recurrent (6, 12, 24, or 32) seizures in "juvenile" (22 days old) rats. This required core temperatures of 42–44°C. These authors described the seizures as limbic (loss of consciousness, facial myoclonus, and head nodding). Indeed, epileptiform discharges were recorded from hippocampal EEGs [concordant with Dube *et al.* (2000)]. Sayin *et al.* (2000) studied electrophysiological changes in hippocampi from rats that sustained three episodes of hyperthermic seizures in 3-day intervals. However, details of the model and of seizure induction were not described.

The model defined by the author's group employs infant rats during the brain development epoch that is equivalent to human infancy and early childhood. The paradigm uses moderately warm air (temperature 42–43°C), and seizures arise at physiological temperatures that closely approximate the threshold temperature for human febrile seizures (Knudsen, 1996). In addition, multiple-depth electrodes have localized the origin of the resulting stereotyped seizures to the limbic circuit (Dube *et al.*, 2000; see also Chapter 15). The paradigm models complex febrile seizures (~20–25 minutes), and is virtually free of mortality and morbidity. The model is described in more detail in Chapter 15.

IV. ANIMAL MODELS: STRENGTHS, LIMITATIONS, AND USES

The preceding discussions described some of the published febrile seizure models, as well as the questions for which they were used. They illustrated the strengths and weaknesses of each model, as well as the advantages and limitations of animal models in general. It is important to highlight that animal models may be suitable, indeed optimal, for investigating certain questions—but not others—regarding febrile seizures.

For example, it is unlikely that febrile seizure models will resolve the issue of the nature, or relative contribution, of genetic factors to the occurrence or consequences of febrile seizures. Whereas genetically engineered animals may be more or less prone to these seizures, this would be expected on manipulation of any gene that is involved in neurotransmission in general. The role of genetic factors is probably best addressed using human studies, as described in Chapters 2 and 17. These human studies have suggested both a significant role for genetic predisposition for having febrile seizures (Chapter 17) and have proved that genetic makeup is not a predominant factor for having febrile seizures or suffering consequences from such seizures (see Jackson *et al.*, 1998). In addition, the mechanisms by which fever generates seizures, or the importance of other parameters associated with the fever (e.g., infection) to the seizures or their consequences, cannot be studied without consideration of the distinction between hyperthermia and fever. Furthermore, precise analysis of the function and regulation of specific genes or gene products, including receptors, channels, or single cell properties, may more appropriately be studied *in vitro*. A powerful approach to these types of studies combines *in vivo* generation of the seizures, followed by *in vitro* investigations of the resulting preparation (see Chapters 14 and 16).

In summary, animal models hold the promise of providing important insights into the mechanisms by which fever or hyperthermia provokes seizures, and the molecular and functional identity of the consequences of these seizures. However, these models provide only an approximation of human febrile seizures, and application of results obtained in the models to the human condition requires caution.

ACKNOWLEDGMENTS

Expert editorial assistance of M. Hinojosa is appreciated. Author's work supported by NIH grants NS28912 and NS35439.

REFERENCES

Baram, T. Z., Hirsch, E., Snead, O. C. III, and Schultz, L. (1992). Corticotropin-releasing hormone-induced seizures in infant rats originate in the amygdala. *Ann. Neurol.* **31**, 488–494.

Baram, T. Z., and Schultz, L. (1994). Corticotropin-releasing hormone receptor antagonist is effective for febrile seizures in the infant rat. *Ann. Neurol.* **36**, 487.

Baram, T. Z., Gerth, A., and Schultz, L. (1997). Febrile seizures: An appropriate-aged model suitable for long-term studies. *Brain Res. Dev. Brain Res.* **246**, 134–143.

Ben-Ari, Y., Khazipov, R., Leinekugel, X., Caillard, O., and Gaiarsa, J. L. (1997). GABAA, NMDA and AMPA receptors: A developmentally regulated "menage à trois." *Trends Neurosci.* **20**, 523–529.

Berg, A. T., Shinnar, S., Hauser, W. A., Alemany, M., Shapiro, E. D., Salomon, M. E., and Crain, E. F. (1992). A prospective study of recurrent febrile seizures. *N. Engl. J. Med.* **327**, 1122–1127.

Bhatnagar, S., and Dallman, M. F. (1999). The paraventricular nucleus of the thalamus alters rhythms in core temperature and energy balance in a state-dependent manner. *Brain Res.* **851**, 66–75.

Carrillo, E., Laorden, M. L., Miralles, F. S., and Puig, M. M. (1990). Dantrolene prevents hyperthermia induced seizures in rat pups [letter]. *Rev. Esp. Fisiol.* **46**, 223–224.

Cartwell, T., Luheshi, G. N., and Rothwell, N. J. (1999). Brain sites of action of endogenous interleukin-1 in the febrile response to localized inflammation in the rat. *J. Physiol.* **518**, 585–94.

Chen, K., Baram, T. Z., and Soltesz, I. (1999). Febrile seizures in the developing brain modify neuronal excitability in limbic circuits. *Nat. Med.* **5**, 888–894.

Chilsolm, J., Kellogg, C., and Frank, J. E. (1985). Developmental hyperthermic seizures alter adult hippocampal benzodiazepine binding and morphology. *Epilepsia* **26**, 151–157.

Dobbing, J., and Sands, J. (1973). Quantitative growth and development of human brain. *Arch. Dis. Child.* **48**, 757–767.

Dube, C., Chen, K., Eghbal-Ahmadi, M., Brunson, K., Soltesz, I., and Baram, T. Z. (2000). Prolonged febrile seizures in the immature rat model enhance hippocampal excitability long term. *Ann. Neurol.* **47**, 336–344.

Eshel, G. M., and Safar, P. (1999). Do standard monitoring sites affect true brain temperature when hyperthermia is rapidly induced and reversed? *Aviation Space Environ. Med.* **70**, 1193–1196.

Fishman, M. A. (1979). Febrile seizures: The treatment controversy. *J. Pediatr.* **94**, 177–184.

Germano, I. M., Zhang, Y. F., Sperber, E. F., and Moshe, S. L. (1996). Neuronal migration disorders increase seizure susceptibility to febrile seizures. *Epilepsia* **37**, 902–910.

Gilbert, M. E., and Cain, D. P. (1985). A single neonatal pentylenetetrazol or hyperthermia convulsion increases kindling susceptibility in the adult rat. *Dev. Brain Res.* **22**, 169–180.

Goddard, G. V., McIntyre, D., and Leech, C. K. (1969). A permanent change in brain function resulting from daily electrical stimulation. *Exp. Neurol.* **25**, 295–330.

Gottlieb, A., Keydor, I., and Epstein, H. T. (1977). Rodent brain growth stages. An analytical review. *Biol. Neonate* **32**, 166–176.

Haas, K. Z., Sperber, E. F., and Moshe, S. L. (1990). Kindling in developing animals: Expression of severe seizures and enhanced development of bilateral foci. *Brain Res. Dev. Brain Res.* **56**, 275–280.

Henker, R. A., Brown, S. D., and Marion, D. W. (1998). Comparison of brain temperature with bladder and rectal temperatures in adults with severe head injury. *Neurosurgery* **42**, 1071–1075.

Hjeresen, D. L., and Diaz, J. (1988). Ontogeny of susceptibility to experimental febrile seizures in rats. *Dev. Psychobiol.* **21**, 261–275.

Holtzman, D., Obana, K., and Olson, J. (1981). Hyperthermia-induced seizures in the rat pup: A model for febrile convulsions. *Science* **213**, 1034–1036.

Ikonomidou-Turski, C., Cavalheiro, E. A., Turski, W. A., Bortolotto, Z. A., and Turski, L. (1987). Convulsant action of morphine, [D-Ala^2, D-Leu^5]-enkephalin and naloxone in the rat amygdala: Electroencephalographic, morphological and behavioral sequelae. *Neuroscience* **20**, 671–686.

Jackson, G. D., McIntosh, A. M., Briellmann, R. S., and Berkovic, S. F. (1998). Hippocampal sclerosis studied in identical twins. *Neurology* **51**, 78–84.

Jiang, W., Duong, T. M., and de Lanerolle, N. C. (1999). The neuropathology of hyperthermic seizures in the rat. *Epilepsia* **40**, 5–19.

Klauenberg, B. J., and Sparber, S. B. (1984). A kindling-like effect induced by repeated exposure to heated water in rats. *Epilepsia* **25**, 292–301.

Knudsen, F. U. (1996). Febrile seizures-treatment and outcome. *Brain Dev.* **18**, 289–293.

Laorden, M. L., Miralles, F. S., and Puig, M. M. (1988). High doses of L-naloxone but neither D-naloxone nor beta-flunaltrexamine prevent hyperthermia-induced seizures in rat pups. *J. Pharm. Pharmacol.* **40**, 223–224.

Liu, Z., Gatt, A., Mikati, M., and Holmes, G. L. (1993). Effect of temperature on kainic acid-induced seizures. *Brain Res.* **631**, 51–58.

Mellergard, P., and Nordstroem, C. (1991). Intracerebral temperature in neurosurgical patients. *Neurosurgery* **28**, 709–713.

Miller, G., Stein, F., Trevino, R., *et al.* (1999). Rectal-scalp temperature difference predicts brain death in children. *Pediatr. Neurol.* **20**, 267–279.

Morimoto, T., Nagao, H., Sano, N., Takahashi, M., and Matsuda, H. (1990). Hyperthermia-induced seizures with a servo system: Neurophysiological roles of age, temperature elevation rate and regional GABA content in the rat. *Brain Dev.* **12**, 279–283.

Morimoto, T., Nagao, H., Sano, N., Takahashi, M., and Matsuda, H. (1991). Electroencephalographic study of rat hyperthermic seizures. *Epilepsia* **32**, 289–293.

Morimoto, T., Nagao, H., Yoshimatsu, M., *et al.* (1993). Pathogenic role of glutamate in hyperthermia induced seizures. *Epilepsia* **34**, 447–452.

Morimoto, T., Kida, K., Nagao, H., Yoshida, K., Fukuda, M., and Takashima, S. (1995). The pathogenic role of the NMDA receptor in hyperthermia-induced seizures in developing rats. *Brain Res. Dev. Brain Res.* **84**, 204–207.

Olson, J. E., Scher, M. S., and Holtzman, D. (1984). Effects of anticonvulsants on hyperthermia-induced seizures in the rat pup. *Epilepsia* **25**, 96–99.

Olson, J. E., Horne, D. S., Holtzman, D., and Miller, M. (1985). Hyperthermia-induced seizures in rat pups with preexisting ischemic brain injury. *Epilepsia* **26**, 360–364.

Palmer, G. C., Borrelli, A. R., Hudzik, T. J., and Sparber, S. (1998). Acute heat stress model of seizures in weanling rats: Influence of prototypic anti-seizure compounds. *Epilepsy Res.* **30**, 203–217.

Pollard, H., Charriaut-Marlangue, C., Cantagrel, S., Represa, A., Robain, O., Moreau, J., and Ben-Ari, Y. (1994). Kainate-induced apoptotic cell death in hippocampal neurons, *Neuroscience* **63**, 7–18.

Ribak, C. E., and Navetta, M. S. (1994). An immature mossy fiber innervation of hilar neurons may explain their resistance to kainate-induced cell death in 15-day-old rats. *Brain Res. Dev. Brain Res.* **79**, 47–62.

Rumana, C. S., Gopinath, S. P., Uzura, M., *et al.* (1998). Brain temperature exceeds systemic temperature in head-injured patients. *Crit. Care Med.* **26**, 562–567.

Sarkisian, M. R., Holmes, G. L., Carmant, L., Liu, Z., Yang, Y., and Stafstrom, C. E. (1999). Effects of hyperthermia and continuous hippocampal stimulation on the immature and adult brain. *Brain Dev.* **21**, 318–325.

Sayin, U., Sutula, T. P., Shanton, J., and Vielhuber, K. (2000). Age-dependence and regional specificity of long-term hippocampal alterations induced by febrile seizures in developing rats. *Epilepsia* **41** (Suppl. 7), 47 (abstract).

Schickerova, R., Mares, P., and Trojan, S. (1984). Correlation between electrocorticographic and motor phenomena induced by pentamethylenetetrazol during ontogenesis in rats. *Exp. Neurol.* **84**, 153–164.

Schwab, S., Spranger, M., Aschof, A., *et al.* (1997). Brain temperature monitoring and modulation in patients with severe MCA infarction. *Neurology* **48**, 762–767.

Sperber, E. F., Stanton, P. K., Haas, K., Ackerman, R. F., and Moshe, S. L. (1992). Developmental differences in the neurobiology of epileptic brain damage. *In* "Molecular Neurobiology of Epilepsy," pp. 67–81. Elsevier, Amsterdam.

Sundgren-Andersson, A. K., Ostlund, P., and Bartfai, T. (1998). Simultaneous measurement of brain and core temperature in the rat during fever, hyperthermia, hypothermia and sleep. *Neuroimmunomodulation* **5**, 241–247.

Swann, J. W., Smith, K. L., Gomez, C. M., and Brady, R. J. (1992). The ontogeny of hippocampal local circuits and focal epileptogenesis. *Epilepsy Res.* (Suppl.) 9, 115–125.

Toth, Z., Yan, X. X., Haftoglou, S., Ribak, C. E., and Baram, T. Z. (1998). Seizure-induced neuronal injury: Vulnerability to febrile seizures in immature rat model. *J. Neurosci.* 18, 4285–4294.

Verity, C. M., Butler, N. R., and Golding, J. (1985). Febrile convulsions in a national cohort followed up from birth. Prevalence and recurrence in the first five years of life. *Br. Med. J.* 290, 1307–1310.

Zhao, D., Wu, X., Pei, Y., and Zuo, Q. (1985). Long-term effects of febrile convulsions on seizure susceptibility in P77PMC rat—Resistant to acoustic stimuli but susceptible to kainate-induced seizures. *Exp. Neurol.* 88, 688–695.

CHAPTER 14

Physiology of Limbic Hyperexcitability after Experimental Complex Febrile Seizures: Interactions of Seizure-Induced Alterations at Multiple Levels of Neuronal Organization

NIKLAS THON, KANG CHEN, ILDIKO ARADI, AND IVAN SOLTESZ

Department of Anatomy/Neurobiology, University of California at Irvine, Irvine, California 92697

Do prolonged experimental febrile seizures cause persistent alterations in neuronal excitability in the limbic system? We combined an hyperthermia-induced seizure model in the immature rat with patch clamp techniques to answer this question. The results demonstrate that experimental complex febrile seizures cause persistent and highly specific alterations in the rat hippocampus at various levels of neuronal organization, from ion channels and synapses to neuronal circuits. © 2002 Academic Press.

I. INTRODUCTION

This chapter summarizes our findings (Chen *et al.*, 1999, 2001) concerning the electrophysiological basis of the long-term modifications in limbic circuits following experimental complex febrile seizures. In all the experiments described below, the hyperthermia-induced seizures lasted for longer than 15 minutes (22.8 minutes on average), and they were induced at postnatal day 10 or 11 in rat pups (see Chapter 15 for description of the hyperthermic seizure model). The electrophysiological experiments were conducted 1 week or months after the seizure episode. Data from rats that experienced prolonged hyperthermia-induced seizures (experimental group) were compared to results from their control littermates, which were either maintained normothermic or underwent the same duration and magnitude of hyperthermia but did not sustain seizures because they were pretreated with a short-acting barbiturate (see Chapter 15). The electrophysiological measurements were conducted in acute brain slices of the hippocampal formation.

II. LIMBIC EXCITABILITY AFTER EXPERIMENTAL COMPLEX FEBRILE SEIZURES

A. LONG-LASTING DECREASE IN THE POPULATION RESPONSES OF CA1 PYRAMIDAL CELLS TO LOW-FREQUENCY AFFERENT STIMULATION

First, field recording experiments were conducted to determine whether experimental complex febrile seizure led to long-lasting alterations in the excitability of the hippocampus. In slices from control animals, low-frequency (0.1 Hz) stimulation of the Schaffer collaterals (originating from CA3 pyramidal cells) evoked the characteristic short-latency, monosynaptic population excitatory postsynaptic potential (EPSP) and population spike discharge in CA1 pyramidal cells. A similar general pattern of response was also observed in rats that experienced hyperthermia-induced seizures 1 week before the electrophysiological experiments. However, the amplitude of the population spikes in the slices from the experimental animals was markedly reduced compared to their normothermic control counterparts (Chen *et al.*, 1999). These experiments, therefore, indicated that the seizures caused long-term (i.e., lasting for at least 1 week) alterations in the excitability of the hippocampus. Additional experiments revealed a similar depression of the perforant path-evoked field responses in the granule cell layer of the dentate gyrus.

What is the mechanism underlying the depression of the population spikes in the CA1 region of the hippocampus after the hyperthermia-induced seizures? To answer this question, the extracellular perfusate was switched to a solution containing the $GABA_A$ receptor antagonist bicuculline. Bicuculline was able to abolish the difference between the population spikes recorded in the experimental and control animals (Chen *et al.*, 1999). These data showed that an enhancement of the $GABA_A$ receptor-mediated inhibitory neurotransmission in the experimental animals was a major factor underlying decreased population spikes in the CA1 region following the experimental febrile seizures.

B. Protein Kinase A-Dependent, Presynaptic Increase in Inhibitory Neurotransmission

Next, whole-cell patch clamp recordings were performed to determine the nature of the enhanced $GABA_A$ receptor-mediated control of CA1 pyramidal cell discharges. The amplitude of the pharmacologically isolated, monosynaptic inhibitory postsynaptic currents (IPSCs), evoked with a stimulating electrode placed close to the pyramidal cell layer, was significantly increased in CA1 pyramidal cells from experimental animals, compared to normothermic controls, 1 week after the induction of seizures. In fact, the potentiation of the evoked IPSCs could also be observed even 10 weeks after the seizures, indicating the long-lasting nature of the alterations in inhibitory synaptic transmission (Chen et al., 1999). The amplitude of the evoked IPSCs in hyperthermic control rats (rats exposed to hyperthermia, but in whom the seizures were blocked with pentobarbital) was not enhanced. Therefore, the potentiation of the IPSCs was due to the hyperthermia-induced seizures, and not to the hyperthermia.

Is the locus of the long-term modification in inhibitory neurotransmission onto the perisomatic region of pyramidal cells pre- or postsynaptic? To answer this question, spontaneously occurring "miniature" IPSCs (mIPSCs) were recorded in the presence of the Na^+ channel antagonists tetrodotoxin and ionotropic glutamate receptor blockers. Miniature IPSCs have been shown to be generated mostly at synapses close to the soma (Soltesz et al., 1995; Cossart et al., 2000). The frequency of the mIPSCs was enhanced in CA1 pyramidal cells from experimental rats, without alterations in the amplitude and kinetics of the synaptic events (Chen et al., 1999). These data are consistent with a presynaptic locus for the long-term enhancement of inhibitory neurotransmission following experimental febrile seizures. Interestingly, when seizures were induced with the prototypic limbic convulsant kainic acid at the same age, and brain slices from the animals that had experienced kainic acid-induced seizures were subjected to electrophysiological studies 1 week later, there was no detectable increase in mIPSC frequency. These findings indicate that the presynaptic alterations after hyperthermia-induced seizures are unique to this seizure type.

Previous data showed that exogenously applied activators of protein kinase A (PKA) and protein kinase C (PKC) can cause a similar increase in mIPSC frequency, without changes in amplitude and kinetics, in pyramidal cells in brain slices from normal animals (Capogna et al., 1995). Therefore, in the next series of experiments, PKC and PKA blockers were tested to determine if the hyperthermic seizure-induced potentiation of inhibitory neurotransmission was due to alterations in molecular pathways involving these protein kinases. Incubation of the brain slices in solutions containing blockers of PKA, but not PKC, abolished the difference in the amplitude of the evoked IPSCs recorded in CA1 pyramidal cells from experimental and control animals. Furthermore, forskolin, which is known to enhance inhibitory synaptic transmission presynaptically through the adenylyl cyclase–PKA system, caused a significantly larger enhancement of the IPSCs in CA1 pyramidal cells from experimental compared to control rats. Taken together, these data demonstrated that experimental complex febrile seizures in the infant rat model lead to a persistent, PKA-dependent, presynaptic potentiation of $GABA_A$ receptor-mediated perisomatic inhibitory neurotransmission (Chen *et al.*, 1999).

The Paradox of Increased Inhibition and Decreased Seizure Threshold

Curiously, both *in vivo* and *in vitro* experiments (see Chapter 15 and Dube *et al.*, 2000) demonstrated that rats experiencing hyperthermia-induced seizures, even though not undergoing spontaneous seizures, did possess a persistently decreased seizure threshold. The decreased seizure threshold was demonstrated both with kainic acid *in vivo*, as well as with tetanic stimulation *in vitro* in combined entorhino–hippocampal slices (Dube *et al.*, 2000). The latter *in vitro* experiments showed that the entorhino–hippocampal circuit in slices from experimental animals started to generate self-sustaining, recurrent seizurelike population discharges after significantly fewer bouts of tetanic stimulation of the Schaffer collaterals than did similar slices taken from control animals (Chapter 15). Therefore, although the circuit does not generate spontaneous seizures, the neuronal circuit becomes less able to resist epileptogenic perturbations after hyperthermia-induced seizures, in spite of the enhanced perisomatic GABAergic inhibition. These seemingly contradictory observations became even more puzzling when additional experiments revealed no obvious alterations in either the evoked or the spontaneous excitatory postsynaptic currents (EPSCs) in CA1 pyramidal cells from seizure-experiencing animals.

Paradoxical increases in GABAergic inhibition in the hippocampus have been reported in several animal models of epilepsy as well (Walker and Kullman, 1999). A lasting increase in amplitude of mIPSCs has been shown to take place in granule cells of the dentate gyrus after kindling (Otis *et al.*, 1994), and subsequent experiments demonstrated that the increased mIPSC amplitude was due to a near-doubling of the number of postsynaptic $GABA_A$ receptors (Nusser *et al.*, 1998). In addition, experimental epilepsy can lead to long-lasting alterations in the subunit composition of $GABA_A$ receptors (Brooks-Kayal *et al.*, 1998; Buhl *et al.*, 1996). Therefore, hyperexcitability in the limbic system can coexist with either postsynaptic (Brooks *et al.*, 1998; Buhl *et al.*, 1996; Otis *et al.*, 1994; Nusser *et al.*, 1998) or presynaptic (Chen *et al.*, 1999) potentiation of

GABA$_A$ receptor-mediated neurotransmission. What is the role of increased inhibition in an ultimately hyperexcitable brain? Could the up-regulated inhibition actually enhance the probability that seizures take place, especially if the stability of the system is tested with repetitive, proconvulsive stimuli? Or, could it be that the enhanced IPSCs are overcome by proexcitatory changes resulting from the seizures? In the next series of experiments, these questions were addressed in the experimental complex febrile seizure model.

C. h-CHANNELS: ALTERATIONS IN A MOLECULAR INHIBITION–EXCITATION CONVERTER

Hyperpolarization-activated mixed-cation channels (h-channels; HCNs) are ubiquitously present in both cardiac and neuronal tissues (Pape and McCormick, 1989; Santoro and Tibbs, 1999). In the heart, h-channels generate the slow pacemaker current, leading to the rhythmic contractions of the heart muscles. In the thalamo-cortical circuits, the current generated by h-channels (I_h) plays a crucial role in sleep rhythms. In principle, h-channels could serve as ideal inhibition–excitation converters, because they are activated by hyperpolarization, and they generate an inward (depolarizing) current. However, in control hippocampal CA1 pyramidal cells, perisomatic IPSPs have not been shown to lead to postinhibitory rebound firing. Furthermore, although h-channels can be potentiated by a variety of neurotransmitter systems, probably all acting through intracellular cAMP, no persistent modulation of I_h has been demonstrated in any cell type. This may be due to the fact that the known forms of h-channel modulation last only as long as the elevated cAMP concentration is present.

To determine whether I_h undergoes a long-lasting modification in its properties after experimental complex febrile seizures, which may enable it to limit the efficacy of the seizure-induced enhancement of inhibitory neurotransmission, the biophysical properties of h-channels were compared in CA1 pyramidal cells from seizure-experiencing and control animals. Whole-cell patch clamp recordings in voltage-clamp mode from CA1 pyramidal cells in slices 1 week after the induction of hyperthermia-induced seizures demonstrated a significant depolarizing shift in the membrane potential for half-maximal activation (V_{50}) of I_h in experimental animals, compared to controls (Chen et al., 2001). These findings were also verified using the noninvasive technique of perforated patch clamp recordings. A small portion of the h-channels is active even around the resting membrane potential, and the probability of h-channel opening is progressively increased as the membrane potential is being hyperpolarized. The depolarizing shift in V_{50} in effect means that the same amount of hyperpolarization opens more h-channels, and, consequently, triggers a stronger depolarizing current. The positive shift in the V_{50} of I_h was present even 9 weeks after the seizures, indicating the long-lasting nature of the alterations in h-channel activation. In addition, the h-channels after the experimental complex febrile seizures also showed slower biexponential activation and deactivation kinetics, without a change in the relative weights of the fast and slow exponential fits to the currents. These results constituted the first demonstration of a persistent change in h-channel properties (Chen *et al.*, 2001).

Additional experiments revealed that the postseizure alterations in I_h could not be explained by a rise in intracellular cyclic AMP levels. Inclusion of cAMP in the recording pipette caused only a small depolarizing shift in the V_{50} of I_h in CA1 cells from control animals. These results were in agreement with previous reports indicating that intracellular cAMP did not cause a large depolarizing shift in the V_{50} of I_h in cells that predominantly express the HCN1 isoform of the h-channel (Santoro and Tibbs, 1999). Intracellular application of cAMP caused similarly small depolarizing shifts in V_{50} of I_h in CA1 pyramidal cells from experimental animals, and the difference between the V_{50} of experimental and control groups was present even at the highest cAMP concentrations. In addition, increased cAMP levels would be expected to accelerate (and not to slow down, as described above) the activation kinetics of I_h after the seizures. Additional experiments also determined that the shift in V_{50} could not be abolished with blockers of PKA or the β-adrenergic receptor. At the present time, the exact mechanism underlying the persistent alteration in h-channels after the hyperthermia-induced seizures is not known. One possibility may include an increase in the relative expression levels of the HCN2 or HCN4 isoforms, which are expressed at relatively low levels in control CA1 pyramidal cells and have a slower kinetics of activation. HCN subunits, including HCN1, HCN2, and HCN4, have been found to be expressed in the hippocampal CA1 region of the P10–11 rat (Bender *et al.*, 2001), so that alteration of the relative expression levels of these subunit isoforms is conceivable. Interestingly, there were no changes after hyperthermia-induced seizures in two potassium currents known to play important roles in neuronal excitability, the slowly inactivating K-current I_D, and the current underlying the slow afterhyperpolarization I_{AHP}, indicating the selectivity of the seizure-induced alterations in intrinsic currents.

D. Interaction of the Potentiated Perisomatic Inhibition with the Altered h-Channels

The shift in V_{50} affected the number of channels open close to the resting membrane potential. For example, there was an increase in the amplitude of I_h even at −70 mV. In addition, the resting membrane potential (recorded in the presence of a $GABA_A$ receptor antagonist) was significantly more depolarized, and the input resistance was decreased, in CA1 pyramidal cells from experimental animals compared to control. The h-channel antagonist ZD-7288 caused a significantly larger hyperpolarization in the resting membrane potential of CA1 pyramidal cells from animals that experienced these seizures. These data showed that the altered properties of h-channels could affect the intrinsic membrane properties of CA1 cells.

The activation curve-shifted I_h in CA1 pyramidal cells from experimental animals opposed hyperpolarizations of the membrane potential to a larger extent, as tested with intracellular injection of negative current pulses. Furthermore, at the end of the current pulse in cells from experimental animals, the membrane potential rose above the baseline, generating a posthyperpolarization depolarizing "hump" that could lead to the firing of action potentials. Both the posthyperpolarization depolarization and the action potentials could be fully blocked with the h-channel antagonist ZD-7288. Similar data were also obtained using short trains of evoked IPSPs in the presence of ionotropic glutamate receptor antagonists. Under these conditions, in control cells, there is no postinhibitory rebound firing. In contrast, in CA1 pyramidal cells from experimental animals, post-IPSP rebound depolarization and firing could be observed, and these postinhibitory events were fully blocked with ZD-7288 (Chen et al., 2001). Therefore, the altered I_h after hyperthermia-induced seizures can limit the effectiveness of the potentiated inhibition, and can even convert it to hyperexcitability.

How can one be sure that a shift in h-channels alone is sufficient to convert the inhibitory inputs to postinhibitory rebound firing? First, the experimental data discussed above showed that ZD-7288 can fully abolish the post-IPSP depolarization and firing in experimental cells. As a further test, multicompartmental computational modeling studies were conducted to determine if a relatively small shift in I_h activation can underlie postinhibitory rebound firing after seizures. Multicompartmental models of CA1 pyramidal cells were constructed based on experimental data, incorporating sodium-currents, delayed rectifier potassium-currents, and h-currents (Chen et al., 2001). Importantly, the model simulated the nonhomogeneous h-channel distribution described in CA1 pyramidal cells (Magee, 1998), a sevenfold linear increase in channel density from the somatic to the most distal dendritic compartment. These computational studies showed that even a small (larger than 2 mV) shift in the V_{50} of I_h channels in the model resulted in post-IPSP rebound depolarization and firing following a short burst of IPSPs, but not after single IPSPs. These simulation data also demonstrated that the depolarizing shift in the activation curve for I_h, even without including the changes in activation and deactivation kinetics, was sufficient to lead to rebound depolarization and firing, whereas slower kinetics alone were not sufficient. These modeling results (Chen et al., 2001) showed that I_h can play a crucial role in limiting the effectiveness of inhibitory inputs, and that the depolarizing shift in I_h activation plays a primary role in this process.

E. Effects on Interneuronal Network Oscillations

The altered I_h can act as an inhibition–excitation converter only if the IPSPs arrive in bursts that are long enough to sufficiently activate the altered h-channels, particularly because the I_h after the seizures showed slower time constants of activation. Single IPSPs, evoked by low-frequency stimulation, never resulted in post-IPSP depolarization and firing. Interestingly, as mentioned above, the overall stability of the circuit was also frequency dependent, because the decreased seizure threshold in population field responses could be readily demonstrated in prior experiments with short tetanic stimulation (Dube *et al.*, 2000), but not when low-frequency stimulation paradigms were used. In the experiments described above, six IPSPs were evoked at 50 Hz, and these IPSPs could trigger considerable postinhibitory firing in CA1 pyramidal cells from seizure-experiencing, but not from control, animals (Chen *et al.*, 2001). Such short bursts of IPSPs are known to occur *in vivo* spontaneously during theta rhythm in the hippocampus (Soltesz and Deschênes, 1993).

Could the experimental complex febrile seizures in the infant rat model alter the degree of synchrony of distributed interneuronal populations within the hippocampal formation? To answer this question, spontaneous IPSCs (sIPSCs) were recorded in the absence of tetrodotoxin (allowing the action potential-dependent GABA release to take place), in control extracellular medium. Under these conditions, sIPSCs in CA1 pyramidal cells can occur either as isolated, individual events, or they can take place in small temporal clusters or bursts. In CA1 cells from animals that experienced hyperthermia-induced seizures, however, the sIPSCs occurred in massive bursts more often than in controls (Chen *et al.*, 2001). Because the amplitude of these sIPSC bursts was much larger than what would be expected to arise from a single interneuron even with multiple release sites, it is likely that the bursts of sIPSCs in CA1 pyramidal cells from experimental animals are generated by the synchronous discharges of many presynaptic interneurons. In addition to the increased sIPSC burst amplitude, the sIPSC bursts took place in CA1 cells from experimental animals more frequently, indicating that experimental complex febrile seizures can persistently alter the temporal properties of synchronized oscillatory discharges in interneuronal networks.

III. CONCLUSIONS AND OUTLOOK

The novel results summarized in this chapter demonstrate that prolonged experimental febrile seizures in the immature rat can lead to robust, long-lasting modifications at the level of channels, synapses, and neuronal networks within the hippocampal formation. Normal development also shapes neuronal networks at all of these levels, and prolonged febrile seizures in infancy can apparently perturb processes at multiple levels of neuronal organization. Interestingly, the long-term effects of prolonged experimental febrile seizures were not independent of each other. Indeed, the seizure-induced alterations in neuronal properties were shown to be able to interact. For example, the effects of the increased perisomatic inhibition (a change with a locus in the interneuronal axon terminal) was found to be significantly modified by another alteration, the change in the activation properties of h-channels (located in the membranes of the postsynaptic pyramidal cells). Therefore, because it is precisely the interactions of the individual changes in cellular and synaptic properties taking place in both principal cells and interneurons that ultimately result in the generation of hyperexcitable responses after a single episode of experimental complex febrile seizures, the net outcome of the febrile seizure-induced modifications can be understood only if all of these individual alterations at multiple levels of organization are delineated and taken into account. The hippocampal circuit after hyperthermia-induced seizures shows a decreased seizure threshold, in spite of an up-regulated inhibitory GABAergic neurotransmission. Our results indicate that the persistently altered gain of I_h neutralizes the increased IPSPs following the seizures. Indeed, the nature of the altered I_h is such that the larger and more frequent the inhibitory hyperpolarizing events become, the more I_h will be activated. The activated I_h opposes the hyperpolarizing inputs, and, at the end of an inhibitory synaptic barrage, the activated I_h can lead to a postinhibitory overshoot and action potential burst firing. This mechanism, perhaps together with other processes (Staley et al., 1995; Buhl et al., 1996), can provide a resolution to the paradox of increased inhibition described in the experimental complex febrile seizure model (Chen et al., 1999), as well as in other models of temporal lobe epilepsy (Walker and Kullman, 1999).

In light of our increased knowledge about the long-term modifications in limbic circuits after hyperthermia-induced seizures, it is interesting to consider the question of whether the potentiated inhibition after experimental febrile seizure is primarily pro- or anticonvulsive in its ultimate net effects. GABAergic inhibitory interneurons can innervate and synchronize thousands of postsynaptic principal cells (Soltesz and Deschênes, 1993; Cobb et al., 1995); therefore, increased inhibition, at least in principle, may lead to hypersynchronous activation of pyramidal cells. Our field recording results indicate that the potentiated inhibitory synaptic transmission induced by the hyperthermic seizures can inhibit pyramidal cell discharges to a greater extent than in controls, as long as the incoming excitatory inputs arrive at low frequencies (Chen et al., 1999). However, when the excitatory pathways are stimulated at higher frequencies, e.g., in tetanic bursts (Dube et al., 2000), the neuronal network shows a significantly decreased ability to inhibit excessive firing in pyramidal cells. The interactions of inhibitory inputs and the modified I_h after experimental complex febrile seizures are also strongly frequency dependent. Therefore, potentiated inhibition can have different, and even opposing, net effects on the control of principal cell firing after hyperthermia-induced seizures. Further research will be necessary to determine the exact conditions of activation of the modified h-channels on various principal cell types by the enhanced inhibitory events generated by the synchronized firing of interneuronal networks. The novel results described in this chapter already suggest that there may be several, hitherto unsuspected opportunities for future therapeutic interventions to control seizures. For example, subunit-specific h-channel antagonists in the future should be tested for their potential to dampen the interactions of enhanced inhibitory inputs and intrinsic currents in pyramidal cells. In addition to h-channels, other "background" conductances, such as extrasynaptic $GABA_A$ receptors and the Na^+/K^+-ATPase, also play prominent roles in the regulation of neuronal excitability (Ross and Soltesz, 2000, 2001; Soltesz and Nusser, 2001). Some of these intrinsic currents have been shown to be altered in a long-lasting manner in hyperexcitable neuronal circuits (Ross and Soltesz, 2000), and they could also be investigated for their therapeutic potential. Furthermore, once the mechanisms underlying the increased frequency and amplitude of the synchronous sIPSC bursts after experimental febrile seizures are understood, novel anticonvulsant therapeutic strategies may be designed to regulate the degree of synchronization among interneurons in the hippocampal neuronal networks (Traub *et al.*, 1998).

ACKNOWLEDGMENTS

The studies summarized in this review were financially supported by NIH grants (NS38580 to I. Soltesz and NS35439 to T. Z. Baram), by the UC Systemwide Biotechnology Research and Education Program (BREP-98-02 to T. Z. Baram and I. Soltesz), by a fellowship from the Studienstiftung des Deutsches Volkes (to N. Thon), and by a postdoctoral fellowship from the Epilepsy Foundation of America (to I. Aradi).

REFERENCES

Bender, R. A., Brewster, A., Santoro, B., Ludwig, A., Hofmann, F., Biel, M., and Baram, T. Z. (2001). Differential and age-dependent expression of hyperpolarization-activated, cyclic nucleotide-gated cation channel isoforms 1–4 suggest evolving roles in the developing rat hippocampus. *Neuroscience,* in press.
Brooks-Kayal, A. R., Shumate, M. D., Jin, H., Rikhter, T. Y., and Coulter, D. A. (1998). Selective changes in single cell $GABA_A$ receptor subunit expression and function in temporal lobe epilepsy. *Nat. Med.* 4, 1166–1172.

Buhl, E. H., Otis, T. S., and Mody, I. (1996). Zinc-induced collapse of augmented inhibition by GABA in a temporal lobe epilepsy model. *Science* **271**, 369–373.

Capogna, M., Gahwiler, B. H., and Thompson, S. M. (1995). Presynaptic enhancement of inhibitory synaptic transmission by protein kinases A and C in the rat hippocampus *in vitro. J. Neurosci.* **15**, 1249–1260.

Chen, K., Baram, T. Z., and Soltesz, I. (1999). Febrile seizures in the developing brain result in persistent modification of neuronal excitability in limbic circuits. *Nat. Med.* **5**, 888–894.

Chen, K., Aradi, I., Thon, N., Eghbal-Ahmadi, M., Baram, T. Z., and Soltesz, I. (2001). Persistently modified h-channels after complex febrile seizures convert the seizure-induced enhancement of inhibition to hyperexcitability. *Nat. Med.* **7**, 331–337.

Cobb, S. R., Buhl, E. H., Halasy, K., Paulsen, O., and Somogyi, P. (1995). Synchronization of neuronal activity in hippocampus by individual GABAergic interneurons. *Nature* **378**(6552), 75–78.

Cossart, R., Hirsch, J. C., Cannon, R. C., Dinoncourt, C., Wheal, H. V., Ben-Ari, Y., Esclapez, M., and Bernard, C. (2000). Distribution of spontaneous currents along the somato-dendritic axis of rat hippocampal CA1 pyramidal neurons. *Neuroscience* **99**, 593–603.

Dube, C., Chen, K., Eghbal-Ahmadi, M., Brunson, K., Soltesz, I., and Baram, T. Z. (2000). Prolonged febrile seizures in the immature rat model enhance hippocampal excitability long term. *Ann. Neurol.* **47**, 336–344.

Magee, J. C. (1998). Dendritic hyperpolarization-activated currents modify the integrative properties of hippocampal CA1 pyramidal neurons. *J. Neurosci.* **18**, 7613–7624.

Nusser, Z., Hájos, N., Somogyi, P., and Mody, I. (1998). Increased number of synaptic GABA(A) receptors underlies potentiation at hippocampal inhibitory synapses. *Nature (London)* **395**, 172–177.

Otis, T. S., De Koninck, Y., and Mody, I. (1994). Lasting potentiation of inhibition is associated with an increased number of gamma-aminobutyric acid type A receptors activated during miniature inhibitory postsynaptic currents. *Proc. Natl. Acad. Sci. U.S.A.* **91**, 7698–7702.

Pape, H. C., and McCormick, D. A. (1989). Noradrenaline and serotonin selectively modulate thalamic burst firing by enhancing a hyperpolarization-activated cation current. *Nature (London)* **340**, 715–718.

Ross, S. T., and Soltesz, I. (2000). Selective depolarization of interneurons in the early post-traumatic dentate gyrus: Involvement of the Na^+/K^+-ATPase. *J. Neurophysiol.* **83**, 2916–2931.

Ross, S. T., and Soltesz, I. (2001). Long-term plasticity in interneurons of the dentate gyrus. *Proc. Natl. Acad. Sci. U.S.A.* **98**(15), 8874–8879.

Santoro, B., and Tibbs, G. R. (1999). The HCN gene family: Molecular basis of the hyperpolarization-activated pacemaker channels. *Ann. N. York Acad. Sci.* **868**, 741–764.

Soltesz, I., and Deschênes, M. (1993). Low- and high-frequency membrane-potential oscillations during theta activity in morphologically identified neurons of the rat hippocampus during ketamine-xylazine anesthesia. *J. Neurophysiol.* **70**, 97–116.

Soltesz, I., and Nusser, Z. (2001). Background inhibition to the fore. *Nature (London)* **409**, 24–27.

Soltesz, I., Smetters, D. K., and Mody, I. (1995). Tonic inhibition originates from synapses close to the soma. *Neuron* **14**, 1273–1283.

Staley, K. J., Soldo, B. L., and Proctor, W. R. (1995). Ionic mechanisms of neuronal excitation by inhibitory $GABA_A$ receptors. *Science* **269**, 977–981.

Traub, R. D., Spruston, N., Soltesz, I., Konnerth, A., Whittington, M. A., and Jeffereys, J.G.R. (1998). Gamma-frequency oscillations: A neuronal population phenomenon regulated by synaptic and intrinsic cellular processes. *Prog. Neurobiol.* **55**, 563–575.

Walker, M. C., and Kullmann, D. M. (1999). Febrile convulsions: A 'benign' condition? *Nat. Med.* **5**, 871–872.

CHAPTER 15

Do Prolonged Febrile Seizures in an Immature Rat Model Cause Epilepsy?

CELINE DUBE

Department of Anatomy/Neurobiology,
University of California at Irvine, Irvine, California 92697

Of all seizures of early childhood, febrile seizures are the most common type. An ongoing controversy about the outcome of these seizures involves the question of whether complex febrile seizures (those that are longer than 15 minutes, recur within a single febrile episode, or have focal features) alter limbic excitability, leading to spontaneous seizures (temporal lobe epilepsy) later in life. Recent data using an immature rat model indicate that prolonged (20 minutes) experimental febrile seizures result in significant structural changes of certain hippocampal neurons and in long-term functional changes of the hippocampal circuit. However, whether these neuroanatomical and electrophysiological changes promote hippocampal excitability and lead to epilepsy have remained unknown. In this chapter, we describe the use of the immature rat model to study this question. The length of the seizures in the model was designed to reproduce "complex" febrile seizures in the human, according to the International League Against Epilepsy (ILAE) classification (Commission, 1981), i.e., those lasting more than 15 minutes. We discuss experiments that use the model to gain insight into long-term consequences of these seizures on susceptibility to further seizures.

Prolonged hyperthermic seizures (21.5 ± 0.9 minutes) were induced in 10- or 11-day-old rats that, as adults, were compared to both hyperthermic and normothermic controls. Prolonged depth hippocampal electroencephalograms (EEGs) and behavioral measures were obtained to determine the presence of spontaneous seizures (epilepsy). To determine susceptibility to limbic seizures, electrophysiological and behavioral effects of subthreshold doses of the *chemical* limbic excitatory agent, kainate, were evaluated. To better define the circuitry influenced by the prolonged febrile seizures early in life, *in vitro* hippocampal–entorhinal cortex (HEnC) slices from febrile seizure-experiencing rats were compared with those from littermate controls. Specifically, the susceptibility of the limbic circuit in animals sustaining experimental febrile seizures early in life to *electrical* excitatory input was determined.

EEGs were normal, and seizures were not observed in adult animals that had experienced prolonged hyperthermic seizures early in life, as well as in normothermic and hyperthermic control animals. Following the administration of very low doses of systemic kainate, a minority of normothermic and hyperthermic controls had one or two brief seizures. In contrast, all of the animals that had experienced early-life "febrile" seizures developed hippocampal seizures, and the majority progressed to status epilepticus. In accord with the *in vivo* results, spontaneous epileptiform discharges were absent in HEnC slices *in vitro*. However, stimulation of Schaffer collaterals led to reverberating, status epilepticus-like discharges exclusively in brain slices from the experimental group. These data suggest that prolonged hyperthermic seizures early in life do not lead to spontaneous limbic seizures, but they markedly reduce seizure threshold to excitatory input *in vivo* (kainate) and *in vitro* (stimulation). These alterations in excitability of the hippocampal network may promote the development of limbic epilepsy.
© 2002 Academic Press.

I. DO HUMAN DATA SUPPORT THE NOTION THAT PROLONGED FEBRILE SEIZURES CAUSE EPILEPSY?

As discussed in previous chapters of this book, febrile seizures are the most common type of childhood seizures, affecting 3–5% of human infants and young children (Verity *et al.*, 1985; Shinnar, 1990; Hauser, 1994). The relationship of childhood febrile seizures to adult temporal lobe epilepsy (TLE) has remained a focus of intense discussion. Although prospective epidemiological studies have not shown a progression of febrile seizures to TLE (Nelson and Ellenberg, 1976; Shinnar, 1998; see also Chapter 7), retrospective analyses of adults with TLE document a high prevalence (30–50%) of a history of febrile seizures during early childhood, suggesting an etiological role for these seizures in the development of TLE (French *et al.*, 1993; Cendes *et al.*, 1993; see also Chapter 6). Proponents of a causal relationship of febrile seizures and TLE have suggested that these seizures result in damage to hippocampal neurons, leading to mesial temporal sclerosis, the pathological hallmark of TLE (Falconer *et al.*, 1964; Sagar and Oxbury, 1987; Theodore *et al.*, 1999). In contrast, the correlation of febrile seizures and TLE can be explained by a preexisting neuronal injury; this, in turn, triggers both the febrile seizures and the subsequent TLE (Toth *et al.*, 1998; Shinnar, 1998; Lewis, 1999). This predisposing injury may be structurally overt, or related to molecular mechanisms such as abnormal ion channels, or signal transduction mechanisms (Dube *et al.*, 2000).

II. USE OF EXPERIMENTAL COMPLEX FEBRILE SEIZURES TO ADDRESS THEIR RELATIONSHIP TO EPILEPTOGENESIS

Because of the difficulty resolving these important questions regarding the causal relationship of febrile seizures and temporal lobe epilepsy using human studies, animal models, permitting induction of febrile seizures, rapid prospective studies, and interventions addressed at dissecting out their mechanisms and consequences, are attractive alternatives. Although animal models using relatively homogeneous populations with a "normal" brain are not suitable to look at issues of genetic susceptibility to the occurrence of complex febrile seizures or their consequences, they can be used to address the effects of such seizures on the developing hippocampus. It should be noted that although genetic predisposition is likely an important element (see Chapter 17), its role is not overwhelming. Thus, identical twin studies have demonstrated that monozygotic twins, with identical genetic makeup, may be discordant for both the occurrence of prolonged febrile seizures as well as for their consequences on hippocampal structure (Jackson *et al.*, 1998). Thus, a significant element of the consequences of prolonged febrile seizures may be independent from genetic makeup, and amenable to study using animal models.

Several models for febrile seizures have been described, and are discussed in detail in Chapters 13 (*in vivo* models) and 16 (*in vitro* preparations). A number of these models have addressed the consequences of these seizures on neuronal excitability, and the potential relationship of febrile seizures to temporal lobe epilepsy and mesial temporal sclerosis (see also Chapter 13). Many parameters differ among models, and it is therefore somewhat difficult to compare the results. For example, animal age, degree and duration of hyperthermia, the length and the number of the seizures, brain temperature, and electroencephalographic (EEG) measurements are highly variable; these are reviewed in Chapters 10 and 13.

This chapter focuses on a model of complex febrile seizures in the immature rat. The model has been characterized (see Chapter 9; Baram *et al.*, 1997; Toth *et al.*, 1998; Chen *et al.*, 1999; Dube *et al.*, 2000) and involves immature rats during a brain development age generally equivalent to that of the human infant and young child (Gottlieb *et al.*, 1977). Thus, hyperthermic seizures are induced in "infant" rats on postnatal day 10 or 11. Increased body and brain temperatures are achieved using warmed air, via a hair dryer (intermediate settings, air temperature ~43°C). The air is directed ~50 cm above the immature rats, which are placed (one or two at a time) on a towel in a 3-liter glass jar. Core temperatures are measured prior to onset of hyperthermia induction, every 2 minutes during it, and at the onset of hyperthermia-induced seizures. Core temperatures have been correlated with brain temperatures. In over 400 animals, raising core and brain temperatures to an average 40.88°C results in hyper-thermic seizures in over 98%. Animals are maintained hyperthermic (39–41.5°C) for 30 minutes, which results in seizure duration of about 20 minutes. After the hyperthermia, animals are moved to a cool surface and maintained normothermic, then returned to their mothers for rehydration. If the hyperthermic controls who are given pentobarbital to block the hyperthermia-induced seizures are still somewhat sedated, they are hydrated orally. Little evidence of dehydration is observed from this mild procedure, animals regain normal activity (including suckling) rapidly, and mortality has been <1% (2/307). The seizures, both behavioral and electrographic, have been characterized and are described below.

This model has been used to look at structural consequences of prolonged febrile seizures, and specifically at the question of whether they induce cell death or lead to functional rewiring of the hippocampal circuit (Chapter 9). In essence, striking cytoskeletal changes in select hippocampal neuronal populations were found to result from experimental prolonged febrile seizures in this model (Toth *et al.*, 1998; see Chapter 9). These changes, in a distribution highly reminiscent of that of the neuronal loss in mesial temporal sclerosis, lasted for several weeks, but were not associated with cell death. However, given their widespread distribution and extent, the question of whether they lead to functional disruption sufficient to influence excitation–inhibition balance in the involved circuits re-quired clarification. This was particularly important, because persistent func-tional modulation of hippocampal circuitry induced by febrile seizures in the im-mature rat model has been demonstrated in an *in vitro* study (Chen *et al.*, 1999; see Chapter 14). In that study, hyperthermia-induced seizures (but not hyper-thermia alone) caused a selective increase in presynaptic inhibitory transmission in the hippocampus that lasted into adulthood. These *in vitro* electrophysiolog-ical data indicated that early-life febrile seizures did powerfully modify the bal-ance of excitation and inhibition within the limbic system.

III. CONSEQUENCES OF PROLONGED EXPERIMENTAL FEBRILE SEIZURES

How do the structural and functional alterations of limbic neurons translate into the development of limbic epilepsy? Do prolonged febrile seizures in this model lead to enhanced epileptic susceptibility long-term? These two questions are the focus of the studies reported in this chapter. These studies were devised to determine whether prolonged febrile seizures in the immature rat resulted in development of spontaneous behavioral and electrophysiological seizures, and if not, whether they altered the susceptibility of the limbic circuit to excitatory input both *in vivo* and *in vitro*, indicating a predisposition to the development of limbic epilepsy.

The methods used in these studies have been described in detail in Dube *et al.* (2000). Briefly, 45 Sprague–Dawley derived rats were used, and all experiments conformed to institutional, federal, and American Association for Laboratory Animal Care (AALAC) guidelines. The overall strategy was to induce complex febrile seizures via hyperthermia, in comparison with hyperthermia alone, in 10-day-old rats. The presence of spontaneous seizures and of EEG abnormalities was determined in adult rats that had experienced complex febrile seizures early in life, compared with littermate normothermic and hyperthermic controls. In addition, to investigate whether these early-life seizures conferred susceptibility to seizures during adulthood, the convulsant threshold of kainic acid for both EEG-assessed and behavioral seizures was determined in all three groups. In parallel, hippocampal–entorhinal cortex sections from experimental and control groups were studied as well.

A. Effects of Hyperthermic Seizures Compared to Hyperthermia without Seizures and Normothermic Controls

Hyperthermic seizures were induced as described above: pups underwent hyperthermia (defined as core temperature higher than 39°C) for 28.2 ± 0.7 minutes. Peak temperature was $41.96 \pm 0.14°C$. Pups developed seizures averaging 21.5 ± 0.9 minutes, at a threshold temperature of $40.88 \pm 0.3°C$. The behavioral features of these seizures consisted of tonic motionless postures with occasional automatisms. The hyperthermic control group sustained the same duration (28.7 ± 0.6 minutes) and magnitude (peak core temperature $41.91 \pm 0.11°C$) of hyperthermia. However, the emergence of seizures was prevented in this group by pretreating them with a short-acting barbiturate (pentobarbital, 30 mg/kg, intraperitoneally), just prior to onset of hyperthermia. This hyperthermic control group thus served to distinguish the effects of hyperthermic (febrile) *seizures* from the potential effects of hyperthermia per se (Toth *et al.*, 1998; Dube *et al.*, 2000). The short-acting barbiturate, the behavioral effects of which disappeared within an hour, was chosen to minimize or obviate potential neuroprotective effects. In addition to the hyperthermic control group, a normothermic control group was evaluated.

Because the goal of these studies required evaluation of hippocampal EEGs later in life, and because hippocampal growth precludes maintaining of chronic electrodes during development, these rats were not implanted with electrodes until adulthood (see below). Therefore, a separate group of animals was studied acutely using hippocampal-depth electrodes, to verify that the hyperthermia did induce epileptic seizures, and that the pentobarbital dose used was sufficient to block these seizures in all animals.

B. Determination of Spontaneous Behavioral and Electrographic Seizures and Altered Sensitivity to Excitation of Temporal Lobe Structures

The potential presence of spontaneous seizures was determined using both behavioral and EEG measures. Starting 2 months after the hyperthermic seizures (on postnatal day 71.4 ± 5.1), rats were prospectively observed for the presence of behavioral limbic seizures. Rats were scored for the presence of established manifestations of limbic seizures: (1) automatisms, including head nodding and bobbing; (2) prolonged (>60 seconds) immobility with fixed staring; (3) rhythmic uni- or bilateral clonic movements (exclusive of grooming); (4) wet-dog shakes; and, (5) rearing and loss of balance (Ben-Ari et al., 1981; Cherubini et al., 1983; Albala et al., 1984; Ikonomidou-Turski et al., 1987; Holmes et al., 1988; Haas et al., 1990). Rats were monitored daily for 3 hours (between 2 and 5 PM) for 7 days.

Electrographic seizures were monitored using hippocampal EEGs. Thus, subsequent to the behavioral monitoring, rats were implanted unilaterally with bipolar twisted-wire electrodes (Baram et al., 1992, 1997; Dube et al., 2000). These recordings served to determine the epileptic nature of any observed behaviors, to localize their origin, and to examine for the possibility of limbic electrographic seizures not associated with behavioral manifestations. All EEG recordings, in both immature and adult rats, were carried out in freely moving animals, via long flexible cables. For the adult rats, hippocampal discharges were recorded and correlated with behavior for 1 hour on each of 7 consecutive days.

To determine whether early-life complex febrile seizures in this model altered the susceptibility to excitatory input into the temporal lobe circuit, both of the control groups, as well as the experimental animals, were subjected to threshold doses of kainic acid. First, a separate group of age- and weight-matched control animals ($n = 10$) was used to determine the threshold dose of kainic acid, defined as one that induces no or very short seizures. In this pilot study, 5 mg/kg of this limbic excitant, given into the peritoneal cavity, was determined to be a threshold dose in naive adult rats of our colony. This dose modified behavior minimally but did not lead to overt seizures. Thus, this dose was chosen to discriminate levels of excitability in the experimental and control groups. Briefly, kainic acid was given to rats carrying hippocampal electrode arrays 3 months after they had sustained hyperthermic seizures, hyperthermia alone, or normothermia. Both behavioral and hippocampal EEGs were monitored, to determine latencies to seizure onset, seizure duration, and both behavioral and EEG seizure severity. Basically, if kainic acid did not lead to (EEG and/or behavioral) seizures, continuous monitoring was performed for 3 hours. If prolonged seizures or status epilepticus resulted, animals were sacrificed after 1 hour allow harvesting of brains. Seizures were defined based on EEG criteria, namely, trains of rhythmic spikes or spike waves with increasing amplitude and decreasing frequency (in samples devoid of movement artifacts). They were confirmed and/or correlated to behavioral measures. Status epilepticus was defined as a prolonged (>30 minutes) and almost continuous series of seizures.

Following the experiments, rats were sacrificed and brains were examined for correct electrode placement as well as for preexisting lesions or those that could have resulted from the surgical manipulations. Because such lesions might alter either the EEG or the susceptibility to seizures, four animals with such lesions (three hemorrhagic infarcts, one hydrocephalus) were excluded, leading to the group sizes described above.

C. IN VIVO AND IN VITRO DETERMINATION OF THE EXCITABILITY OF THE LIMBIC CIRCUIT

To obtain a clearer understanding of the precise circuits and cellular mechanisms involved in the effects of complex febrile seizures on long-term limbic excitability, in vitro electrophysiology was carried out, using the hippocampal–entorhinal cortex (HEnC) slice preparation. [Preparation of the slices, modified from Rafiq et al. (1993, 1995) and Coulter et al. (1996), can be found in Dube et al. (2000).] Briefly, on postnatal days 17–18, rats that experienced hyperthermia-induced seizures and their littermate controls were anesthetized with halothane and decapitated, and their brains were removed and cooled in 4°C oxygenated sucrose artificial cerebral spinal fluid (ACSF). After 2 minutes of incubation, brain slices (450 mm) were sectioned along a 12° inclined transverse, yielding one to three slices per brain. The slices were then preincubated, submerged in 32°C oxygenated ACSF for a minimum of 1 hour. A reduced magnesium concentration of 0.5 mM, compared to a normal concentration of 1–2 mM, was employed to promote polysynaptic interactions. Following incubation, individual slices were placed in a recording chamber perfused with warmed ACSF (35°C) and humidified 95% O_2/5% CO_2; recordings were made using an Axopatch-200A amplifier (Axon Instruments, Foster City, CA), digitized at 88 kHz (Neurocorder, NeuroData, Delaware Water Gap, PA), then stored in pulse-code-modulated form. Stimulating electrodes were placed in the CA1 stratum radiatum, to generate a 2-second, 60-Hz train of stimuli to the Schaffer collaterals, with a pulse width of 100 μsec. Stimulus intensities were adjusted to four times the minimal intensity required to evoke a population spike of 0.5 mV (~3.5–5 mA). Stimulating trains were applied 10 times with a

10-minute interval, except when sustained epileptiform activity developed. The occurrence of sustained epileptiform activity was virtually an all-or-none event (lasting either >30 minutes or <1.5 minutes), so that data were not normally distributed and required nonparametric analysis (Mann–Whitney Rank Sum Test).

IV. CONSEQUENCES OF EXPERIMENTAL PROLONGED FEBRILE SEIZURES IN THIS MODEL

A. ADULT SPONTANEOUS SEIZURES

Hyperthermic seizures on postnatal day 10 did not result in spontaneous seizures later in life, as evident from both behavioral and *in vivo* electrophysiology analyses. In essence, EEGs from adult rats experiencing complex febrile seizures early in life were indistinguishable from those of the control groups, and neither electrographic nor behavioral spontaneous limbic seizures were noted.

B. ALTERATION OF LIMBIC EXCITABILITY

Early-life experimental complex febrile seizures in the rat model resulted in long-term alteration of limbic excitability *in vivo.* They significantly increased the susceptibility of these rats to develop severe and prolonged seizures in response to threshold doses of kainic acid. As shown in Figure 1, the low threshold dose of systemic kainic acid led to short, mild seizures in a minority of normothermic or hyperthermic control rats. Specifically, control rats developed transient hyperactivity interspersed with immobility after administration of the drug, and in most animals, no seizures developed during the 3-hour recording and monitoring session. When observed, the seizures in the control groups were short, lasting less than a minute. In contrast, all of the adult rats who had experienced prolonged febrile seizures early in life developed prolonged limbic seizures, and most went on to develop status epilepticus (Figure 1A). Thus, rats in the experimental group rapidly developed hyperactivity, immobility, and frank electrographic limbic seizures (Figure 1B). In addition, the latency to the development of these electrographic seizures was short, as typical for seizure induction by much higher (10–14 mg/kg) kainic acid doses (Sperk *et al.,* 1983; Cronin and Dudek, 1988). Finally, as would be expected for the effects of high doses of kainic acid, these seizures progressed to status epilepticus in 8 of 11 animals. The EEGs in Figure 1B are typical in that they demonstrate the almost all-or-none effect of kainic acid on experimental and control groups, respectively. Thus, kainic acid induced hippocampal spike and wave discharges that increased in duration with

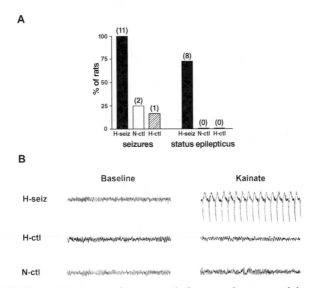

FIGURE 1   (A) Differential induction of seizures and of status epilepticus in adult rats by low-dose kainic acid as a function of prolonged hyperthermic seizures early in life. Three groups of adult rats were investigated: those experiencing prolonged hyperthermic seizures on postnatal days 10–11 (H-seiz; $n = 11$); a control group subjected to similar hyperthermia, but in which seizures were blocked (H-ctl; $n = 6$); and a control group kept normothermic (N-ctl; $n = 8$). Kainic acid led to seizures in all adult H-seiz animals and to status epilepticus in most, whereas only 2/8 and 1/6 of the normothermic and hyperthermic control groups, respectively, developed brief seizures. (B) Hippocampal EEGs from adult rats before (left) and 45 minutes after administration of low-dose (5 mg/kg) kainic acid (right). (Left) Normal EEGs in rats that had sustained hyperthermic seizures early in life (H-seiz), in hyperthermic controls in which early-life seizures were prevented (H-ctl), and in normothermic controls (N-ctl). (Right) Differential effects of low doses of kainic acid in these groups. Prolonged trains of spikes (top), leading to status epilepticus, developed in H-seiz animals (8/11), whereas the EEG remained normal in the large majority of hyperthermic and normothermic controls. Calibration: vertical, 1 mV; horizontal, 1 second. [Modified from C. Dube, K. Chen, M. Eghbal-Ahmadi, K. Brunson, I. Soltesz, and T. Z. Baram (2000). Prolonged febrile seizures in the immature rat model enhance hippocampal excitability long term. *Ann Neurol.* 47, 336–344, with permission.]

time. In addition, it should be emphasized that this experimental design distinguished between the effects of hyperthermia and of hyperthermic seizures. This is essential, because hyperthermia per se may exacerbate glutamate-mediated neuronal injury at least in adult brain (Liu *et al.*, 1993).

C. IN VITRO EVIDENCE FOR INCREASED EXCITABILITY IN THE LIMBIC CIRCUIT

Early-life complex febrile seizures in the rat model resulted in a long-term increase of excitability of the hippocampal–entorhinal cortex circuit *in vitro*. In

224 Celine Dube

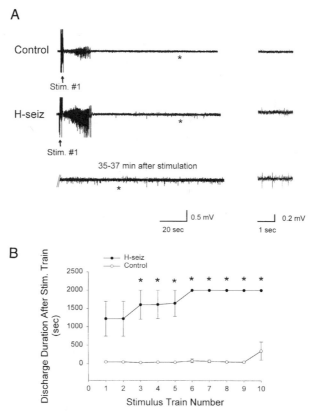

FIGURE 2 Epileptiform activity that was recurrent and self-sustaining was evoked by repeated stimulus trains only in hippocampal–entorhinal cortex slices derived from animals who had experienced hyperthermic seizures 1 week before the experiment (experimental, H-seiz), but not in slices from control littermates. (A) Tracings recorded from the CA1 pyramidal cell layer from slices of a control rat compared with those derived from an experimental animal. Beyond the immediate after-discharge, no spontaneous epileptiform activity followed the first stimulus train in the control slice. In contrast, the first stimulus train evoked recurrent, self-sustaining field discharges in the H-seiz slice that usually lasted for the duration of the experiment (>30 minutes). Tracing segments from the time points indicated by the asterisks are depicted in an expanded time scale on the right. (B) A plot of the number of the stimulation train of the Schaffer collaterals against the duration of the after-discharge evoked by the train. Again, the HEnC slices from the experimental (H-seiz) rats were far more prone to prolonged discharges, compared to controls. Tracings were obtained for 30 minutes (1800 seconds), the maximal duration plotted on the graph (control, $n = 4$; H-seiz, $n = 5$). [Modified from C. Dube, K. Chen, M. Eghbal-Ahmadi, K. Brunson, I. Soltesz, and T. Z. Baram (2000). Prolonged febrile seizures in the immature rat model enhance hippocampal excitability long term. *Ann Neurol.* 47, 336–344, with permission.]

essence, HEnC slices from both control and experimental rats did not manifest spontaneous abnormal activity. However, whereas control slices did not develop longer duration, self-sustaining activity even after repeated stimulus trains, a 2-second, 60-Hz train stimulation of the Schaffer collaterals triggered not only a short (20–70 seconds) after-discharge, but often prolonged, self-sustaining epileptiform activity, lasting for the duration of the experiment (>30 minutes). This was evident with the first (Figure 2A) or after a few stimulus trains. This self-sustaining epileptiform field discharge activity was evident in CA1 (Figure 2), as well as in other regions of the slice, including CA3 and dentate gyrus (not shown).

V. FUNCTIONAL CONSEQUENCES OF FEBRILE SEIZURES

What do these *in vivo* and *in vitro* data indicate about the functional consequences of experimental complex febrile seizures in the immature rat model? First, they clearly demonstrate that a single, prolonged febrile seizure does not lead to epilepsy, i.e., spontaneous recurrent unprovoked seizures. However, the hippocampal circuit of animals experiencing these seizures early in life was no longer "normal." Indeed, the limbic circuit, both *in vivo* and *in vitro*, was far less stable, and prone to excitatory input of either chemical or electrical nature. These alterations in excitability of the hippocampal network may thus be considered proepileptogenic.

Although long-term changes in neuronal excitability have been demonstrated after many (25) recurrent seizures in the immature rat (Holmes *et al.*, 1998), these changes have rarely been shown with a single seizure of limited duration. In addition, unlike chemical or electrical models of seizures early in life, the experimental approach used here has the advantage of approximating the scenario of early-life febrile seizures. In this context, it should be noted that none of the effects of the febrile seizures could be attributed to the hyperthermia per se. The hyperthermic control group, i.e., adult rats exposed to hyperthermia early in life, but in whom seizures were prevented using barbiturates, demonstrated a sensitivity to the low dose of kainic acid that was quite similar to that of the normothermic control group (16 and 25%, respectively). This clearly indicates that hyperthermic seizures, and not the actual rise in brain and core temperature, were the cause of these changes.

It should be noted that the duration of the hyperthermic seizures in this study (21.5 ± 0.9 minutes) was relatively long compared with that of most febrile seizures in the human: the vast majority of febrile seizures last less than 10 minutes, and only 6–7% last longer than 15 minutes (Nelson and Ellenberg, 1976; Offringa, 1994). Thus, seizures in this model may be considered prolonged or complex. Indeed, it is these prolonged seizures in the human that have been associated with subsequent temporal lobe epilepsy (French *et al.*, 1993; Cendes *et al.*, 1993; Theodore *et al.*, 1999; Harvey *et al.*, 1995).

VI. MECHANISMS FOR THE ENHANCED EXCITABILITY AFTER PROLONGED EXPERIMENTAL FEBRILE SEIZURES

Specific changes in select currents and neurotransmitters involved in the modulation of the hippocampal circuit in this model are described in Chapter 14. Single-cell electrophysiological studies *in vitro* revealed that hippocampi from animals experiencing hyperthermic seizures on postnatal days 10–11 were distinguished by a selective presynaptic increase in inhibitory synaptic transmission. These changes were clearly established by a week following the seizures, and lasted into adulthood (Chen *et al.*, 1999). They indicate a novel GABAergic mechanism for the altered inhibition/excitation balance that is specific to the early-life hyperthermic seizure (Chen *et al.*, 1999). The single-cell recording indicated enhanced release of the inhibitory neurotransmitter GABA after the hyperthermic seizures. Subsequent data, described in Chapter 14, provide the clue to the transformation of this apparent enhancement of inhibitory drive into enhanced excitability, as shown here both *in vitro* and *in vivo*.

Indeed, the strength of the data shown here derives from the fact that the changes observed occurred both *in vitro*, allowing precise analysis of the molecular mechanisms involved, and *in vivo*, validating the significance of these changes in the whole organism. Thus, in the hippocampal–entorhinal cortex slice preparation that encompasses the principal components of the limbic circuit (Rafiq *et al.*, 1993, 1995), prolonged hyperthermia-induced seizures in the immature rat promoted self-sustaining status epilepticus-like activity in response to electrical stimulation. These results correlated well with the enhanced potency of chemical stimulation (activation of glutamate receptors by kainic acid), as demonstrated *in vivo*. Thus, the combined data indicate that prolonged febrile seizures in the immature rat model increase the probability of hippocampal seizure induction later in life. However, because spontaneous seizures did not develop, we conclude that these seizures did not result in epilepsy. In other words, febrile seizures in this model constitute a *required* but not a *sufficient* step in a multistage process by which such seizures contribute to the development of an epileptic limbic circuit.

As is the case for all extrapolations from rodent models to the human situation, great caution is required in interpreting the results presented here in perspective with the clinical arena. In addition, it is fully recognized that hyperthermia may not fully replicate the setting of a febrile illness in an infant or child. Nevertheless, application of these results may provide insight into mechanisms of human epileptogenesis. Thus, it is considered that in analogy to the finding in the immature rat, human prolonged febrile seizures may enhance excitability and susceptibility to further limbic seizures. This may facilitate the development of epilepsy in the event of additional excitatory insults (which would be analogous to the electrical stimulation or the kainic acid administration used here).

It should also be considered that the experiments described here were based on "normal" immature rats with "normal" brains, and that seizures were induced by hyperthermia in virtually all animals. However, in the setting of a previously injured or genetically compromised central nervous system, when a previous proexcitant event had already occurred, the results of prolonged febrile seizures may differ, as discussed in Chapter 10. In this predisposed brain, prolonged febrile seizures might be sufficient to complete the epileptogenic process.

VII. SUMMARY

Evidence from both *in vivo* and *in vitro* studies argues for long-term alterations in limbic excitability caused by prolonged early-life febrile seizures in the immature rat model. Spontaneous seizures did not occur during adulthood, and spontaneous neuronal activity in hippocampal EEGs or in slice recordings were unaltered; therefore, these early-life prolonged experimental febrile seizures, by themselves, did not lead to epilepsy in the setting of a normal limbic circuit. However, the profound and persistent changes in excitability in these animals resulted in overall increased propensity to the generation of limbic seizures. This may be a first and critical step in the epileptogenic process.

REFERENCES

Albala, B. J., Moshe, S. L., and Okada, R. (1984). Kainic acid-induced seizures: A developmental study. *Brain Res.* 315, 139–148.

Baram, T. Z., Hirsch, E., Snead, O. C. III, and Schultz, L. (1992). Corticotropin-releasing hormone-induced seizures in infant rats originate in the amygdala. *Ann. Neurol.* 31, 488–494.

Baram, T. Z., Gerth, A., and Schultz, L. (1997). Febrile seizures: An age appropriate model. *Dev. Brain Res.* 246, 134–143.

Ben-Ari, Y., Tremblay, E., Riche, D., Ghilini, G., and Naquet, R. (1981). Electrographic, clinical and pathological alterations following systemic administration of kainic acid, bicuculline or pentetrazole: Metabolic mapping using the deoxyglucose method with special reference to the pathology of epilepsy. *Neuroscience* 6, 1361–1391.

Cendes, F., Andermann, F., Dubeau, F., Gloor, P., Evans, A., Jones-Gotman, M., Olivier, A., Andermann, E., Robitaille, Y., and Lopes-Cendes, I. (1993). Early childhood prolonged febrile convulsions, atrophy and sclerosis of mesial structures, and temporal lobe epilepsy: An MRI volumetric study. *Neurology* 43, 1083–1087.

Chen, K., Baram, T. Z., and Soltesz, I. (1999). Febrile seizures in the developing brain modify neuronal excitability in limbic circuits. *Nature Med.* 5, 888–894.

Cherubini, E., De Feo, M. R., Mecarelli, O., and Ricci, G. F. (1983). Behavioral and electrographic patterns induced by systemic administration of kainic acid in developing rats. *Brain Res.* 285, 69–77.

Commission on Classification and Terminology of the International League Against Epilepsy (1981). Proposal for revised clinical and electroencephalographic classification of epileptic seizures. *Epilepsia* **22**, 489–501.

Coulter, D. A., Rafiq, A., Shumate, M., Gong, Q. Z., DeLorenzo, R. J., and Lyeth, B. G. (1996). Brain injury-induced enhanced limbic epileptogenesis: Anatomical and physiological parallels to an animal model of temporal lobe epilepsy. *Epilepsy Res.* **26**, 81–91.

Cronin, J., and Dudek, F. E. (1988). Chronic seizures and collateral spouting of dentate mossy fibers after kainic acid treatment in rats. *Brain Res.* **474**, 181–184.

Dube, C., Chen, K., Eghbal-Ahmadi, M., Brunson, K., Soltesz, I., and Baram, T. Z. (2000). Prolonged febrile seizures in the immature rat model enhance hippocampal excitability long term. *Ann. Neurol.* **47**, 336–344.

Falconer, M. A., Serafetinides, E. A., and Corsellis, J.A.N. (1964). Etiology and pathogenesis of temporal lobe epilepsy. *Arch. Neurol.* **10**, 233–248.

French, J. A., Williamson, P. D., Thadani, V. M., Darcey, T. M., Mattson, R. H., Spencer, S. S., and Spencer, D. D. (1993). Characteristics of medial temporal lobe epilepsy. I. Results of history and physical examination. *Ann. Neurol.* **34**, 774–780.

Gottlieb, A., Keydar, Y., and Epstein, H. T. (1977). Rodent brain growth stages: An analytical review. *Biol. Neonate* **32**, 166–176.

Haas, K. Z., Sperber, E. F., and Moshe, S. L. (1990). Kindling in developing animals: Expression of severe seizures and enhanced development of bilateral foci. *Dev. Brain Res.* **56**, 275–280.

Harvey, A. S., Grattan-Smith, J. D., Desmond, P. M., Chow, C. W., and Berkovic, S. F. (1995). Febrile seizures and hippocampal sclerosis: Frequent and related findings in intractable temporal lobe epilepsy of childhood. *Pediatr. Neurol.* **12**, 201–206.

Hauser, W. A. (1994). The prevalence and incidence of convulsive disorders in children. *Epilepsia* **35**, (Suppl. 2), S1–S6.

Holmes, G. L., and Thompson, J. L. (1988). Effects of kainic acid on seizure susceptibility in the developing brain. *Dev. Brain Res.* **39**, 51–59.

Holmes, G. L., Gairsa, J. L., Chevassus-Au-Louis, N., and Ben-Ari, Y. (1998). Consequences of neonatal seizures in the rat: Morphological and behavioral effects. *Ann. Neurol.* **44**, 845–857.

Ikonomidou-Turski, C., Cavalheiro, E. A., Turski, W. A., Bortolotto, Z. A., and Turski, L. (1987). Convulsant action of morphine, [D-Ala^2, D-Leu^5]-enkephalin and naloxone in the rat amygdala: Electroencephalographic, morphological and behavioral sequelae. *Neuroscience* **20**, 671–686.

Jackson, G. D., McIntosh, A. M., Briellmann, R. S., and Berkovic, S. F. (1998). Hippocampal sclerosis studied in identical twins. *Neurology* **51**, 78–84.

Lewis, D. V. (1999). Febrile convulsions and mesial temporal sclerosis. *Curr. Opin. Neurol.* **12**, 197–201.

Liu, Z., Gatt, A., Mikati, M., and Holmes, G. L. (1993). Effect of temperature on kainic acid-induced seizures. *Brain Res.* **631**, 51–58.

Nelson, K. B., and Ellenberg, J. H. (1976). Predictors of epilepsy in children who have experienced febrile seizures. *N. Engl. J. Med.* **295**, 1029–1033.

Offringa, M., Bossuyt, P. M., Ellenberg, J. H., Nelson, K. B., Knudsen, F. U., Annegers, J. F., el-Radhi, A. S., Habbema, J. D., Derksen-Lubsen, G., *et al.* (1994). Risk factors for seizure recurrence in children with febrile seizures: A pooled analysis of individual patient data from five studies. *J. Pediatr.* **124**, 574–584.

Rafiq, A., DeLorenzo, R. J., and Coulter, D. A. (1993). Generation and propagation of epileptiform discharges in a combined entorhinal cortex/hippocampal slice. *J. Neurophysiol.* **70**, 1962–1974.

Rafiq, A., Zhang, Y. F., DeLorenzo, R. J., and Coulter, D. A. (1995). Long-duration self-sustained epileptiform activity in the hippocampal-parahippocampal slice: A model of status epilepticus. *J. Neurophysiol.* **74**, 2028–2042.

Sagar, H. J., and Oxbury, J. M. (1987). Hippocampal neuron loss in temporal lobe epilepsy: Correlation with early childhood convulsions. *Ann. Neurol.* **22**, 334–340.

Shinnar, S. (1990). Febrile seizures. *In* "Current Therapy in Neurological Disease" (R. T. Johnson, ed.), pp. 29–32. Decker, Philadelphia.

Shinnar, S. (1998). Prolonged febrile seizures and medial temporal sclerosis. *Ann. Neurol.* **43**, 411–412.

Sperk, G., Lassmann, H., Baran, H., Kish, S. J., Seitelberger, F., and Hornykiewicz, O. (1983). Kainic acid-induced seizures: Neurochemical and histopathological changes. *Neuroscience* **10**, 1301–1315.

Theodore, W. H., Bhatia, S., Hatta, J., Fazilat, S., DeCarli, C., Bookheimer, S. Y., and Gaillard, W. D. (1999). Hippocampal atrophy, epilepsy duration, and febrile seizures in patients with partial seizures. *Neurology* **52**, 132–136.

Toth, Z., Yan, X. X., Haftoglou, S., Ribak, C. E., and Baram, T. Z. (1998). Seizure-induced neuronal injury: Vulnerability to febrile seizures in immature rat model. *J. Neurosci.* **18**, 4285–4294.

Verity, C. M., Butler, N. R., and Golding, J. (1985). Febrile convulsions in a national cohort followed up from birth. I. Prevalence and recurrence in the first five years of life. *Br. Med. J.* **290**, 1307–1310.

CHAPTER 16

Basic Electrophysiology of Febrile Seizures

ROBERT S. FISHER* AND JIE WU[†]

*Department of Neurology, Stanford University School of Medicine, Stanford, California 94305, and [†]Department of Neurology, Barrow Neurological Institute/St. Joseph's Hospital and Medical Center, Phoenix, Arizona 85013

Temperature affects multiple processes in brain relevant to brain excitability, and no one simple mechanism is likely to account for febrile seizures. Possible mechanisms range from effects on ion channels to effects on complex networks giving rise to seizures. Kinetics of sodium and calcium ion channel activation and deactivation change so as to increase excitability of tissue. Action potentials narrow with increasing temperature, which could enhance excitation or inhibition, depending on underlying circuitry. Few studies have looked at changes in synaptic potentials with hyperthermia; however, excitatory postsynaptic potentials (EPSPs) are altered in the hippocampal slice model system and so is paired-pulse inhibition. Post-burst after-hyperpolarizations, generated by outward potassium currents in response to inward calcium currents, decrease with higher temperature. Hyperpolarizing sodium–potassium pumps are temperature-sensitive, decreasing with cooling, but information is not available as to whether the pumps are altered in hyperthermia.

Neurotransmitter systems change in complex ways with temperature. Activity of glutamic acid decarboxylase, the synthetic enzyme for GABA, decreases considerably with increased temperature. A variety of other potentially excitatory effects of temperature are observed on glutamate, acetylcholine, opiates, serotonin, and vasopressin neurotransmitter systems.

Febrile seizures have been linked to several different genes, some of which code for ion channels. It therefore is reasonable to consider that functional disturbances of ion balance may underlie some febrile seizures. One such functional disturbance is spreading depression. Experiments in hippocampal slices from young rats demonstrate that hyperthermia consistently provokes spreading depressions. These are accompanied by negative DC shifts and large increases in extracellular potassium activity. During the depolarizing phase of the spreading depression, neurons generate synchronous bursting. Whether clinical febrile seizures involve a component of spreading depression will await further studies in whole animal neural systems.

Behavioral and electroencephalographic febrile seizures can be modeled in the laboratory by artificial heating techniques applied to a rat or guinea pig. Hyperthermic seizures in young rats have been shown to alter long-term brain excitability, perhaps challenging the clinical impression of their benign long-term course. Given the high incidence of febrile seizures and their disturbing nature, it is to be hoped that they will become the subject of much more intense physiological investigation in the future. © 2002 Academic Press.

I. INTRODUCTION

Mammals maintain their body temperature within a narrow range. One possible reason for the survival advantage conferred by temperature regulation is avoidance of physiological dysfunction that can result from temperatures that are either too low or too high. Febrile seizures are an example of an age-specific disorder resulting from excess temperature. Because many processes in the brain are affected by temperature, it is difficult to speculate as to which ones might be involved in febrile seizures. Table 1 presents a nonexclusive list of neurophysiological properties dependent in part on temperature.

The difficulty arises not in showing a temperature dependence of various physiological properties, but in knowing the relevance of such changes to the physiology of clinical febrile seizures. As a starting point, we will consider what is known about how increased temperature affects excitability of brain tissue. It is worth mentioning in passing that a considerable body of literature also exists on the effects of cooling, which usually reduces brain excitability (Lundgren et al., 1994; Vastola et al., 1969). Discussion of the effects of cooling is beyond the scope of this chapter.

TABLE 1 Neuronal Processes Sensitive to Temperature

Passive membrane properties

Action potential

Transmitter release

Transmitter uptake

Channel kinetics

Extracellular diffusion

Metabolic pumps

Long-term potentiation

Neuronal survival

Neuronal synchrony

II. NEURONAL PROCESSES SENSITIVE TO TEMPERATURE

A. CHANNEL KINETICS

Ion fluxes through neuronal channels underlie changes in neuronal excitability. Evidence now is accumulating that certain familial febrile seizures represent channelopathies. The syndrome known as "generalized epilepsy with febrile seizures plus" (GEFS+) (Scheffer and Berkovic, 1997) is associated with a sodium channel deficit (Wallace *et al.*, 1998). GEFS+, type 1, is linked to chromosome 19q13, resulting in a mutation in the β1 subunit of the voltage-gated sodium channel (Alekov *et al.*, 2000). The type 2 GEFS+ mutation affects the α subunit of the sodium channel (Alekov *et al.*, 2000). The change in channel function in the type 2 mutation results in a 50% delay in sodium inactivation. This change could imbalance a neuronal network and cause seizures.

Kinetics of ion channel opening and closing can change with environmental variables, including temperature (Bernardi *et al.*, 1994; Petracchi *et al.*, 1994; Silver *et al.*, 1996). An interesting example can be found in studies of locust neurons (Ramirez *et al.*, 1999). Locusts cannot fly well in the heat. A heat shock almost immediately alters membrane properties of locust ganglion neurons such that outward neuronal potassium currents inactivate rapidly. Action potentials then become broader and disrupt the precise neuronal circuitry involved in driving wing movements.

In bullfrog sympathetic neurons, whole-cell calcium currents increased about 60% when temperature was increased from 20 to 30°C (van Lunteren *et al.*, 1993). In chick cultured dorsal root ganglion neurons, high voltage-activated, dihydropyridine-sensitive calcium currents increased with increased temperature (Acerbo and Nobile, 1994). The rise phase of the calcium current became faster, with less of an effect on the decay phase of the current. A non-dihydropyridine-sensitive calcium current in this same system showed increase of both activation and inactivation to increased temperature. Therefore, different ionic currents in the same system may demonstrate heterogeneous responses to hyperthermia.

Mathematical models can simulate excitatory postsynaptic currents, and the effects of temperature. Wahl and colleagues (1996) simulated excitatory postsynaptic currents by modeling release of 4000 neurotransmitter molecules simultaneously from a point source centered 15 nm above a rectangular grid of 196 postsynaptic receptors. The channel "open" probability can be plotted as a function of time after neurotransmitter release. When temperature was changed from 22 to 37°C, the rise time from 10 to 90% of peak open probability declined from 0.28 to 0.07 msec, the peak open probability increased from 0.27 to 0.56, and the decay time constant decreased from 2.33 to 0.70 millisec. The net effect of heat in the model was to lower the peak open probability, but maintain excitatory postsynaptic currents for a longer interval of time. Rate constants for opening and decay of channels play greater roles at low concentrations of neu-rotransmitter (Trussel and Fischbach 1989).

B. The Action Potential

Effects of temperature on action potentials are known to all electromyogra-phers. Limbs must be near normal temperature to accurately measure conduc-tion velocity in the nerves. During warming of a peripheral nerve from 18 to 36°C, nerve conduction velocity increases and synchrony of firing increases (Franssen and Wieneke, 1994).

The depolarizing phase of the action potential is dominated by increased sodi-um conductance through the voltage-dependent sodium channel. Repolariza-tion occurs when the sodium channel "gates" begin to swing shut, and when the delayed inward rectifier potassium current causes influx of positive potassium ions. Increased heat affects the opening of the sodium gates, but less so the potas-sium and sodium inactivation processes. The net result is narrowing of the ac-tion potential (Figure 1). In itself, it is impossible to predict whether this would be epileptogenic or antiepileptogenic, because it would be highly dependent on the details of circuitry in which a particular set of action potentials was involved. However, 4-aminopyridine, which blocks certain types of potassium currents, causes broadening of the action potentials, and can lead to seizures.

Hibernating animals, such as hamsters, increase body temperature at the end of hibernation. Hypothalamic neurons in hibernators are intrinsically suscep-tible to temperature variations. For such neurons, temperature is a signal to indicate time for hibernation. Hypothalamic neurons are less sensitive in non-hibernating species (Shen and Schwartzkroin, 1988). Sensitivity is additional-ly a function of age. Rewarming hippocampal slices from hamsters produced

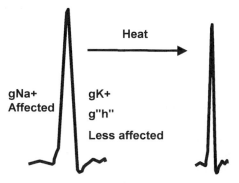

FIGURE 1 Schematic of effect of increased temperature on the action potential. The sodium gate current, gNa+, is more affected than in gK+, the delayed rectifier current, or g"h," the inactivation of the sodium current. The net result is a narrower action potential.

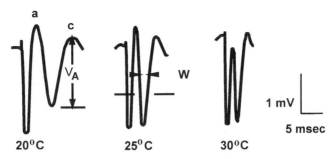

FIGURE 2   Population spikes in the hippocampus at different temperatures. Adapted from Eckerman *et al.* (1990). *Am J. Physiol.* **258**, R1140–R1146, with permission.

a decreased population spike amplitude (Gabriel *et al.*, 1998). Rats showed a biphasic effect on warming, with decrease of the population spike, followed by an increase. The decrease was mediated by adenosine because adenosine blockers reversed the depression (Masino and Dunwiddie, 1999).

Extracellular recordings from region CA1 of *in vitro* hippocampus demonstrate population spikes (Figure 2), which are known to reflect synchronous action potentials in a very densely packed region of neurons. Increasing temperature from 20 to 30°C in a hamster hippocampal slice leads to narrowing of the population spikes evoked by shocking afferent fibers (Eckerman *et al.*, 1990). This finding is consistent with the prior findings in action potentials measured in isolation.

C. Synaptic Potentials

Little information is available on temperature dependence of synaptic potentials. Schiff and Somjen (1985) compared synaptic potential sizes at 29, 33, and 37°C in the submerged hippocampal slice. At 33°C, population spikes and excitatory postsynaptic potentials (EPSPs) were increased in amplitude. At 37°C, population spikes disappeared, but paradoxically the EPSP increased. This finding was believed by the authors to be consistent with cell hyperpolarization, moving the EPSP away from its equilibrium potential and thereby increasing its amplitude, while simultaneously moving the membrane potential below action potential threshold. Hyperpolarization can occur as a consequence of hypoxia (Hyllienmark and Brismar, 1999), so relative hypoxia in the submerged slice at high temperature could play a role in these findings.

Inhibition can be studied via extracellular recordings in the hippocampus using the paired-pulse method. If a stimulating pulse is followed by a second pulse delivered 20–50 msec after the first, the second pulse is smaller because of recurrent inhibition generated by the first pulse. Hyperthermia decreased this so-called paired-pulse inhibition in region CA1 of the hippocampus in urethane-

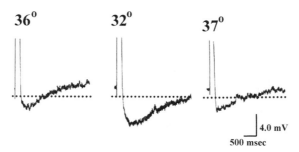

36° 32° 37°

4.0 mV
500 msec

FIGURE 3   An after-hyperpolarization (AHP) is evoked in a neuron from a guinea pig hippocampal slice. The six evoked action potentials are truncated by the high gain. At higher temperatures, the AHP is smaller. [Adapted with permission from S. M. Thompson, L. M. Masukawa, and D. A. Prince (1985). *J. Neurosci.* **5**, 817–824. Copyright 1985 by the Society for Neuroscience.]

anesthetized rats (Liebregts *et al.*, 1999). However opposite effects were found in the dentate gyrus during hyperthermia.

Postburst after-hyperpolarizations are of key importance in regulating excitability of potentially epileptogenic circuits. Thompson *et al.* (1985) evaluated effects of temperature changes from 37 to 30°C on guinea pig hippocampal region CA1 neurons (Figure 3). The following properties were evident at higher temperature: decreased input resistance, decreased amplitude and duration of action potentials, decreased postburst after-hyperpolarizations, and decreased spike frequency adaptation. Similar findings occurred in the locust ganglion, in which raising the temperature from 10 to 40°C produced significant changes in action potentials (Burrows, 1989). These changes present a complex mix of both excitatory and inhibitory actions.

Field potential recordings from region CA1 of hippocampal slices harvested from 2- to 28-day-old Wistar rats showed epileptiform bursting at high bath temperatures (Tancredi *et al.*, 1992). No such bursting was seen in slices from animals older than 28 days.

Metabolic hyperpolarizing pumps provide another level of functional inhibition after extensive periods of neuronal excitation. Local application of glutamate to neurons induces a period of excitation and depolarization, followed by hyperpolarization. The hyperpolarization results from an energy-dependent sodium–potassium exchange pump that carries two potassium ions into the neurons for each three sodium ions extruded. Pump hyperpolarizations are attenuated when temperature is reduced from 37 to 32°C. Looked at conversely, hyperpolarization after excitation can be enhanced by higher temperature.

D. ELECTROLYTES

Hydrated ions carry currents in the brain, across neuronal membranes through channels, and along the axes of the extracellular matrix. Increased temperature has been associated with a variety of changes in ions and electrolytes. The usual experimental paradigm has been to compare serum or cerebrospinal fluid (CSF) concentration of an ion in children with and without febrile seizures. Findings vary with the nature of the control group, i.e., children with nonfebrile seizures or children with no history of seizures, and with the timing of the measurement in relation to the febrile seizure. In these circumstances a causative relationship can be difficult to establish, even with a strong correlation.

Fever produces a 3.5% decline ($p < 0.01$) in CSF sodium concentration and osmolality, and this decline stands at 3.8% among children who recently had a febrile seizure (Kivaranta et al., 1996). Therefore, water balance changes during febrile illness, but not differentially in children with or without febrile seizures. However, children with complicated or multiple febrile seizures have lower baseline sodium levels than do children with simple febrile convulsions (Kiviranta and Airaksinen, 1995). In a study of 69 children with a history of febrile convulsions, 52% had baseline levels less than 135 mM (Hugen et al., 1995). Lower sodium levels correlated with increased probability for having a subsequent febrile seizure. Low serum sodium in a setting of febrile seizures usually is a secondary phenomenon resulting from inappropriate secretion of antidiuretic hormone (Rutter and O'Callaghan, 1978).

Temperature also affects glucose levels. Fever increases CSF and blood glucose concentrations, but not differentially for children with and without febrile seizures (Kiviranta et al., 1995).

Zinc is an endogenous N-methyl-D-aspartate (NMDA) antagonist, so decreasing levels of zinc could activate NMDA receptors (Izumi et al., 1990). Zinc concentrations are enriched in the mossy fiber terminal fields of hippocampus, and may play a role in regulating excitability in this and other central nervous system (CNS) pathways. Serum and CSF zinc concentrations are about one-third lower in patients with febrile convulsions than in patients with meningitis or controls (Burhanoglu et al., 1996). In contrast, concentrations of serum and CSF copper, magnesium, and protein are not decreased in patients with febrile seizures. In children with febrile seizures, between seizures, zinc serum levels remain less than those of control children, but the discrepancy is not as pronounced as it is immediately after a febrile seizure (Gunduz et al., 1996). The correlation of low zinc levels and tendency toward febrile seizures is intriguing and worthy of prospective evaluation.

E. NEUROTRANSMITTERS

Modulations of neurotransmitter function play key roles in epileptogenesis and protection against seizures (Fisher and Coyle, 1991). Therefore, it is necessary to consider how a temperature increase might affect neurotransmitter systems.

γ-Aminobutyric acid (GABA) has been the most studied neurotransmitter pertaining to epilepsy. Several years ago, Loscher and associates (Loscher *et al.*, 1981) found lower CSF GABA in 23 children with febrile seizures, compared to 16 seizure-free controls. However, differences in subject ages can produce large differences in CSF GABA levels (Schmiegelow *et al.*, 1990). CSF GABA levels do not differ in age-matched children with febrile and afebrile seizures or in controls (Knight *et al.*, 1985; Rating *et al.*, 1983; Schmiegelow *et al.*, 1990).

GABA is synthesized by glutamic acid decarboxylase (GAD), which is a temperature-dependent enzyme. GAD activity can be estimated by observing the rate of transfer of $^{14}CO_2$ from glutamate to GABA in brain homogenates. When 2- to 5-day-old rats were subjected to hyperthermia, resulting in febrile seizures, brain homogenate GAD activity declined 37–48% (Arias *et al.*, 1992). Homogenates from 10- to 15-day-old rats, which did not seize in response to hyperthermia, showed no decline in GABA. By way of contrast, choline acetyltransferase and lactic dehydrogenase did not change after hyperthermic seizures. However, whole-brain GABA activity was not altered. GABA concentration in brain declines in response to hyperthermia (Morimoto *et al.*, 1990). One study produced hyperthermic seizures in young rats by heating brain with infrared radiation (Fukuda *et al.*, 1997). GABA antagonists lowered, and GABA agonists increased, the threshold for seizures. Although the authors conclude that "these results support the hypothesis that reduced GABAergic system activity underlies febrile seizures," it is possible that GABAergic alterations could alter expression of febrile seizures without being part of febrile seizure pathophysiology. Chen *et al.* (1999) observed increased GABAergic inhibition, consistent with increased GABAergic terminals, chronically after a hyperthermic seizure.

GABA manipulation provides a possible therapeutic approach to febrile seizures. The GABA agonists muscimol and progabide, and also valproic acid and γ-hydroxybutyric acid, all produced dose-dependent increases in latency to onset of microwave-provoked hyperthermic seizures (Pedder *et al.*, 1988). Elevation of brain GABA concentrations by the GABA transaminase metabolism inhibitor, vigabatrin, reduced hyperthermic seizures in epileptic chickens (Johnson *et al.*, 1985). Phenobarbital, which is an allosteric modulator of the GABA receptor, has been used for prophylaxis of clinical febrile seizures (Rantala *et al.*, 1997).

Glutamate is the primary excitatory neurotransmitter in the forebrain. Hyperthermia causes a rapid increase in the extracellular concentration of glutamate (Morimoto *et al.*, 1993). Glutamate activation of cortex via the NMDA receptor may play a role in genesis of febrile seizures. The noncompetitive NMDA-associated channel blocker, MK-801, causes a dose-dependent increase in the temperature required to produce a hyperthermic behavioral seizure in rats (Morimoto *et al.*, 1995). Both competitive and noncompetitive NMDA antagonists inhibit hyperthermic seizures in chicks (Pedder *et al.*, 1990).

Hyperthermia-induced convulsions in rats produce a complex pattern of changes on nicotinic and cholinergic acetylcholine (ACh) receptors (McCaughran *et al.*, 1984). Muscarinic receptors decreased in frontal cortex, but increased in cerebellum in the wake of a seizure. Synthetic and catabolic ACh enzymes both increased after a seizure. Immediately after a seizure produced by placing 15-day-old rat pups in 40°C ambient temperature (Carrillo *et al.*, 1992), brain methionine-enkephalin was elevated. CSF levels of the serotonin metabolite 5-hydroxyindoleacetic acid (5-HIAA) were reduced both at times 2 hours and 3–6 days after febrile seizures (Giroud *et al.*, 1990). This suggests that a decrease in 5-HIAA may be a marker for susceptibility to febrile convulsions. The lateral septal region of the hypothalamus produces an endogenous antipyretic, in the form of arginine vasopressin (Veale *et al.*, 1984). However, vasopressin is itself a potentially seizurogenic substance (Croiset and DeWeid, 1997; Veale *et al.*, 1984), and could in theory contribute to the genesis of a febrile seizure.

Benzodiazepines are a mainstay of emergency therapy for essentially any type of seizure. Hyperthermic seizures induced in 15-day-old rats alter hippocampal benzodiazepine binding and induce a long-term decrease in responsiveness to benzodiazepines (Chisholm *et al.*, 1985).

In summary, hyperthermia has not yet been shown to produce a dominant neurotransmitter change. Several changes, including reduction of GABA synthesis, increased extracellular concentrations of glutamate, reduction in serotonin, and release of hypothalamic vasopressin, could, however, contribute to a reduced seizure threshold during hyperthermia.

F. SPREADING DEPRESSION

Genetic studies of febrile seizures suggest that some forms of febrile seizures result from channelopathies. The "generalized epilepsy with febrile seizures plus" syndrome (Singh *et al.*, 1999) is associated with a mutation in the gene coding for a voltage-sensitive sodium channel (Wallace *et al.*, 1998). Ion channels control movement of ions across neuronal membranes. It therefore is reasonable to consider whether febrile seizures might result in part from loss of regulation of ionic homeostasis.

Spreading depression, first described by Leao (1986), represents a disturbance of control of potassium concentration in neuronal tissue. Normal extracellular potassium concentration is approximately 3 mM. During spreading depression the extracellular potassium concentration may increase 10-fold. Spreading depressions may be induced experimentally by potassium application to the brain, glutamate application, puffs of air to the brain, trauma, and a variety of other methods. In clinical practice, spreading depression has been hypothesized to be involved in the pathophysiology of migraine aura (Lauritzen,

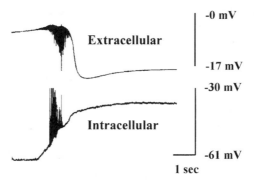

FIGURE 4   Spreading depression in a hippocampal slice from a 37-day-old rat, in response to bath temperature increase from 34.0 to 36.3°C. A massive depolarization results, with transient firing of the cell.

1994) and in mediation of postischemic neuronal injury (Nedergaard, 1996). The etiology and mechanism of spreading depression remain uncertain, but attention has focused on disturbances of the sodium–potassium pump that restores ion balance after neuronal excitation.

Our laboratory has investigated a possible role for spreading depression in the pathogenesis of febrile seizures (Wu and Fisher, 2000). We studied the effects of increased temperature on hippocampal slices from 53 rats that were 1 week to several months of age. Using the temperature control devices on the slice recording chamber, temperatures were raised from 34 to 40°C over 10–20 minutes. Temperature increase produced hyperthermic spreading depressions (Figure 4) in an age-dependent manner. We defined hyperthermic spreading depressions as at least a 10-mV depolarization and at least a 10 mM increase in extracellular potassium concentration, sustained for at least 10 seconds, and reversible within 30 minutes. Actual mean intracellular depolarization was 38.6 $\pm$ 0.2 mV ($n = 29$). Extracellular potassium activity rose from a mean baseline of 6.4 $\pm$ 0.2 mM to a mean peak of 43.8 $\pm$ 10.9 mM ($n = 6$, $p < 0.000001$). Mean duration of the spreading depression was 35.6 $\pm$ 4.0 seconds ($n = 29$).

The likelihood of temperature provoking a spreading depression was dependent on age of the animals from which the slice was harvested. Among animals 8–16 days old, 0 of 12 showed spreading depressions. In contrast, 29 of 30 rats 21–59 days old, and 8 of 12 in animals over 60 days of age, showed spreading depressions. This age dependence parallels the clinical tendency of febrile seizures to occur in children, although there is no direct numerical correlation between maturity in humans and rodents in this model, because rats are substantially mature by 1 month of age.

In our spreading depression hypothesis of febrile seizures, seizure activity

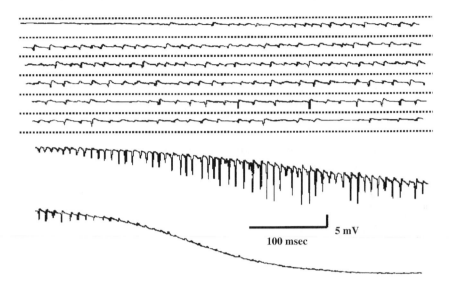

FIGURE 5   Spreading depression in a hippocampal slice from a 19-day-old rat, with a bath temperature increase to 39.5°C. The tracings show field recordings, recorded continuously line-to-line over a total time span of 5.9 seconds. Dotted lines portray the baseline extracellular voltage. A negative extracellular voltage shift occurs, with accompanying transient paroxysmal discharges.

occurs on the depolarizing phase of the spreading depression. When spreading depression is in full force, the high extracellular potassium concentration depolarizes neurons to the point of sodium channel inactivation. However, prior to that point of inactivation, neurons are transiently depolarized and excited.

Figure 5 illustrates an excitatory component of a hyperthermic spreading depression. The spreading depression can occur independent of bursting activity, because the sodium channel blocker tetrodotoxin prevents the epileptiform bursting without inhibiting the spreading depression.

We hypothesized the following sequence. Increased temperature accelerates the rates of many chemical reactions in the brain, thereby consuming more oxygen and high-energy phosphates. After a febrile seizure, there is evidence of intracellular glucose deficit and failure of electrolyte pumps, in the form of increased ketones, lactate, and uric acid (Aiyathurai *et al.*, 1989). As the energy substrates of the cell decline, the energy-dependent sodium–potassium pump fails and potassium exits the neurons. Accumulated extracellular potassium concentration transiently depolarizes and excites neurons. During this time, there is a seizure. Subsequent progression of the spreading depression then inhibits them by over-depolarization. During the latter phases of the hyperthermic spreading depression, the child would evidence postictal manifestations.

When energy is sufficiently repleated to reactivate the pump, balance and normal neuronal excitability is restored.

Applicability of *in vitro* slice data to the human condition of febrile seizures can be debated. Hippocampal slices are relatively hypoxic, and spreading depression might be a nonspecific response to hypoxia or injury in this preparation, rather than to a temperature increase. Nevertheless, the spreading depression hypothesis opens different avenues of thought for treatment of febrile seizures, because spreading depressions do not respond to the usual antiepileptic medications. A search for spreading depression-like events in live animal models of febrile seizures should help to judge the relevance of this hypothesis.

III. WHOLE-ANIMAL STUDIES OF HYPERTHERMIA

Data on membrane and synaptic properties will not necessarily give answers to the practical questions faced by clinicians, such as whether a febrile seizure predisposes to epilepsy, and whether treatment of febrile seizures is useful in preventing future epilepsy, issues considered elsewhere in this book. A more direct answer to such questions can be based on longitudinal study of animal models for febrile seizures, which have been available for at least 20 years (Holtzman *et al.*, 1981). Such animal models usually produce seizures by physically heating baby rats, via a variety of methods. Hyperthermic rats can have behavioral seizures, including myoclonus and generalized clonic convulsions, with associated EEG spikes, or rapid spike-wave bursts (Morimoto *et al.*, 1992; Dube *et al.*, 2000). Hyperthermic seizures often are preceded by long runs of high-voltage slow waves, analogous to EEG changes seen in clinical febrile seizures (Morimoto *et al.*, 1991).

Baby rats subject to hyperthermic seizures do not have spontaneous seizures as adults (Dube *et al.*, 2000). However, hyperthermic seizures alter susceptibility to later seizures, such as chemically induced seizures (McCaughran and Manetto, 1983). The reverse relationship also holds true: chemically induced seizures with pentylenetetrazol lower the threshold for induction of hyperthermic seizures (McCaughran and Manetto, 1983). Hippocampal slices from rats made hyperthermic in the first weeks of life show prolonged epileptiform discharges in response to chemical or electrical stimulation (Dube *et al.*, 2000).

Repeated hyperthermic seizures in 30-day-old rats can produce kindling-like long-term changes in brain excitability (Zhao *et al.*, 1985). Chen and colleagues (1999) found that febrile seizures induced in 10-day-old rats resulted in persistent hyperexcitability of limbic circuits for at least 9 weeks after the induced seizure (Figure 6 and Chapter 14). In this study, core temperature was raised to 41.0°C, by using warmed air. Approximately 98% of the animals developed

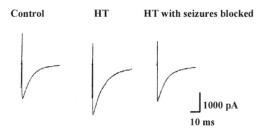

FIGURE 6   Intracellular potentials to afferent shock from hippocampal slices from controls and a 10-day-old rat made hyperthermic (HT) to 41.0°C a week before. Modified and reprinted with permission from K. Chen, T. Z. Baram, and I. Soltesz (1999). *Nature Med.*

acute tonic seizures. Hippocampal slices, harvested a week after the seizure, showed enhanced inhibitory postsynaptic potentials (IPSPs) in response to stimulation. The physiological significance of these IPSP changes, which would be expected to be anticonvulsant, remains open for interpretation (see also Chapter 14). However, it is interesting that a single hyperthermic seizure can have long-lasting effects on brain physiology.

The mechanisms of long-term excitability changes after hyperthermic seizures remain largely undefined. Prolonged febrile seizures in childhood have been argued to produce hippocampal cell loss (Sloviter, 1999; see also Toth *et al.*, 1998, and Chapter 9). Two hypotheses have been offered to explain excitability of subsequent hippocampal circuits. One posits the selective loss of inhibitory interneurons. The other hypothesis focuses on growth of aberrant excitatory connections. Sarkisian *et al.* (1999) raised the question of whether hyperthermia alone can affect excitability and histology of subsequent brain, or whether hyperthermia needed to be coupled with electrical stimulation of the tissue. Neither hyperthermia (Sarkisian *et al.*, 1999; Toth *et al.*, 1998) nor hyperthermia plus continuous hippocampal stimulation (Sarkisian *et al.*, 1999) produced histological changes in hippocampus. The group receiving continuous hippocampal stimulation, but not those receiving hypothermia alone, developed subsequent seizures. In this model, hyperthermic seizures did not lead to a mesial temporal sclerosis picture. However, when hyperthermia-induced seizures developed into status epilepticus, then neurodegeneration occurred in a pattern similar to that of mesial temporal sclerosis (Jiang *et al.*, 1999).

IV. CONCLUSION

Studies in simple systems demonstrate significant temperature dependence of ion channel kinetics, action potentials, excitatory postsynaptic currents, inhibitory postsynaptic potentials, postburst after-hyperpolarizing potentials, hyperpolarizations due to ionic pumps, and neurotransmitter systems. Changes resulting from these phenomena are both excitatory and inhibitory in varying circumstances. Additionally, effects of hypoxia may confound studies in isolated tissue explants, which could be more severe at higher temperatures. Consequently, no straightforward explanation for febrile seizure emerges from studies on simple systems.

Evaluation of temperature effects in mammalian brain is even more difficult than it is in isolated neuronal systems. Temperature dependence differs among different species, at different ages of experimental animals, and under different experimental conditions. Effects of seizures resulting from hyperthermia may be difficult to distinguish from primary effects of hyperthermia (see Chapter 15).

Rapid advances presently are being made in understanding the genetics of febrile seizures. Multiple genes appear to be involved in different families, again highlighting the diversity of mechanisms by which high temperature can influence brain excitability. At least some of these genes appear to code for ion channels. It is relatively plausible that disturbances of ionic balance—for example, loss of potassium control seen during spreading depression—may play a role in hyperthermic seizures.

Febrile seizures are the most common nonidiopathic type of seizure in the world, affecting from 3 to 6% of the world's children. Therefore, it is surprising that more is not known about the physiology of febrile seizures. Relatively recent development of suitable animal models and multidisciplinary physiological, neurochemical, and genetic studies may soon rectify this deficit of understanding.

ACKNOWLEDGMENTS

Dr. Fisher was supported by NIH Grant RO1 NS39344, by the Sandra Solheim Aiken Fund for Epilepsy, and by the James Anderson and Maslah Saul M.D. Research Fund. Dr. Wu was supported by the Womens' Board of the Barrow Neurological Institute.

REFERENCES

Acerbo, P., and Nobile, M. (1994). Temperature dependence of multiple high voltage activated Ca^{2+} channels in chick sensory neurones. *Eur. Biophys. J.* **23**, 189–195.

Aiyathurai, E. J., Low, P. S., and Jacob, E. (1989). Hyperpolarization and short-circuiting as mechanisms of seizure prevention following febrile convulsions. *Brain Dev.* **11**, 241–246.

Alekov, A., Rahman, M. M., Mitrovic, N., Lehmann-Horn, F., and Lerche, H. (2000). A sodium channel mutation causing epilepsy in man exhibits subtle defects in fast inactivation and activation *in vitro*. *J. Physiol.* **529**, 533–539.

Arias, C., Valero, H., and Tapia, R. (1992). Inhibition of brain glutamate decarboxylase activity is related to febrile seizures in rat pups. *J. Neurochem.* 58, 369–373.

Bernardi, P., D'Inzeo, G., and Pisa, S. (1994). A generalized ionic model of the neuronal membrane electrical activity. *IEEE Trans. Biomed. Eng.* 41, 125–133.

Burhanoglu, M., Tutuncuoglu, S., Coker, C., Tekgul, H., and Ozgur, T. (1996). Hypozincaemia in febrile convulsion. *Eur. J. Pediatr.* 155, 498–501.

Burrows, M. (1989). Effects of temperature on a central synapse between identified motor neurons in the locust. *J. Comp. Physiol.* 165, 687–695.

Carrillo, E., Fuente, T., and Laorden, M. L. (1992). Hyperthermia-induced seizures alter the levels of methionine-enkephalin in immature rat brain. *Neuropeptides* 21, 139–142.

Chen, K., Baram, T. Z., and Soltesz, I. (1999). Febrile seizures in the developing brain result in persistent modification of neuronal excitability in limbic circuits. *Nat. Med.* 5, 888–894.

Chisholm, J., Kellogg, C., and Franck, J. E. (1985). Developmental hyperthermic seizures alter adult hippocampal benzodiazepine binding and morphology. *Epilepsia* 26, 151–157.

Croiset, G., and DeWied, D. (1997). Proconvulsive effect of vasopressin; mediation by a putative V2 receptor subtype in the central nervous system. *Brain Res.* 759, 18–23.

Dube, C., Chen, K., Eghbal-Ahmadi, M., Brunson, K., Soltesz, I., and Baram, T. Z. (2000). Prolonged febrile seizures in the immature rat model enhance hippocampal excitability long term. *Ann. Neurol.* 47, 336–344.

Eckerman, P., Scharruhn, K., and Horowitz, J. M. (1990). Effects of temperature and acid–base state on hippocampal population spikes in hamsters. *Am. J. Physiol.* 258, R1140–R1146.

Fisher, R. S., and Coyle, J. T. (1991). "Neurotransmitters and Epilepsy: Frontiers of Clinical Neuroscience," Vol. 11, pp. 1–260. Wiley-Liss, New York.

Franssen, H., and Wieneke, G. H. (1994). Nerve conduction and temperature: Necessary warming time. *Muscle Nerve* 17, 336–344.

Fukuda, M., Morimoto, T., Nagao, H., and Kida, K. (1997). The effect of GABAergic system activity on hyperthermia-induced seizures in rats. *Brain Res. Dev. Brain Res.* 104, 197–199.

Gabriel, A., Klussmann, F. W., and Igelmund, P. (1998). Rapid temperature changes induce adenosine-mediated depression of synaptic transmission in hippocampal slices from rats (non-hibernators) but not in slices from golden hamsters (hibernators). *Neuroscience* 86, 67–77.

Giroud, M., Dumas, R., Dauvergne, M., D'Athis, P., Rochette, L., Beley, A., and Bralet, J. (1990). 5-Hydroxyindoleacetic acid and homovanillic acid in cerebrospinal fluid of children with febrile convulsions. *Epilepsia* 31, 178–181.

Gunduz, Z., Yavuz, I., Koparal, M., Kumandas, S., and Saraymen, R. (1996). Serum and cerebrospinal fluid zinc levels in children with febrile convulsions. *Acta Paediatr. Jpn.* 38, 237–241.

Holtzman, D., Obana, K., and Olson, J. (1981). Hyperthermia-induced seizures in the rat pup: A model for febrile convulsions in children. *Science* 213, 1034–1036.

Hugen, C. A., Oudesluys-Murphy, A. M., and Hop, W. C. (1995). Serum sodium levels and probability of recurrent febrile convulsions. *Eur. J. Pediatr.* 154, 403–405.

Hyllienmark, L., and Brismar, T. (1999). Effect of hypoxia on membrane potential and resting conductance in rat hippocampal neurons. *Neuroscience* 91, 511–517.

Izumi, Y., Ishii, K., Akiba, K., and Hayashi, T. (1990). Hypozincemia during fever may trigger febrile convulsion. *Med. Hypotheses* 32, 77–80.

Jiang, W., Duong, T. M., and de Lanerolle, N. C. (1999). The neuropathology of hyperthermic seizures in the rat. *Epilepsia* 40, 5–19.

Johnson, D. D., Wilcox, R., Tuchek, J. M., and Crawford, R. D. (1985). Experimental febrile convulsions in epileptic chickens: The anticonvulsant effect of elevated gamma-aminobutyric acid concentrations. *Epilepsia* 26, 466–471.

Kiviranta, T., and Airaksinen, E. M. (1995). Low sodium levels in serum are associated with subsequent febrile seizures. *Acta Paediatr.* 84, 1372–1374.

Kiviranta, T., Airaksinen, E. M., and Tuomisto, L. (1995). The role of fever on cerebrospinal fluid glucose concentration of children with and without convulsions. *Acta Paediatr.* **84**, 1276–1279.

Kiviranta, T., Tuomisto, L., and Airaksinen, E. M. (1996). Osmolality and electrolytes in cerebrospinal fluid and serum of febrile children with and without seizures. *Eur. J. Pediatr.* **155**, 120–125.

Knight, M., Ebert, J., Parish, R. A., Berry, H., and Fogelson, M. H. (1985). Gamma-aminobutyric acid in CSF of children with febrile seizures. *Arch. Neurol.* **42**, 474–475.

Lauritzen, M. (1994). Pathophysiology of the migraine aura. The spreading depression theory. *Brain* **117**, 199–210.

Leao, A. A. (1986). Spreading depression. *Funct. Neurol.* **1**, 363–366.

Liebregts, McLachlan, and Leung (1999). *Soc. Neurosci.* 643.9.

Loscher, W., Rating, D., and Siemes, H. (1981). GABA in cerebrospinal fluid of children with febrile convulsions. *Epilepsia* **22**, 697–702.

Lundgren, J., Smith, M. L., Blennow, G., and Siesjo, B. K. (1994). Hyperthermia aggravates and hypothermia ameliorates epileptic brain damage. *Exp. Brain. Res.* **99**, 43–55.

Masino, S. A., and Dunwiddie, T. V. (1999). Temperature-dependent modulation of excitatory transmission in hippocampal slices is mediated by extracellular adenosine. *J. Neurosci.* **19**, 1932–1939.

McCaughran, J. A. Jr., and Manetto, C. (1983). Potentiation of hyperthermia-induced convulsions in the developing rat by previous treatment with pentylenetetrazol. *Exp. Neurol.* **79**, 287–292.

McCaughran, J. A., Jr., Edwards, E., and Schechter, N. (1984). Experimental febrile convulsions in the developing rat: Effects on the cholinergic system. *Epilepsia* **25**, 250–258.

Morimoto, T., Nagao, H., Sano, N., Takahashi, M., and Matsuda, H. (1990). Hyperthermia-induced seizures with a servo system: Neurophysiological roles of age, temperature elevation rate and regional GABA content in the rat. *Brain Dev.* **12**, 279–283.

Morimoto, T., Nagao, H., Sano, N., Takahashi, M., and Matsuda, H. (1991). Electroencephalographic study of rat hyperthermic seizures. *Epilepsia* **32**, 289–293.

Morimoto, T., Yoshimatsu, M., Nagao, H., and Matsuda, H. (1992). Three types of hyperthermic seizures in rats. *Brain Dev.* **14**, 53–57.

Morimoto, T., Nagao, H., Yoshimatsu, M., Yoshida, K., and Matsuda, H. (1993). Pathogenic role of glutamate in hyperthermia-induced seizures. *Epilepsia* **34**, 447–452.

Morimoto, T., Kida, K., Nagao, H., Yoshida, K., Fukuda, M., and Takashima, S. (1995). The pathogenic role of the NMDA receptor in hyperthermia-induced seizures in developing rats. *Brain Res. Dev. Brain Res.* **84**, 204–207.

Nedergaard, M. (1996). Spreading depression as a contributor to ischemic brain damage. *Adv. Neurol.* **71**, 75–83.

Pedder, S. C., Wilcox, R., Tuchek, J., Johnson, D. D., and Crawford, R. D. (1988). Protection by GABA agonists, gamma-hydroxybutyric acid, and valproic acid against seizures evoked in epileptic chicks by hyperthermia. *Epilepsia* **29**, 738–742.

Pedder, S. C., Wilcox, R. I., Tuchek, J. M., Johnson, D. D., and Crawford, R. D. (1990). Attenuation of febrile seizures in epileptic chicks by N-methyl-D-aspartate receptor antagonists. *Can. J. Physiol. Pharmacol.* **68**, 84–88.

Petracchi, D., Pellegrini, M., Pellegrino, M., Barbi, M., and Moss, F. (1994). Periodic forcing of a K^+ channel at various temperatures. *Biophys. J.* **66**, 1844–1852.

Ramirez, J. M., Elsen, F. P., and Robertson, R. M. (1999). Long-term effects of prior heat shock on neuronal potassium currents recorded in a novel insect ganglion slice preparation. *J. Neurophysiol.* **81**, 795–802.

Rantala, H., Tarkka, R., and Uhari, M. (1997). A meta-analytic review of the preventive treatment of recurrences of febrile seizures. *J. Pediatr.* **131**, 922–925.

Rating, D., Siemes, H., and Loscher, W. (1983). Low CSF GABA concentration in children with febrile convulsions, untreated epilepsy, and meningitis. *J. Neurol.* **230**, 217–225.

Rutter, N., and O'Callaghan, M. J. (1978). Hyponatraemia in children with febrile convulsions. *Arch. Dis. Child.* 53, 85–87.

Sarkisian, M. R., Holmes, G. L., Carmant, L., Liu, Z., Yang, Y., and Stafstrom, C. E. (1999). Effects of hyperthermia and continuous hippocampal stimulation on the immature and adult brain. *Brain Dev.* 21, 318–325.

Scheffer, I. E., and Berkovic, S. F. (1997). Generalized epilepsy with febrile seizures plus. A genetic disorder with heterogeneous clinical phenotypes. *Brain* 120, 479–490.

Schiff, S. J., and Somjen, G. G. (1985). The effects of temperature on synaptic transmission in hippocampal tissue slices. *Brain Res.* 345, 279–284.

Schmiegelow, K., Johnsen, A. H., Ebbesen, F., Mortensen, T., Berg, A. M., Thorn, I., Skov, L., Ostergaard, J. R., and Sorensen, O. (1990). Gamma-aminobutyric acid concentration in lumbar cerebrospinal fluid from patients with febrile convulsions and controls. *Acta Paediatr. Scand.* 79, 1092–1098.

Shen, K. F., and Schwartzkroin, P. A. (1988). Effects of temperature alterations on population and cellular activities in hippocampal slices from mature and immature rabbit. *Brain Res.* 475, 305–316.

Silver, R. A., Cull-Candy, S. G., and Takahashi, T. (1996). Non-NMDA glutamate receptor occupancy and open probability at a rat cerebellar synapse with single and multiple release sites. *J. Physiol.* 494, 231–250.

Singh, R., Scheffer, I. E., Crossland, K., and Berkovic, S. F. (1999). Generalized epilepsy with febrile seizures plus: A common childhood- onset genetic epilepsy syndrome. *Ann. Neurol.* 45, 75–81.

Sloviter, R. S. (1999). Status epilepticus-induced neuronal injury and network reorganization. *Epilepsia* 40(Suppl. 1),S34–S39.

Tancredi, V., D'Arcangelo, G., Zona, C., Siniscalchi, A., and Avoli, M. (1992). Induction of epileptiform activity by temperature elevation in hippocampal slices from young rats: An *in vitro* model for febrile seizures? *Epilepsia* 33, 228–234.

Thompson, S. M., Masukawa, L. M., and Prince, D. A. (1985). Temperature dependence of intrinsic membrane properties and synaptic potentials in hippocampal CA1 neurons *in vitro. J. Neurosci.* 5, 817–824.

Toth, Z., Yan, X. X., Haftoglou, S., Ribak, C. E., and Baram, T. Z. (1998). Seizure-induced neuronal injury: Vulnerability to febrile seizures in an immature rat model. *J. Neurosci.* 18, 4285–4294.

Trussel, L. O., and Fischbach, G. D. (1989). Glutamate receptor desensitization and its role in synaptic transmission. *Neuron* 3, 209–218.

van Lunteren, E., Elmslie, K. S., and Jones, S. W. (1993). Effects of temperature on calcium current of bullfrog sympathetic neurons. *J. Physiol.* 466, 81–93.

Vastola, E. F., Homan, R., and Rosen, A. (1969). Inhibition of focal seizures by moderate hypothermia. A clinical and experimental study. *Arch. Neurol.* 20, 430–439.

Veale, W. L., Cooper, K. E., and Ruwe, W. D. (1984). Vasopressin: Its role in antipyresis and febrile convulsion. *Brain Res. Bull.* 12, 161–165.

Wahl, L. M., Pouzat, C., and Stratford, K. J. (1996). Monte Carlo simulation of fast excitatory synaptic transmission at a hippocampal synapse. *J. Neurophysiol.* 75, 597–608.

Wallace, R. H., Wang, D. W., Singh, R., Scheffer, I. E., George, A. L., Jr., Phillips, H. A., Saar, K., Reis, A., Johnson, E. W., Sutherland, G. R., Berkovic, S. F., and Mulley, J. C. (1998). Febrile seizures and generalized epilepsy associated with a mutation in the Na^+-channel beta1 subunit gene SCN1β. *Nat. Genet.* 19, 366–370.

Wu, J., and Fisher, R. S. (2000). Hyperthermic spreading depressions in the immature rat hippocampal slice. *J. Neurophysiol.* 84, 1355–1360.

Zhao, D. Y., Wu, X. R., Pei, Y. Q., and Zuo, Q. H. (1985). Kindling phenomenon of hyperthermic seizures in the epilepsy-prone versus the epilepsy-resistant rat. *Brain Res.* 358, 390–393.

CHAPTER 17

The Genetics
of Febrile Seizures

DAVID A. GREENBERG[1] AND GREGORY L. HOLMES

*Departments of Psychiatry and Biomathematics, Mt. Sinai School of Medicine
and the Columbia University Genome Center, New York, New York 10029,
and Department of Neurology, Harvard Medical School, Children's Hospital,
Boston, Massachusetts 02115*

The importance of genetic factors in the occurrence of febrile seizures
has long been recognized. Population studies have demonstrated that
febrile seizures occur at a much higher than expected incidence in first- and
second-degree relatives of children with febrile seizures. Family history also
has a role in determining whether children have febrile seizure recurrences
and subsequently develop afebrile seizures. We discuss the methods used
to study the genetics of febrile seizures. Segregation analyses have not yielded clear evidence of a single mode of inheritance and the evidence taken together demonstrates extensive heterogeneity in the genetic contribution to
febrile seizures. Linkage studies have yielded evidence of genes on chromosomes 2, 5, 8, 19p, and 19q, but almost always in single large pedigrees.
Other large pedigrees show no evidence of linkage to any of these loci.
Thus, febrile seizures are a common condition strongly influenced by genetic factors, but specific genes that affect the majority of febrile seizure
cases have yet to be identified. © 2002 Academic Press.

I. INTRODUCTION

The literature concerning the genetics of febrile seizures is voluminous and
somewhat controversial but it is generally recognized that the risk for developing febrile seizures is higher in some families than in others (Bethune *et al.*,
1993; Doerfer and Wasser, 1987; Fukuyama *et al.*, 1979; Jennings and Bird,
1981; Offringa *et al.*, 1994; Suanami *et al.*, 1988; Tsuboi, 1977; Tsuboi and Okada, 1985). However, there is no agreement regarding the magnitude of the con-

[1]Current affiliations: Mathematical Genetics Unit, Department of Biostatistics and Psychiatry,
Division of Clinical-Genetic Epidemiology, New York State Psychiatric Institute, New York, New
York 10032; and Division of Statistical Genetics, Department of Biostatistics, Mailman School of
Public Health, Columbia University, New York, New York 10029.

tribution of genetic factors to the risk of developing febrile seizures. The reasons for controversy over the genetics of febrile seizures reflect our ignorance of mechanisms that lead to epilepsy, the existence of clear environmental influences that cause fever, the systems unrelated to epilepsy that come into play as a result of infection, and the methodological problems of studying the genetics of complex disease.

In the current review, we discuss the methodologies that have been applied to the study of the genetics of febrile seizures and the results that have been obtained from these methods. Our hope is that a discussion of the results will demonstrate that studying the genetics of febrile seizures can be fruitful and, at the same time, warn those interested that genetic methodology is anything but easy and straightforward.

We discuss two main topics: (1) population, family, and twin studies of febrile seizure, all of which show strong evidence of genetic influences, and (2) the techniques of studying the genetic contribution to disease applied to febrile seizures. The techniques include segregation analysis, a now mostly moribund method, although not without its uses, and linkage analysis, the most powerful method for finding genes of moderate to large effect.

II. POPULATION, FAMILY, AND TWIN STUDIES OF FEBRILE SEIZURES

A. INCIDENCE OF FEBRILE SEIZURES

The reported incidence of febrile seizures has varied widely. In a review of the literature in 1984, Tsuboi (1984) found the reported prevalence of febrile seizures to range from 0.1 to 15.1%. According to the case ascertainment method, the mean prevalence rate was 2.7% (range, 1.5–4.8%) by questionnaire survey, 4.3% (0.1–14%) by reports of general practitioners or medical record reviews, and 8.1% (2.5–15%) by examination. The differences were largely influenced by the methods employed to identify cases and definitions used by the authors. In Tsuboi's report (1984), boys were found to be more prone than girls to febrile seizures.

The most accurate figures are those derived from populations of children followed longitudinally. Using the 1958 British birth cohort, Ross and colleagues (1980) found 2.4% of children to have febrile seizures; and Verity and associates (1985), reporting the results of the Child Health and Education Survey, found a cumulative incidence rate of 2.5% of 13,038 children followed from birth. In a longitudinal study in the United States, Nelson and Ellenberg (1978) found a cumulative incidence of febrile seizures at 7 years to be 3.5% in white children and 4.2% in black children. It should be noted that most of the incidence studies are of European or North American populations. There are fewer studies from other parts of the world.

B. FAMILY STUDIES

The first step in investigating the genetics of almost any condition is to show that it occurs more frequently in families. The vast majority of studies examining genetic factors in febrile seizures have reported a higher than expected (expectation based on population frequencies) number of family members with febrile seizures. For example, Nelson and Ellenberg (1990) in the Collaborative Perinatal Project of the National Institute of Neurological Disorders and Strokes (NINDS) found that family history was the most important of the few identified factors that made a substantial contribution to vulnerability to febrile seizures.

A positive family history for febrile seizures can be elicited in 25–40% of patients with febrile seizures (Annegers *et al.*, 1979; Frantzen *et al.*, 1970; Hauser *et al.*, 1985). The reported frequency in siblings of children with febrile seizures has ranged from 9 to 22% (Annegers *et al.*, 1979; Frantzen *et al.*, 1970; Fukuyama *et al.*, 1979; Jennings and Bird, 1981; Metrakos and Metrakos, 1970; Tsuboi, 1977). Between 8 and 14% of parents of children with febrile seizures have a history of febrile seizures (Frantzen *et al.*, 1968, 1970; Tsuboi, 1977).

Tsuboi (1982) evaluated 16,806 children receiving routine health care examinations at the Health Center in Fuchu City, Japan. In this population 1123 children (5.7%) had at least one febrile seizure. The incidence of febrile seizures was 20.7% among siblings, 10.9% among parents, and 14.1% among first-degree relatives of the probands. These numbers were compared with the incidence of febrile seizures in relatives of the control population: 8.4% in siblings, 1.6% in parents, and 3.8% among first-degree relatives of the controls. Similar figures from Japan were reported by Fukuyama *et al.* (1979), who found an incidence of febrile seizures in 19.9% of siblings, 13.9% in parents, 3.9% in uncles and aunts, and 0.7% in grandparents of children with febrile seizures. Of the 229 relatives with a history of febrile seizures, over 95% were parents, siblings, aunts, and uncles. Hauser *et al.* (1985) found an 8% incidence of febrile seizures in siblings of patients with febrile seizures. The relative risk for febrile seizures in siblings was 3.7% with a 95% confidence interval (CI) of 3.0–4.6. In the Hauser *et al.* (1985) study, the risk of febrile seizures in the children of the probands was 8.4%, or 4.4 times that expected (CI 2.5–7.3) in the normal population. An increased risk in second-degree relatives, i.e., cousins, aunts, and uncles of children with febrile seizures, has been reported (Hauser *et al.*, 1985; Tsuboi, 1982). For example, Hauser *et al.* (1985) found that nieces or nephews of the probands had a 2.7% greater risk than that expected in the control population (CI 1.7–4.1).

A higher rate of febrile seizures was found in a Japanese population (Fukuyama *et al.*, 1979) than in the American population (Hauser *et al.*, 1985). The risk of febrile seizures among siblings of the probands was also higher in the Japanese population (Fukuyama *et al.*, 1979) than in the American population

(Hauser *et al.*, 1985). The percentage of siblings with febrile convulsions in the Japanese population (19.9%) was more than twice as great as in the American population (8.0%); however, the percentage of febrile seizures in the Japanese control population (6.7%) was also more than twice as great as in the American population (2.4%). Thus, despite the large differences in incidence, when the heritability of febrile seizures is compared in the two groups, the genetic contribution for febrile seizures among siblings (60–80%) is comparable in the two populations.

The risk to siblings of probands increases substantially if more than one family member has a history of febrile seizures. Tsuboi (1982) found the incidence among siblings to be highest (45%) if two members of a family had prior febrile seizures, second highest (16%) among children with one febrile seizure relative, and lowest (0.8%) if no family member had febrile seizures. Likewise, the incidence among siblings was highest (38.9%) if both parents had febrile seizures, intermediate (31.4%) if one parent had febrile seizures, and lowest (17.8%) if neither parent had a prior febrile seizure. In an American study, Hauser *et al.* (1985) found that if neither parent of a child with febrile seizures had a history of febrile seizures, the risk to siblings was 2.7% (CI 2.0–3.6). When one parent was affected, the relative risk in siblings was 10.0% (CI 6.3–15); when both parents were affected, the relative risk was 20% (CI 9.6–36.8).

The number of febrile seizures in a child also affects the risk of febrile seizures in siblings. Siblings of children with more than four febrile seizures were more likely to have febrile seizures than were those of children with fewer than three seizures (Tsuboi, 1982). Hauser *et al.* (1985) also found that the greater the number of febrile seizures in probands, the higher the risk in the siblings, nieces, nephews, and children. Fukuyama *et al.* (1979), Wadhwa *et al.* (1992), and Rich *et al.* (1987) all suggest that the more seizures seen in the index case, the higher the risk for family members. Whether the seizures are simple or complex may relate to familial risk. Wadhwa *et al.* (1991) report that the familial prevalence of febrile seizures was the same whether the family was identified through complex or simple febrile seizure, but Hauser *et al.* (1985) found that the presence of complex features of febrile seizures in probands (including focal seizures, the occurrence of multifocal seizures in a single day, and/or postictal or Todds paralysis) was associated with an increased risk for febrile seizures in siblings. However, the difference in results is not entirely clear because Wadhwa *et al.* (1991) also report that the prevalence of afebrile seizures was much higher in the complex group (6% vs. 29%). The question of whether only simple febrile seizures or both simple and complex febrile seizures are associated with a familial risk is important for genetic analysis because it will influence which type of proband is most suitable for linkage studies.

A number of other factors were identified in determining risk to relatives of children with febrile seizures. In the Hauser *et al.* study (1985), age of seizure onset in the proband played a role in seizure risk in siblings. Siblings, but not children, nieces, or nephews of probands having their first febrile seizure at age 4 years or older were at significantly higher risk for febrile seizures than were siblings of probands with a first febrile seizure prior to age 4. A prolonged febrile seizure (longer than 10 minutes) in the absence of other complex features was also associated with an increased risk for febrile seizures in siblings when compared with that expected.

C. Twin Studies

Population-based twin registries provide a valuable tool for examining the importance of genetic and environmental factors in the etiology of disorders such as epilepsy. Febrile seizures have been studied in several large twin studies. As with population studies comparing the familial incidence of febrile seizures, these studies have had varying results. Again, these differences relate to varying methods of case ascertainment and definition of febrile seizures. Lennox-Buchthal (1971) found a concordance rate of 80% for febrile seizures in monozygotic twins matched for similar neurological development. Other authors found a lower rate. Tsuboi (1982) reported a concordance rate of febrile seizures in monozygotic twins of 46% and observed that the rate was much higher than the rate for dizygotic twin pairs (13%). Schittz-Christensen (1972) found a pairwise concordance rate of only 28% in monozygotics, compared with a rate of 11% in dizygotic twins. Based on these numbers, the authors postulated that factors responsible for febrile seizures are genetic in nature only to a limited extent. Tsuboi and Endo (1991) examined 46 twin pairs. The reported concordance rate was much higher in monozygotic than in dizygotic twins (69% vs. 20%, respectively).

A large difference in monozygotic vs. dizygotic concordance suggests a strong genetic component is present, especially when the rate in monozygotic twins is three- to fourfold greater in monozygotic than in dizygotic twins. Note also that the rate in dizygotic twins in the Tsuboi and Endo study is about the same as in siblings, which is what one should observe if there is no particular bias in data collection, which can often occur if one collects twins based on the presence of disease rather than for twin-ness.

Among 14,352 twin pairs collected in Virginian and Norwegian twin panels in whom questionnaire information was available, 257 pairs had febrile seizures (Corey et al., 1991). Proband concordance rates for febrile seizures were 33% in monozygotic twins and 11% in dizygotic twins. The rates were similar in boys and girls.

One way of controlling for genetic influences is to examine discordant monozygotic twin pairs. Because monozygotic twins share the same genes, phenotypic differences between the twins of a pair must be due to environmental or random factors. Two reports from Australia used discordant twins to try and answer the question whether hippocampal sclerosis was causally related to prolonged febrile seizures (Jackson *et al.*, 1998; Breillman *et al.*, 1998). These investigators examine three sets of monozygotic twin pairs; one twin of the pair had temporal lobe epilepsy and the co-twin did not. They examined both affected and unaffected twins using magnetic resonance imaging (MRI). The most important historical finding was that in all three cases, the affected twin had prolonged febrile seizures in childhood and the unaffected co-twin did not. Hippocampal sclerosis was present in the affected twins but not in the unaffected twins.

III. GENETIC ANALYSIS METHODS

A. SEGREGATION ANALYSIS

Segregation analysis is a technique for determining the mode of transmission of a trait. "Mode of transmission" refers to how the trait is passed from one generation to the next—whether one allele or two at the trait locus is necessary for trait expression, whether more than one locus is involved, whether there is a "major gene" as opposed to many genes of small effect, etc. In segregation analysis, one calculates a statistic based on the affectedness pattern in the family— that is, which classes of relatives are affected and how frequently. That statistic is then compared with what one would expect assuming some known model of inheritance. For example, an investigator might ascertain a series of families and note that a high proportion of siblings has the trait. In testing whether the observed pattern of inheritance in the families is compatible with, say, dominant inheritance, the investigator could count the proportion of siblings affected and statistically test whether that proportion was different from 0.5, which is the expected proportion assuming dominant inheritance at low gene frequency. If the observed proportion is statistically significantly different from 0.5, then a dominant mode of inheritance is rejected. One can then go on to test other modes of inheritance [e.g., recessive inheritance, dominant with reduced penetrance, inheritance due to two loci, or polygenic inheritance (i.e., the accumulated effect of many genes, each exerting a small influence), etc.]. ("Penetrance" is defined as the probability of showing the disease phenotype given that an individual, in fact, has the disease genotype.) If a mode of inheritance cannot be rejected, it does not prove that the assumed mode of inheritance is correct, only that it cannot be rejected with the data in hand.

Segregation analysis has the advantage that one needs nothing other than family structures to be able to draw conclusions. It has the substantial disadvantage that, like many purely statistical techniques, it can reject an assumed mode of inheritance but cannot prove that the assumed mode of inheritance is, in fact, operating in the trait under study. A further disadvantage is that a large number of families must be included if one is to get reliable results. Most problematically for studies of common disease—and this is true of virtually all genetic techniques—it assumes that the phenotypes, the very definition of affected, reflect a unitary underlying cause, i.e., etiological homogeneity. In common disease, this is seldom the case.

Thus, the information that one obtains from segregation analysis is often quite limited and is also affected by issues of ascertainment, which may affect the reliability of results even more than in epidemiological studies.

There are few segregation analysis studies of febrile seizures in the literature. However, all find an increased familial risk. Wadhwa *et al.* (1992) studied 95 "typical" (or simple) and 49 "atypical" (or complex) families. The "familial prevalence" was 29.1% overall, with the complex group showing far higher values for familial risk than the simple group (41 vs. 23%). In addition, about 13% of seizures were afebrile, with the "complex" group far outnumbering the "simple" (27 vs. 6%). These figures for "familial prevalence" do not represent a true segregation analysis, but demonstrate that febrile seizures are more common in certain families. Because the details of the ascertainment are not reported, it is possible that these families, with their high reported density of affected members, were identified *because* they were particularly dense, thus raising the specter of biased ascertainment. A reported segregation analysis revealed no clear pattern of inheritance, which the authors interpret as suggesting polygenic inheritance. However, they apparently do not explicitly test for a polygenic pattern (Hodge *et al.*, 1989).

Although Tsuboi and Endo (1991) do not report the results of a formal segregation analysis, they remark that a segregation analysis showed maternal preponderance. However, they do report that the morbidity risk was high in siblings (32%) and lower in aunts and uncles (14%) and lower still in cousins (6%). Like the Wadhwa *et al.* (1992) study, sibling risk appeared to be quite high (23%) and was also high in parents (17%).

In an often-cited study, Rich *et al.* (1987) performed a complex segregation analysis of 467 nuclear families ascertained through febrile seizure probands. These probands were identified as having had their first febrile seizure while residing in Rochester, Minnesota during the years 1935–1964. After ascertaining the probands, both first- and second-degree relatives were then identified through the Olmsted County, Minnesota records. This information on how the probands were identified suggests that ascertainment was so-called "truncate," that is, the probability of a family being identified was the same for all families, regardless how many family members were affected. (We mention the possible effect of this ascertainment scheme below.) Other affected family members were then identified from a review of medical records. These investigators took cognizance of the possible role of heterogeneity and its effect on segregation analysis by dividing the families into two groups based on the number of seizures observed in the proband.

The authors found that in families in which the proband had two or more seizures, the evidence for a single major gene increased. In families in which the proband had only a single seizure, the polygenic model could not be rejected, although other models could. Also rejected was the hypothesis of "no genetic component."

The authors discuss possible sources of ascertainment bias, including complications such as parents preventing further febrile seizures in a child by treatment with medication to lower fever. Another source of possible ascertainment problems lay in the program used for the analysis. This program corrects for ascertainment in pedigrees by an idiosyncratic method that, to our knowledge, has never been fully investigated or tested. In addition, a "polygenic" mode of inheritance means that there are many genes contributing to trait expression, each gene contributing a small effect. It has never been shown whether this model can be distinguished from a two-, three-, or four-locus genetic model in which the loci interact, a model now much invoked in studies of some of the common epilepsies. Thus, finding that polygenic inheritance cannot be rejected tells us little about the probability of finding loci via linkage analysis, nor does it support or reject the effect of genetic heterogeneity, or of a mixture of genetic and nongenetic causes.

Sources of error notwithstanding, the finding of a stronger genetic effect in families in which probands have multiple seizures suggests that genetic factors play a more major role in such families. This kind of finding is important in the design of linkage studies, which seek to find the actual genes involved, because it suggests how one could subdivide the data to produce a more genetically homogeneous phenotype for analysis. Because heterogeneity is one of the major factors that make it difficult to find disease-related loci, any analysis that increases knowledge of possible heterogeneity is of help in identifying genes for the trait.

B. LINKAGE ANALYSIS

Segregation analysis is purely statistical. It compares observed patterns of affectedness seen in families with patterns predicted assuming some theoretical model. The method does not use other biological data. Linkage and association analyses, on the other hand, use markers that exist throughout the genome to look for those markers whose presence, in some way, correlates with disease. However, linkage and association use that marker information in quite different ways. These differences are important to bear in mind when examining marker evidence for the involvement of a gene in febrile seizures.

Linkage analysis works by looking for cosegregation of disease with marker alleles in families. A "linkage marker" is any known locus on the genome in which the specific sequences on the two DNA strands at that locus can be different in different people. Marker loci with many alleles, such as the HLA loci, are good for linkage analysis because the large number of alleles means that one can usually unambiguously trace the movement of marker alleles from one generation to the next. Theoretically, now that so-called single nucleotide polymorphisms (SNPs) can be used as markers, the precision with which we can examine the genome is almost unlimited (but see Hodge *et al.*, 1999).

An important point is that in linkage analysis, it does not matter which allele of the marker locus is transmitted with the disease. It is likely to be a different marker allele in different families. However, if there is linkage, alleles of the marker will consistently cosegregate with the disease within families. If no linkage exists, one will see families in which there is no correlation between the marker genotypes in sibs and presence of disease. (In association analysis, the same allele is seen together with the disease at the population level, but not necessarily within families.)

In common diseases such as febrile seizures, the phenotype–genotype correlation in families is not usually as obvious as in Mendelian diseases such as Huntington's disease. Common diseases present us with problematic complicating factors. One of those is likely to be reduced penetrance, which is the probability of being affected given that the disease genotype is present. However, although reduced penetrance has the effect of reducing the power for detecting linkage, it will not, by itself, lead to either false positives or false negatives as long as it is allowed for in the analysis. Depending on how the analysis is performed, even if the penetrance is misspecified in the analysis, it will often have little effect on the final evidence for linkage (Greenberg, 1989).

The major complicating factors in linkage analysis that can lead to failure to find a disease-influencing locus are heterogeneity and incorrect phenotype definition. When two or more traits cannot be distinguished clinically, families collected for genetic analysis will represent a mixture of the different diseases. A form of disease that is linked to a marker locus will become undetectable because the form(s) that are not linked to that locus will overwhelm the evidence for linkage.

Probably the best method for determining the existence of linkage and heterogeneity is to stratify the sample on clinical characteristics that enrich the data for one particular form of disease. For example, Durner *et al.* (1999) found evidence of linkage to idiopathic generalized epilepsy of adolescent onset on chromosome 8. However, this evidence emerged only after stratifying the sample into those families in which juvenile myoclonic epilepsy was present and those in which it was not. When the families without juvenile myoclonic epilepsy were analyzed as a group, strong evidence of linkage emerged that had been censored in the analysis of the entire data set. Analysis of the entire data set but assuming heterogeneity produced some evidence of linkage, but it was far from strong. This example is a clear demonstration that stratifying the families based on clinical characteristics can not only yield evidence for linkage, but can also validate clinical etiological differentiation based on particular symptoms.

However, although clinical features may reflect genetic heterogeneity, they may merely reflect variable expression of the same gene, and clinically identical patients may have differing genetic etiologies. If one can delineate the genetic component to a disease, this can lead to information about the disease that can have clinical applications.

IV. KNOWN LINKAGES FOR FEBRILE SEIZURES

Five areas of the genome have been shown to be linked to febrile seizure in some way. Two of those, *FEB1* and *FEB2*, have been suggested on chromosomes 8 and 19p, respectively, and involve only febrile seizures. Three others, on chromosomes 2, 19q, and 5, involve the generalized epilepsy with febrile seizures (GEFS) syndrome. For the most part these linkages have been observed in just one or two, or at most a few, large, unique families (Table 1). The linkage on chromosome 8 has not yet been replicated, nor have candidate genes been reported (Wallace *et al.*, 1996).

Chromosome 19 appears to harbor at least two loci related to febrile seizures. Linkage on 19p was seen in an extended pedigree (Johnson *et al.*, 1998) and this linkage was replicated in another single large family (Kugler *et al.*, 1998). Wallace *et al.* (1998) found linkage in 19q in a single large family in which a variety of seizure types were observed. The phenotypes in this family included febrile seizure, generalized epilepsy, and a continuation of febrile seizures beyond the age in which they usually cease, termed GEFS+ (Scheffer and Berkovic, 1997). Wallace *et al.* (1998) report that in this family, the actual mutation is in a sodium channel subunit, SCN1B. The authors also show that the mutated protein exhibits altered electrophysiologic characteristics. These investigators genotyped 24 individuals in this pedigree who have some form of epilepsy, including febrile seizures, GEFS, febrile seizures + absence, and myoclonic–astatic epilepsy. Among these, 7 affected individuals, including one member of an affected sib pair, do not have the SCN1B mutation seen in the other affected members. Another affected member, although untyped, cannot share the SCN1B mutation identical by descent. The authors suggest that these

TABLE 1   Reported Linkages in Febrile Seizures

Chromosomal location	Report	Identified locus	Replication	Type of family data
2q	Baulac et al. (1999)	SCN1A	Peiffer et al. (1999); Escayg et al. (2000); Lopez-Cendes et al. (2000); Wallace et al. (2001)	Mostly individual large pedigrees
5q	Nakayama et al. (2000)	?		Large pedigree + nuclear families
5q	—	?	?Durner et al. (2001)	Nuclear families; same marker as Nakayama et al. but IGE phenotype
5	Wallace et al. (2001)	GABA$_A$ receptor γ-2 subunit	—	Single large pedigree
8p	Wallace et al. (1996)	?	—	Large pedigree
19p	Johnson et al (1998)	?	Kugler et al. (1998)	Large pedigrees
19q	Wallace et al. (1998)	?SCN1B	—	Large pedigree

affected individuals are phenocopies and that possible family history of epilepsy in the marrying-in individuals explains the fact that they do not share the SCN1B mutation. The presence of many apparent phenocopies in a single large pedigree and the failure to find the same linkage in 25 other families may suggest that one or more other genes besides the SCN1B are required for disease expression and that further evidence that SCN1B is the causative mutation is necessary.

Indirect evidence supporting the sodium channel SCN1B mutation comes from studies of chromosome 2. Linkage has been suggested to chromosome 2q21–33, a region in which a number of sodium channel subunits exist (Alekov et al., 2000). This is the one locus in which linkage has been found by a number of different groups, although always in single, large pedigrees (Baulac et al., 1999; Peiffer et al., 1999; Moulard et al., 1999; Lopez-Cendes et al., 2000; Wallace et al., 2001). All these studies suggest linkage to the same area, but localization is not exact. It is possible that all these linkages are to the same locus, but that differences in classification, pedigree structures and informativeness, and other technical factors lead to evidence for linkage in different locations. Escayg *et al.* (2000) suggest that a mutation in the SCN1A subunit of the sodium channel is the mutation in the family they study. Alekov *et al.* (2000) expressed a mutated chromosome 2 sodium channel gene *in vitro* and found subtle changes in inactivation of the sodium channel, although the changes were much more subtle than in the SCN4A receptor in muscle. Wallace *et al.* (2001) found three different mutations in the SCN1A gene in three out of 36 GEFS+ families. Three other families showed mutations in the SCN1B locus (chromosome 19q). These authors did not find any evidence of a mutation at these loci in 30 other families they studied and also no mutations in 17 sporadic GEFS+ cases. From this work, it appears that the sodium channel mutations that lead to febrile seizures in rare, highly penetrant families do not account for the genetic contribution to febrile convulsions.

The evidence on chromosome 5q is somewhat different. The linkage, reported thus far only in the Japanese population (Nakayama *et al.*, 2000), was observed using a data set identified through febrile seizures families. The investigators performed linkage in a single large family and found evidence for linkage on 5q, and then went on to test the linkage in a set of nuclear families, which also showed evidence for linkage. Because the authors analyzed their data using a method that does not take heterogeneity into account, they did not test for the existence of heterogeneity. An association analysis also showed evidence of association with one of the alleles of D5S644, the same marker at which he maximum evidence for linkage occurred. This suggests that the disease locus is quite close to this marker. Although this linkage and association have not yet been replicated in febrile seizures families, a report by Durner *et al.* (2001) found significant evidence of linkage to the same chromosome 5 marker in families with generalized epilepsy but grouped for the presence of absence epilepsy in any family member. This confluence of findings suggests that the same locus may produce different phenotypes in genetically different populations. It also suggests that investigators searching for epilepsy genes should test known epilepsy loci for linkage, even if the original phenotype for the known locus is different from what one is studying.

Interestingly, another linkage report also implicates the long arm of chromosome 5. Wallace *et al.* (2001) found strong evidence for linkage to chromosome 5 markers in a single family ascertained through febrile seizures and absence epilepsy. These authors report a mutation in a GABA receptor subunit, GABRG2, which codes for the γ subunit. This locus is apparently not close to D5S644 reported by Nakayama *et al.* (2000) and Durner *et al.* (2001), but it could suggest a group of related genes in the region.

Racacho *et al.* (2000) examined linkages to a number of reported epilepsy loci in two large Canadian kindreds, including loci discussed above, and found no evidence of linkage to any. Thus, although genes can be found in individual large families, these findings have not yet given us even the range of possible genetic causes for febrile convulsions.

V. SUMMARY

Four facts emerge from the genetics literature on febrile seizures.

1. The evidence from epidemiology, family studies, and twin studies is that there is a strong genetic component to febrile seizures. Further, other forms of epilepsy are seen more frequently in febrile seizure families than is expected.

2. The segregation analyses and the linkage studies of febrile seizures thus far show evidence of heterogeneity. Almost all linkage findings in febrile seizures (with the exception of the Japanese population on chromosome 5) have involved single or a few large families. The strongest evidence has emerged on chromosome 2, with several independent large families showing evidence of linkage.

3. The linkages have been replicated on chromosome 2 in an area of sodium channel receptors. The linkage on chromosome 19q also shows evidence that a sodium channel is involved in the disease.

4. There is as yet no evidence that any of these loci play a role in the common forms of febrile seizure seen in the clinic, with the exception of the chromosome 5 locus identified in the Japanese population. A linkage seen in the Japanese population in families identified through febrile seizure patients has also been observed in families identified through absence patients. If confirmed, this finding would suggest that the genetic background differences, as represented by ethnic group, may produce different phenotypes for the same genetic locus.

Finally, what emerges from all the genetic studies is that the febrile seizure is a genetically heterogeneous condition. It is likely that the interaction of multiple genes and environment is necessary for the expression of febrile seizures, that different genes can produce the same phenotype, and that the ethnic background plays a role in the observed phenotype. Thus, despite the recent identification of loci in individual families, we still appear to be a long way from understanding the genetic influences in febrile seizures.

ACKNOWLEDGMENTS

Supported by grants from the NIH (DK31775, NS27941, and MH48858) to DAG and the Emily P. Rogers Research Fund and a grant to GLH from the NINDS (NS27984).

REFERENCES

Alekov, A., Rahman, M. M., Mitrovic, N., Lehmann-Horn, F., and Lerche, H. (2000). A sodium channel mutation causing epilepsy in man exhibits subtle defects in fast inactivation and activation in vitro. *J. Physiol.* **529** (Pt. 3), 533–539.

Anderson, V. E., Hauser, W. A., and Rich, S. S. (1986). Genetic heterogeneity in the epilepsies. In "Basic Mechanisms of the Epilepsies. Molecular and Cellular Approaches" (A. V. Delgado-Escueta, A. A. Ward, Jr., D. M. Woodbury, and R. J. Porter, eds.), pp. 59–75. Raven Press, New York.

Annegers, J. F., Hauser, W. A., Elveback, L. R., and Kurland, L. T. (1979). The risk of epilepsy following febrile convulsions. *Neurology* **29**, 297–303.

Annegers, J. F., Blakley, S. A., Hauser, W. A., and Kurland, L. T. (1990). Recurrence of febrile convulsions in a population-based cohort. *Epilepsy Res.* **5**, 209–216.

Baulac, S., Gourfinkel-An, I., Picard, F., Rosenberg-Bourgin, M., Prudhomme, J. F., Baulac, M., Brice, A., *et al.* (1999). A second locus for familial generalized epilepsy with febrile seizures plus maps to chromosome 2q21-q33. *Am. J. Hum. Genet.* **65**, 1078–1085.

Bethune, P., Gordon, K., Dooley, J., Camfield, C., and Camfield, P. (1993). Which child will have a febrile seizure? *Am. J. Dis. Child.* **147**, 35–39.

Briellmann, R. S., Jackson, G. D., Torn-Broers, Y., and Berkovic, S. F. (1998). Twins with different temporal lobe malformations: Schizencephaly and arachnoid cyst. *Neuropediatrics* **29**, 284–286.

Corey, L. A., Berg, K., Pellock, J. M., Solass, M. H., Nance, W. E., and DeLorenzo, R. J. (1991). The occurrence of epilepsy and febrile seizures in Virginian and Norwegian twins. *Neurology* **41**, 1433–1436.

Doerfer, J., and Wasser, S. (1987). An epidemiologic study of febrile seizures and epilepsy in children. *Epilepsy Res.* **1**, 149–151.

Durner, M., Zhou, G., Fu, D., Abreu, P., Shinnar, S., Resor, S. R., Moshe, S. L., *et al.* (1999). Evidence for linkage of adolescent-onset idiopathic generalized epilepsies to chromosome 8 and genetic heterogeneity. *Am. J. Hum. Genet.* **64**, 1411–1419.

Durner, M., Keddache, M. A., Tomasini, L., Shinnar, S., Resor, S. R., Cohen, J., Harden, C., *et al.* (2001). Genome scan of idiopathic generalized epilepsy evidence for major susceptibility gene and modifying genes influencing the seizure type. *Ann. Neurol.* **49**, 328–335.

Escayg, A., MacDonald, B. T., Meisler, M. H., Baulac, S., Huberfeld, G., An-Gourfinkel, I., Brice, A., *et al.* (2000). Mutations of SCN1A, encoding a neuronal sodium channel, in two families with GEFS+2. *Nat. Genet.* **24**, 343–345.

Frantzen, E., Lennox-Buchtal, M., and Nygaard, A. (1968). Longitudinal EEG and clinical study of children with febrile convulsions. *Electroencephalogr. Clin. Neurophysiol.* **24**, 197–212.

Frantzen, E., Lennox-Buchtal, M., Nygaard, A., and Stene, J. (1970). A genetic study of febrile seizures. *Neurology* **20**, 909–917.

Fukuyama, Y., Kagawa, K., and Tanaka, K. (1979). A genetic study of febrile convulsions. *Eur. Neurol.* **18**, 166–182.

Gardiner, R. M. (1990). Genes and epilepsy. *J. Med. Genet.* **27**, 537–544.

Greenberg, D. A. (1989). Inferring mode of inheritance by comparison of lod scores. *Am. J. Med. Genet.* **34**, 480–486.

Hauser, W. A., and Hersdorffer, D. C. (1990). "Epilepsy: Frequency, Causes and Consequences." Demos, New York.

Hauser, W. A., Annegers, J. F., Anderson, V. E., and Kurland, L. T. (1985). The risk of seizure disorders among relatives of children with febrile convulsions. *Neurology* **35**, 1268–1273.

Hodge, S. E., Greenberg, D. A., Durner, M., Delgado-Escueta, A. V., and Janz, D. (1989). Is juvenile myoclonic epilepsy polygenic? In "Genetics of the Epilepsies" (G. Beck-Mannagetta, V. E. Anderson, H. Doose, and D. Janz, eds.), pp. 62–66. Springer-Verlag, Berlin.

Hodge, S. E., Goehnke, M., and Spence, M. A. (1999). Loss of information due to ambiguous hap-lotyping of SNPs. *Nat. Genet.* **21**, 360–361.

Jackson, G. D., McIntosh, A. M., Briellmann, R. S., and Berkovic, S. F. (1998). Hippocampal scle-rosis studied in identical twins. *Neurology* **51**, 78–84.

Jennings, M. T., and Bird, T. D. (1981). Genetic influences in the epilepsies. *Am. J. Dis. Child.* **135**, 450–457.

Johnson, W. G., Kugler, S. L., Stenroos, E. S., Meulener, M. C., Rangwalla, I., Johnson, T. W., and Mandelbaum, D. E. (1996). Pedigree analysis in families with febrile seizures. *Am. J. Med. Genet.* **61**, 345–352.

Johnson, E. W., Dubovsky, J., Rich, S. S., O'Donovan, C. A., Orr, H. T., Anderson, V. E., Gil-Nagel, A., *et al.* (1998). Evidence for a novel gene for familial febrile convulsions, FEB2, linked to chro-mosome 19p in an extended family from the Midwest. *Hum. Mol. Genet.* **7**, 63–67.

Kugler, S. L., Stenroos, E. S., Mandelbaum, D. E., Lehner, T., McKoy, V. V., Prossick, T., Sasvari, J., *et al.* (1998). Hereditary febrile seizures: Phenotype and evidence for a chromosome 19p locus. *Am. J. Med. Genet.* **79**, 354–361.

Lennox-Buchtal, M. (1971). Febrile and nocturnal convulsions in monozygotic twins. *Epilepsia* **12**, 147–156.

Lopes-Cendes, I., Scheffer, I. E., Berkovic, S. F., Rousseau, M., Andermann, E., and Rouleau, G. A. (2000). A new locus for generalized epilepsy with febrile seizures plus maps to chromosome 2. *Am. J. Hum. Genet.* **66**, 698–701.

Metrakos, J. D., and Metrakos, K. (1970). Genetic factors in epilepsy. In "Epilepsy: Modern Prob-lems in Pharmacopsychiatry" (E. Niedermeyer, ed.), pp. 71–86. Karger, Basel.

Moulard, B., Guipponi, M., Chaigne, D., Mouthon, D., Buresi, C., and Malafosse, A. (1999). Iden-tification of a new locus for generalized epilepsy with febrile seizures plus (GEFS+) on chro-mosome 2q24-q33. *Am. J. Hum. Genet.* **65**, 1396–1400.

Nakayama, J., Hamano, K., Iwasaki, N., Nakahara, S., Horigome, Y., Saitoh, H., Aoki, T., *et al.* (2000). Significant evidence for linkage of febrile seizures to chromosome 5q14-q15. *Hum. Mol. Genet.* **9**, 87–91.

Nelson, K. B., and Ellenberg, J. H. (1978). Prognosis in children with febrile seizures. *Pediatrics* **61**, 720–727.

Nelson, K. B., and Ellenberg, J. H. (1990). Prenatal and perinatal antecedents of febrile seizures. *Ann. Neurol.* **27**, 127–131.

Offringa, M., Bossuyt, P. M., Lubsen, J., Ellenberg, J. H., Nelson, K. B., Knudsen, F. U., Annegers, J. F., el-Radhi, A. S., Habbema, J. D., Derksen-Lubsen, G., *et al.* (1994). Risk factors for seizure recurrence in children with febrile seizures: A pooled analysis of individual patient data from five studies. *J. Pediatr.* **124**, 574–584.

Peiffer, A., Thompson, J., Charlier, C., Otterud, B., Varvil, T., Pappas, C., Barnitz, C., *et al.* (1999). A locus for febrile seizures (FEB3) maps to chromosome 2q23-24. *Ann. Neurol.* **46**, 671–678.

Racacho, L. J., McLachlan, R. S., Ebers, G. C., Maher, J., Bulman, D. E. (2000). Evidence favoring genetic heterogeneity for febrile convulsions. *Epilepsia* **41**, 132–139.

Rich, S. S., Annegers, J. F., Hauser, W. A., and Anderson, V. E. (1987). Complex segregation analy-sis of febrile convulsions. *Am. J. Hum. Genet.* **41**, 249–257.

Ross, E. M., Peckham, C. S., West, P. B., and Butler, N. R. (1980). Epilepsy in childhood: Findings from the National Child Development Study. *Br. Med. J.* **280**, 207–210.

Scheffer, I. E., and Berkovic, S. F. (1997). Generalized epilepsy with febrile seizures plus. A genet-ic disorder with heterogeneous clinical phenotypes. *Brain* **120**, 479–490.

Schiitz-Christensen, E. (1972). Genetic factors in febrile convulsions. An investigation of 64 same-sexed twin pairs. *Acta Neurol. Scand.* **48**, 538–546.

Suanami, K., Hayashi, N., and Endo, S. (1988). A twin study of febrile convulsions in the general population. *J. J. Psychiatr. Neurol.* **42**, 549–551.

Tsuboi, T. (1977). Genetic aspects of febrile convulsions. *Hum. Genet.* **38**, 169–173.

Tsuboi, T. (1982). Febrile convulsions. *In* "Genetic Basis of the Epilepsies" (V. E. Anderson, W. A. Hauser, J. K. Penry, *et al.*, eds.), pp. 123–134. Raven Press, New York.

Tsuboi, T. (1984). Epidemiology of febrile and afebrile convulsions in children in Japan. *Neurology* **34**, 175–181.

Tsuboi, T., and Endo, S. (1991). Genetic studies of febrile convulsions: Analysis of twin and family data. *In* "Genetic Strategies in Epilepsy Research" (V. E. Anderson, W. A. Hauser, I. E. Leppik, J. L. Noebels, and S. S. Rich, eds.), pp. 119–128. Elsevier, Amsterdam.

Tsuboi, T., and Okada, S. (1985). Exogenous causes of seizures in children: A population study. *Acta Neurol. Scand.* **71**, 107–113.

van den Berg, B. J. (1974). Studies on convulsive disorders in young children. *Dev. Med. Child Neurol.* **16**, 457–464.

Verity, C. M., Butler, N. R., and Goldring, J. (1985). Febrile convulsions in a national cohort followed up from birth. I. Prevalence and recurrence in the first five years of life. *Br. Med. J.* **290**, 1307–1310.

Wadhwa, N., Bharucha, B., Chablani, U., and Contractor, N. (1992). An epidemiological study of febrile seizures with special reference to family history and HLA linkage. *Indian Pediatr.* **29**, 1479–1485.

Wallace, R. H., Berkovic, S. F., Howell, R. A., Sutherland, G. R., and Mulley, J. C. (1996). Suggestion of a major gene for familial febrile convulsions mapping to 8q13-21. *J. Med. Genet.* **33**, 308–312.

Wallace, R. H., Wang, D. W., Singh, R., Scheffer, I. E., George, A. L., Jr., Phillips, H. A., Saar, K., *et al.* (1998). Febrile seizures and generalized epilepsy associated with a mutation in the Na^+-channel beta 1 subunit gene SCN1B. *Nat. Genet.* **19**, 366–370.

Wallace, R. H., Scheffer, I. E., Barnett, S., Richards, M., Dibbens, L., Desai, R. R., Lerman-Sagie, T., *et al.* (2001). Neuronal sodium-channel alpha 1-subunit mutations in generalized epilepsy with febrile seizures plus. *Am. J. Hum. Genet.* **68**, 859–865.

CHAPTER 18

Evaluation of the Child with Febrile Seizures

N. PAUL ROSMAN

Floating Hospital for Children, Boston, Massachusetts 02111

Febrile seizures result from age-dependent brain hyperexcitability that is induced by fever. Though there are important genetic influences that render a child with fever more likely to develop seizures, it is the fever per se that causes the seizure. Of primary importance in the diagnostic assessment of such children are efforts directed to finding the cause of the fever. Once found, the cause should be treated specifically (e.g., antibiotics for otitis media) and/or symptomatically (e.g., antipyretics for viral pharyngitis). It is essential to exclude underlying meningitis in all children with febrile seizures, either clinically or, if any doubt remains, by lumbar puncture. In as many as one child in six with meningitis, seizures are the presenting sign and in one-third of these cases, meningeal signs and symptoms may be lacking. The great majority of such cases of meningitis are bacterial in origin, and delay in diagnosis can result in serious neurological morbidity and even death.

In the child who convulses with fever, it is important always to consider that something in addition to the fever has caused the child to have a seizure. Unnoted infection such as meningitis or encephalitis, as well as a systemic illness, head trauma, intoxication, electrolyte imbalance, low blood sugar, or a phakomatosis can cause seizures. One must also consider the possibility that the child with a febrile seizure has epilepsy and that fever has simply triggered a seizure recurrence in a child who also experiences unprovoked seizures.

Thus, based on the specifics of each case, the diagnostic evaluation of the child with a febrile seizure can be very limited or moderately comprehensive. Imaging studies are necessary only in selected cases. The electroencephalogram is of limited value. The primary concern is always the need to exclude meningitis. Therefore, a lumbar puncture should be done except in those cases where the possibility of central nervous system infection seems truly remote. © 2002 Academic Press.

I. INTRODUCTION

A febrile seizure is defined as a seizure in association with a febrile illness in the absence of a central nervous system (CNS) infection or acute electrolyte imbalance in children without prior afebrile seizures (ILAE, 1993; see also Chapter 1). The definition implies that in order to make the diagnosis of a febrile seizure in a child who presents with a seizure and a fever, one must exclude meningitis, encephalitis, serious electrolyte imbalance, and other acute neurological illnesses as well as prior unprovoked seizures. The diagnostic evaluation is therefore aimed at addressing the cause of the fever and deciding whether there are other potential causes for the seizure besides the fever per se. The most common issue confronted in the emergency room is whether a lumbar puncture is necessary to exclude meningitis. This chapter reviews the diagnostic evaluation of the child who presents with a seizure in the context of a febrile illness.

II. DIAGNOSTIC EVALUATION

A. HISTORY

The patient history should focus on three main areas:

1. What is the illness that triggered the febrile seizure, and, most importantly, is there anything to suggest meningitis? Seizures occur frequently in bacterial meningitis and can be the heralding sign. Because children with bacterial meningitis are almost always febrile, the possibility of meningitis must always be considered in the child with fever who experiences a seizure. One must also consider the possibility of encephalitis, in which the majority of seizures are complex (see below) (Green et al., 1993). Because bacterial meningitis is a very serious illness, particularly in young children, it is essential to make that diagnosis promptly. If treatment is delayed, the likelihood of serious neurological sequellae and even death is greatly increased.

2. Is the child at substantially increased risk for later development of afebrile seizures, including those that recur (epilepsy)? That risk increases if the child's febrile seizure was complex rather than simple. Simple febrile seizures (80–85% of all febrile seizures) are generalized and last less than 10 or 15 minutes and do not recur within 24 hours. Complex febrile seizures (15–20% of all febrile seizures) are longer than 10 or 15 minutes or focal in nature or recurrent within a day. The risk of later unprovoked seizures is also increased if the child was neurologically abnormal before the first febrile seizure. Additionally, the risk of later afebrile seizures is greater when there is a family history of epilepsy in the child's parents or siblings (Rosman, 2001) (see Chapter 5).

3. Could something other than (or in addition to) fever have caused the seizure? Examples include anticholinergic medications (such as diphenhydramine or amitriptyline) (Ellenhorn and Barceloux, 1988), toxins, discontinuance of previously prescribed anticonvulsants, head trauma, hypoglycemia, electrolyte imbalance, or a phakomatosis (such as tuberous sclerosis, Sturge–Weber disease, or neurofibromatosis).

B. EXAMINATION

The most important part of the examination is to look for the source of the child's fever, with meningitis (usually bacterial) of primary importance in that regard. Very often in young children with meningitis and occasionally in older ones, meningeal signs may be absent. Bacterial meningitis in children is almost always accompanied by signs of acutely increased intracranial pressure. These include an altered mental state, vomiting, strabismus (cranial nerve VI, or less often cranial nerve III, palsies), a "setting sun" sign of the eyes, change in vital signs (increased blood pressure, decreased or increased pulse rate, decreased respirations), and, in the infant, a full and nonpulsatile fontanelle and occasionally separated sutures. In the older child, if bacterial meningitis is accompanied by an intracranial abscess (extradural, subdural, or brain), vascular thrombosis with brain infarction, or hydrocephalus, papilledema may be seen. Signs of accompanying illnesses, such as an otitis media, pharyngitis, viral exanthem, or gastroenteritis should be sought, along with evidence of trauma (especially to the head) and any skin lesions (brown, white, and red) that can indicate a phakomatosis. An identification bracelet can provide evidence of an established seizure disorder. The classic neurologic examination in the child with a febrile seizure often discloses transient abnormalities that in this circumstance lack localizing value.

C. LABORATORY INVESTIGATIONS

Many laboratory studies have been shown to be unhelpful in the management of the child with febrile seizures, except when specific symptoms or signs (e.g., vomiting or diarrhea) exist. Laboratory studies include a complete blood count, blood sugar, serum electrolytes, serum calcium, phosphorus, magnesium, blood urea nitrogen levels, and urinalysis (Asnes et al., 1975; Rutter and Smales, 1977; Gerber and Berliner, 1981; Wallace, 1988; AAP, 1996).

In the presence of fever in the child who has experienced a seizure, the decision about laboratory testing should be directed primarily to identifying the source of the fever. Thus, a complete blood count, blood culture, urine culture, and (less often) stool culture (particularly for *Shigella*) are not uncommonly indicated. It is of note that the incidence of occult bacteremia in children less than 2 years of age with simple febrile seizures is not different than the risk of occult bacteremia in same age children with fever alone (about 5% in either instance) (Chamberlain and Gorman, 1988). In children with diarrhea, vomiting and particularly with evidence of dehydration, serum electrolytes should be measured. Other studies that may be helpful include anticonvulsant blood levels (if the child is being treated for a seizure disorder) and a blood sugar level when there is prolonged postictal obtundation, with vomiting and ketosis, or if the cerebrospinal fluid is to be examined (Rosman, 1987).

D. Brain Imaging

There are some circumstances in which neuroimaging (a cranial computed tomograph or magnetic resonance image) is indicated in a child who has had a febrile seizure: (1) when the history or examination indicates possible or definite head trauma (e.g., scalp swelling and discoloration, hemotympanum); (2) if the examination points to a possible structural brain lesion (e.g., microcephaly, spasticity); or (3) with evidence of increased intracranial pressure (persisting irritability or drowsiness, recurrent vomiting, fullness of the anterior fontanelle in the young child, cranial nerve VI palsies, or papilledema in the older child). In the great majority of children with febrile seizures, however, such clinical features are lacking and there is no need to do neuroimaging (Rosman, 2001). In particular, as discussed below, unless these clinical features are present, there is no need to perform an imaging study before performing a lumbar puncture.

III. SHOULD THE CHILD WITH A FEBRILE SEIZURE HAVE A LUMBAR PUNCTURE?

Underlying meningitis is present in 2–5% of children with apparent febrile seizures (Shinnar, 1999). Because in the great majority of such cases the cause is bacterial, and because bacterial meningitis is a very serious disease especially in young children, the threshold for doing a lumbar puncture must be low in the child who convulses with fever. In 13–16% of children with meningitis, seizures are the presenting sign of disease; in approximately 30–35% of these children (mostly children younger than 18 months), meningeal signs and symptoms may be absent (AAP, 1996). In a retrospective review of 42 cases of acute bacterial meningitis with complicating seizures in children and adults, 60% of the seizures began within the first 2 days of the illness (Rosman *et al.*, 1985).

A lumbar puncture routinely done in 96% of 328 children with a first febrile seizure led to the detection of four cases of unsuspected meningitis; one of the four was bacterial (*Haemophilus influenzae*). Following an initial negative lumbar puncture, two additional children continued to be febrile; both went on to develop meningeal signs within 48 hours and a repeat lumbar puncture disclosed meningococcal meningitis in both (Rutter and Smales, 1977). Thus, if one decides to do a lumbar puncture in a child with a febrile seizure and it is normal, but the suspicion of meningitis remains, a follow-up lumbar puncture must be done. By contrast, in a retrospective review of 503 cases of meningitis (97% bacterial) in children from 2 months to 15 years of age, seizures or suspected seizures occurred in 115 cases before the diagnosis of meningitis. In none of these cases, however, was seizure the sole presenting feature (Green *et al.,* 1993). It is important to stress that an identified source of fever (e.g., otitis media) does not exclude the presence of meningitis. In a retrospective review of 325 children with meningitis, 43 (13%) presented with seizures. Fifteen of these 43 lacked signs of meningeal irritation; of these, four had additional sources of infection outside the central nervous system (two had otitis media, one had pharyngitis, and one had otitis media and pharyngitis) and three had a history of a prior febrile seizure. Five of the 15 patients were more than 2 years of age. In eight of the 15, the meningitis was bacterial (including three of the five who were more than 2 years of age). The seizures were usually brief and generalized (Ratcliffe and Wolf, 1977).

In 1990, guidelines for doing a lumbar puncture in the child who convulses with fever were developed at a workshop in London, England under the joint auspices of the Royal College of Physicians and the British Paediatric Association. They concluded that the indications for lumbar puncture were clinical signs of meningism, complex febrile convulsions, the child who is unduly drowsy or irritable or systemically ill, *probably* children less than 18 months of age, and *certainly* children less than age 12 months (Addy, 1991). Subsequently, the American Academy of Pediatrics (AAP) has developed a Practice Parameter for the Neurodiagnostic Evaluation (including lumbar puncture) of the child with a first simple febrile seizure. Their recommendations for lumbar puncture are equally applicable if the child's febrile seizure is complex. With complex febrile seizures, however, the criteria for performing a lumbar puncture should be even more liberal because complex febrile seizures are much more frequently associated with meningitis than are simple ones (Green *et al.,* 1993).

The AAP recommends that a lumbar puncture be strongly considered in infants younger than 12 months after a first seizure with fever (because the clinical signs and symptoms associated with meningitis may be minimal or absent in this age group). In children *between 12 and 18 months,* lumbar puncture should be considered (because clinical signs and symptoms of meningitis may be subtle). *Beyond 18 months* of age, lumbar puncture is not routinely indicated (because clinical signs of meningitis are more reliable at this age), but lumbar puncture is recommended in the presence of meningeal signs and symptoms (neck stiffness; Kernig and Brudzinski signs) or for any child when the history or examination suggests the presence of an intracranial infection. In infants and children with febrile seizures who have had prior antibiotic treatment, lumbar puncture should be strongly considered (because prior antibiotic treatment can mask signs and symptoms of meningitis) (AAP, 1996). As discussed above, there is no need to perform an imaging study prior to performing a lumbar puncture unless there are specific indications for imaging.

Cerebrospinal fluid is more likely to be abnormal in children with febrile seizures who have had (1) suspicious findings on physical and/or neurological examinations (particularly meningeal signs); (2) complex febrile seizures, because the majority of febrile seizures associated with bacterial meningitis are complex (Green *et al.*, 1993); (3) physician visits within 48 hours before the febrile seizure; (4) febrile seizures on arrival to emergency departments; (5) prolonged postictal states, because most children with simple febrile seizures recover quickly; and (6) initial febrile seizures after 3 years of age, because most febrile seizures occur between 18 and 22 months of age (Hirtz, 1989), with initial febrile seizures after 4 years of age seen in only 15% of children (Aicardi, 1994). Failure to diagnose meningitis occurs more often in children (1) younger than 18 months, who may show no signs or symptoms of meningitis, (2) children who are evaluated by less experienced healthcare providers, and (3) children who may be unavailable for follow-up.

IV. ELECTROENCEPHALOGRAPHY IN THE MANAGEMENT OF FEBRILE SEIZURES

Electroencephalography (EEG) is of limited value in the management of febrile seizures despite the fact that epileptiform activity on an EEG is seen in 2–86% (average 25%) of these children (Millichap, 1968). The EEG is probably most helpful in those children in whom it is uncertain whether a febrile seizure has occurred. EEGs done on the same day of the seizure have been abnormal in as many as 88% of cases, usually with bilateral posterior slow wave activity. The same type of abnormality is present in about one-third of children during the first 6 days after a febrile seizure and usually disappears by 7 to 10 days (Frantzen *et al.*, 1968; Rosman, 1987). Thus, the presence of an EEG abnormality that later disappears serves to confirm the clinical impression of seizure. Ictal EEGs have rarely been recorded in children with febrile seizures. If obtained, generalized or lateralized rapid spiking can be seen (Lennox-Buchthal, 1973).

In 676 children with febrile seizures, EEGs were done from 7 to 20 days after the illness, when the patients were afebrile. Abnormal EEGs were found in 22%. The most common abnormalities were rapid spike waves. Less often seen, in decreasing frequency, were spike and sharp waves, other abnormalities, slow spike waves, and polyspikes. When the initial febrile seizure was focal or prolonged, it was more likely to be associated with paroxysmal abnormalities on the EEG. Additional predictors of paroxysmal activity on the EEG were older age, numbers of previous febrile seizures, and preexisting motor abnormalities (Sofijanov et al., 1992).

Serial EEGs over several years in children with febrile seizures are often abnormal, with an increase in these abnormalities over time. The most frequent abnormalities seen are bilateral slowing; generalized spike wave discharges (unusual before 2 years of age) at rest, with hyperventilation, or after photic stimulation; focal spikes or sharp waves; and hypnagogic paroxysmal spike waves (Stores, 1991).

Thus, EEG abnormalities accompanying febrile seizures can be seen ictally, postictally, and in sequential tracings over several years, yet none of these abnormalities has been convincingly associated with increased risk of febrile seizure recurrence (Stores, 1991; AAP, 1996; Kuturec et al., 1997) or with greater likelihood of later development of epilepsy (Stores, 1991). The Practice Parameter of the AAP also found the EEG not to be predictive of later epilepsy (1) in children with simple febrile seizures, (2) in children in whom febrile seizures are complex, and/or (3) in those with febrile seizures and preexisting neurological disease (a group at higher risk for later epilepsy) (AAP, 1996). Therefore, at the present time the EEG is not considered part of the routine diagnostic evaluation of the child with either simple or complex febrile seizures.

REFERENCES

Addy, D. P. (Chairman), et al. (1991). Guidelines for the management of convulsions with fever. Joint Working Group of the Research Unit of the Royal College of Physicians and the British Paediatric Association. BMJ 303, 634–636.

Aicardi, J. (1994). Febrile convulsions. In "Epilepsy in Children" (J. Aicardi, ed.), 2nd Ed., pp. 253–275. Raven Press, New York.

American Academy of Pediatrics Practice Parameter (1996). The neurodiagnostic evaluation of the child with a first simple febrile seizure. Provisional Committee on Quality Improvement, Subcommittee on Diagnosis and Treatment of Febrile Seizures. Pediatrics 97, 769–775.

Asnes, R. S., Novick, L. F., Nealis, J., et al. (1975). The first febrile seizure: A study of current pediatric practice. J. Pediatr. 87, 485–488.

Chamberlain, J. M., and Gorman, R. L. (1988). Occult bacteremia in children with simple febrile seizures. Am. J. Dis. Child. 142, 1073–1076.

Commission on Epidemiology and Prognosis, International League Against Epilepsy (1993). Guidelines for epidemiologic studies on epilepsy. Epilepsia 34, 592–596.

Ellenhorn, M. J., and Barceloux, D. G. (eds.). (1988). "Medical Toxicology–Diagnosis and Treatment of Human Poisoning," 1st Ed. Elsevier Science Publishers, New York.

Frantzen, E., Lennox-Buchthal, M., and Nygaard, A. (1968). Longitudinal EEG and clinical study of children with febrile convulsions. *Electroenceph. Clin. Neurophysiol.* 24, 197–212.

Gerber, M. A., and Berliner, B. C. (1981). The child with a "simple" febrile seizure. *Am. J. Dis. Child.* 135, 431–433.

Green, S. M., Rothrock, S. G., Clem, K. J., *et al.* (1993). Can seizures be the sole manifestation of meningitis in febrile children? *Pediatrics* 92, 527–534.

Hirtz, D. G. (1989). Generalized tonic-clonic and febrile seizures. *Pediatr. Clin. N. Am.* 36, 375–382.

Kuturec, M., Emoto, S. E., Sofijanov, N., *et al.* (1997). Febrile seizures: Is the EEG a useful predictor of recurrences? *Clin. Pediatr.* 36, 31–36.

Lennox-Buchthal, M. A. (1973). "Febrile Convulsions—A Reappraisal," pp. 1–138. Elsevier, Amsterdam.

Millichap, J. G. (1968). "Febrile Convulsions," pp. 1–222. Macmillan, New York.

Ratcliffe, J. C., and Wolf, S. M. (1977). Febrile convulsions caused by meningitis in young children. *Ann. Neurol.* 1, 285–286.

Rosman, N. P. (1987). Febrile seizures. *Emerg. Med. Clin. North Am.* 5, 719–737.

Rosman, N. P. (2001). Febrile seizures. *In* "Pediatric Epilepsy: Diagnosis and Therapy" (J. M. Pellock, W. E. Dodson, and B.F.D. Bourgeois, eds.), 2nd Ed., pp. 163–175. Demos Medical Publishing, Inc., New York.

Rosman, N. P., Peterson, D. B., Kaye, E. M., *et al.* (1985). Seizures in bacterial meningitis: Prevalence, patterns, pathogenesis and prognosis. *Pediatr. Neurol.* 1, 278–285.

Rutter, N., and Smales, R. C. (1977). Role of routine investigations in children presenting with their first febrile convulsion. *Arch. Dis. Child.* 52, 188–191.

Shinnar, S. (1999). Febrile seizures. *In* "Pediatric Neurology: Principles and Practice" (K. F. Swaiman and S. Ashwal, eds.), 3rd Ed. pp. 676–682. Mosby, St. Louis.

Sofijanov, N., Emoto, S., Kuturec, M., *et al.* (1992). Febrile seizures: Clinical characteristics and initial EEG. *Epilepsia* 33, 52–57.

Stores, G. (1991). When does an EEG contribute to the management of febrile seizures? *Arch. Dis. Child.* 66, 554–557.

Wallace, S. J. (1988). "The Child with Febrile Seizures," pp. 1–182. John Wright, London.

CHAPTER 19

Practical Management Approaches to Simple and Complex Febrile Seizures

FINN URSIN KNUDSEN

Paediatric Department, Glostrup University Hospital, DK-2600 Glostrup, Denmark

Febrile seizures are the most common form of childhood seizures. Although generally benign, they are extremely upsetting to the parents, the recurrence rate is high, there is a slightly increased risk of subsequent epilepsy, and in very rare cases febrile status epilepticus may damage the brain. Even complex febrile seizures often have a benign outcome. Prophylactic continuous daily antiepileptic drug therapy is no longer routinely recommended. Daily phenobarbital and valproate, but not phenytoin or carbamazepine, are effective in preventing seizure recurrence, but due to their potential adverse effects should only be used in rare cases, if at all. Intermittent phenobarbital with fever is ineffective and obsolete. Valproate treatment during febrile episodes has doubtful efficacy. Chloral hydrate with fever appears to be effective, but only few data exist. Intermittent diazepam prophylaxis at times of fever reduces the risk of seizure recurrence if sufficient doses are given, compliance is optimized and very low-risk children are left untreated. The treatment is not recommended as a routine management for simple febrile seizures, but may be considered in multiple simple febrile seizures, complex febrile seizures, and febrile status epilepticus. An attractive alternative is immediate anticonvulsant treatment with rectal diazepam or lorazepam, which offer the opportunity for rapid, safe, simple, and effective seizure cessation. It is considered a first-line treatment of febrile seizures and is useful for parents, caretakers, and professionals, in and outside of the hospital. Some clinicians prefer a "wait and see" policy. Two major targets of treatment are rapid seizure cessation with rectal diazepam or lorazepam in cases of potential febrile status epilepticus and careful parental counseling. © 2002 Academic Press.

I. INTRODUCTION

Although in recent years many new data on the treatment and prognosis of febrile seizures have emerged, many controversies remain. We are still unable to offer evidence-based treatment for the entire spectrum of children with febrile seizures. Six important aspects may influence the approach to treatment:

1. Febrile seizures are benign in most cases.
2. They are extremely upsetting to the parents (see Chapter 20).
3. The recurrence rate is high (30–40%) (see Chapter 3).
4. There is a slightly increased risk of subsequent epilepsy (see Chapter 5).
5. Febrile status epilepticus (duration ∼30 minutes) may, in very rare cases, damage the brain.
6. A small group of children with focal febrile status epilepticus are at some risk of developing hippocampal sclerosis and temporal lobe epilepsy (see Chapter 6–8).

The following treatment strategies are available:

1. Continuous prophylaxis, i.e., daily antiepileptic medication with phenobarbital, valproate, primidone, phenytoin, or carbamazepine.
2. Intermittent prophylaxis with benzodiazepines, phenobarbital, valproate, or chloral hydrate given at time of fever.
3. Immediate therapy of ongoing seizures with benzodiazepines administered rectally, orally, or by the nasal route.
4. Antipyretic treatment during fever.
5. A "wait and see" policy.

A survey of prescribing strategies for febrile seizures in a number of European countries (Baldy-Moulinier *et al.*, 1998) documented a lack of consensus on which treatment strategy should be used. Continuous or intermittent prophylaxis with antiepileptic agents was prescribed by a relative minority of the respondents, whereas intermittent prophylaxis with rectal or oral diazepam was used by an appreciable proportion of the clinicians. Only 50% did not advocate drugs to prevent febrile seizures. In an older survey, Millichap and Colliver (1991) asked 909 North American physicians, including pediatricians and pediatric neurologists, how they treated simple and complex febrile seizures. Even for simple febrile seizures, almost 50% of the respondents prescribed chronic prophylaxis with phenobarbital for 12–24 months and about 20% recommended diazepam for intermittent use during febrile episodes. A total of 89% prescribed long-term phenobarbital for the prevention of complex febrile seizures. This approach is now outdated (American Academy of Pediatrics, 1995, 1999).

This chapter looks at the pros and cons for the available treatment modalities for both simple and complex febrile seizures in various clinical settings. A summary of the data is given in Table 1. Reviews or points of view on the topic include those by Millichap *et al.* (1960), Lennox-Buchthal (1973), Nelson and Ellenberg (1976, 1978, 1981), Knudsen (1979), Consensus Development Panel (1980), Wallace (1988), Freeman (1990), Maytal and Shinnar (1990), Rosman *et al.* (1993), Camfield *et al.* (1995), and Knudsen *et al.* (1996). Other relevant surveys have been reported by Knudsen and Vestermark (1978), Wolf (1979), Addy (1981), Deonna (1982), Wright (1987), Newton and McKinlay (1988), Knudsen (1988, 1991, 1996, 2000), Freeman (1992), Aicardi (1994), Smith (1994), and Freeman and Vining (1995). The British guidelines for the management of convulsions with fever were published in 1991 (Research Unit of the Royal College of Physicians and the British Paediatric Association). Guidelines for the long-term treatment of simple febrile seizures have recently been published by the American Academy of Pediatrics (1999), and a Japanese consensus report is also available (Fukuyama *et al.,* 1996).

TABLE 1   Effect of Treatment on the Recurrence Rate of Febrile Seizures

Treatment	Effect
Continuous prophylaxis	
Phenytoin	No documented efficacy
Carbamazepine	No documented efficacy
Phenobarbital	Effective
Valproate	Effective
Primidone	Few data
Intermittent prophylaxis with fever	
Phenobarbital	Ineffective and obsolete
Valproate	Dubious efficacy
Chloral hydrate	Appears to be effective, but few data
Diazepam (oral or rectal)	Effective
Other benzodiazepines (lorazepam, nitrazepam, clonazepam, midazolam)	Probably effective, but few data
Immediate anticonvulsant therapy	
Rectal diazepam (in solution or gel)	Effective in uncontrolled studies
Rectal diazepam as suppository	Effective only after 20–30 minutes
Rectal lorazepam in solution	Probably effective, but few data
Rectal clonazepam in solution	Probably effective, but few data
Midazolam (nasal, oral, buccal)	Probably effective, but few data
Rectal chloral hydrate	Probably effective, but few data
Antipyretic drugs during fever	Not effective
No treatment	Recurrence rate 30–40%

II. CONTINUOUS PROPHYLAXIS

Continuous prophylaxis, most commonly with phenobarbital, was a common therapeutic approach to febrile seizures in the past (Millichap and Colliver 1991). Some antiepileptic drugs, notably phenobarbital and valproate, can be effective in reducing the risk of recurrent febrile seizures. However, with the increasing recognition of the benign nature of most febrile seizures and the adverse effects of antiepileptic drugs on cognition and behavior (American Academy of Pediatrics, 1995), continuous prophylaxis is no longer used except in very selected cases (American Academy of Pediatrics, 1999; Knudsen, 2000).

A. PHENYTOIN

Several clinical trials have found that phenytoin is not effective in preventing recurrent febrile seizures. In a prospective, open, "odd and even dates" randomized trial, 218 children were given either phenytoin as continuous prophylaxis or no treatment following a first febrile seizure. The recurrence rate over 12–36 months was low and almost identical in the two groups (19 vs. 18%), but the phenytoin doses were only 5–8 mg/kg/day (Frantzen et al., 1964; Lennox-Buchthal, 1973). Continuous phenytoin prophylaxis with higher doses, adjusted to maintain a therapeutic serum level of 10–20 µg/ml, was also found ineffective in preventing new febrile seizures (Melchior et al., 1971). The recurrence rate was even somewhat higher in the phenytoin group (29%), as compared to the control group (19%). Four children had new febrile seizures despite proved high or toxic serum levels of phenytoin at the time of the seizure. Phenytoin was an ineffective prophylactic agent in a placebo-controlled, randomized study containing 138 children with febrile seizures. The 12-month recurrence rate was 35% in the placebo group and 34% in the phenytoin group. The drug is considered unsuitable for prophylaxis because of lack of efficacy, adverse effects, compliance problems, and the saturation kinetics of the drug (Bacon et al., 1981).

B. CARBAMAZEPINE

In the few available trials, carbamazepine has not demonstrated efficacy in preventing recurrent febrile seizures. Two trials have compared the prophylactic efficacy of carbamazepine with phenobarbital against febrile seizures (Monaco et al., 1980; Antony and Hawke 1983). In both trials, the recurrence rates in the carbamazepine group were comparable with no treatment and significantly higher as compared to children taking phenobarbital. In a small study, 16 children who had recurrent febrile seizures while on phenobarbital were given carbamazepine and 13 had recurrences (Camfield *et al.*, 1982). Therefore, carbamazepine is not recommended as a prophylactic agent for the treatment of febrile seizures.

C. Phenobarbital

Phenobarbital is the most widely used drug for continuous prophylaxis of febrile seizures. Five randomized double-blind, controlled clinical trials have studied the efficacy of phenobarbital as a prophylactic agent. Four of the trials documented a significant difference in the incidence of recurrences between children receiving phenobarbital and those given placebo: 5 vs. 25% (Camfield *et al.*, 1980), 19 vs. 33% (Ngwane and Bower, 1980), 9 vs. 44% in children younger than 14 months (Bacon *et al.*, 1981), and 7 vs. 53% (Thilothammal *et al.*, 1993). The fifth study found no effect of chronic phenobarbital prophylaxis but had a high rate of noncompliance with the therapeutic regimen (Farwell *et al.*, 1990). In addition, a number of open, randomized or quasirandomized (Campbell *et al.*, 1998), controlled studies (Wolf *et al.*, 1977; Knudsen and Vestermark, 1978; Wallace and Smith, 1980) and nonrandomized studies (Færø *et al.*, 1972; Thorn, 1975, 1981; Wallace, 1975; Minagawa and Miura, 1981) all documented a significant chronic seizure control. Only a single unblinded, quasirandomized study reported failure of phenobarbital to prevent febrile seizures (Heckmatt *et al.*, 1976). In a meta-analysis, Newton (1988) pooled the results from six small British trials and analyzed them on an intention-to-treat basis. Sixty-six of 296 (22%) treated children had recurrences compared with 58 of 236 (25%) controls. The meta-analysis concluded that although phenobarbital per se may prevent as many as half the recurrences, the treatment is hardly effective from an intention-to-treat point of view (Newton, 1988).

Phenobarbital has frequent and substantial side-effects and may adversely influence cognition, behavior, sleep, and quality of life for the child and the family. Common problems include fussiness, sleep problems with insomnia or inverted sleep pattern, mood changes with irritability, stubbornness, aggressive behaviour, and attention deficit/hyperactivity disorder (ADHD)-like symptoms, including hyperactivity and attention deficits, but also drowsiness and lethargy (Wallace, 1988). These side-effects occur in about 40–50% of the children treated, and are only partly dose dependent (Wolf and Forsythe, 1978; Newton, 1988). Chronic phenobarbital treatment may be detrimental to the child's IQ (Byrne *et al.*, 1987; Farwell *et al.*, 1990) and may induce major depressive disorder and suicidal ideation in adolescents (Brent *et al.*, 1987). Less severe adverse effects were found by Camfield *et al.* (1979). Psychological and behavioral side-effects of chronic phenobarbital treatment have been verified in a well-designed, double-blind, cross-over study (Vining *et al.*, 1987).

In summary, daily phenobarbital is effective in preventing further febrile seizures, especially if serum levels above 15 g/ml are maintained. However, if the results are analyzed on an intention-to-treat basis, the efficacy is less impressive or even questionable. Chronic prophylaxis does not appear to prevent the few cases of later epilepsy. Virtually all trials have reported compliance problems. Consensus has been reached that because of its unsatisfactory adverse effect profile, especially on behavior and cognition (American Academy of Pediatrics, 1995) (see Chapter 4), phenobarbital should no longer be used as a first-line drug, but is only to be applied in rare cases, if at all.

D. PRIMIDONE

Only few data are available. However, because primidone is metabolized to phenobarbital along with other metabolites, the prophylactic efficacy in febrile seizures is probably similar to that of phenobarbital (Cavazzuti, 1975; Minagawa and Miura, 1981). The type and severity of side-effects are also similar to those of phenobarbital. The drug has not been used extensively and is not recommended for routine prophylaxis of febrile seizures.

E. VALPROATE

Several studies have confirmed the efficacy of daily valproate in preventing recurrent febrile seizures. In a well-designed, but small, double-blind, randomized, controlled trial (Ngwane and Bower, 1980) a total of 64 children with their first febrile seizure were given either sodium valproate (30–60 mg/kg, $n = 18$), phenobarbital (3–6 mg/kg, $n = 21$), or no treatment ($n = 21$). The 12-month recurrence rates were 5, 19, and 33%, respectively, suggesting that valproate in rather high doses affords effective seizure control. An open, randomized, therapeutic trial comparing chronic prophylaxis with valproate, phenobarbital, or placebo after a first febrile seizure confirmed these results (Mamelle et al., 1984). The 24-month recurrence rates were 4, 19, and 35%, respectively. Two controlled, but not randomized or blinded, studies compared the prophylactic efficacy of phenobarbital, sodium valproate, and primidone. In 141 children with simple febrile seizures treated with valproate (20 mg/kg), phenobarbital (5 mg/kg), or primidone (25 mg/kg), the 12-month recurrence rates were 4, 4, and 4%, respectively, as compared to 55% among untreated controls (Cavazzuti, 1975). A Japanese study made a comparison between phenobarbital, primidone, and valproate in children with at least two febrile seizures. The recurrence rates in the three groups were 17, 14, and 13%, respectively (Minagawa and Miura, 1981). Valproate and diazepam were found to be equally effective in reducing the risk of a recurrence in children having a high risk of further febrile seizures (Lee *et al.*, 1986). In a meta-analysis, four published or unpublished British valproate trials were identified. Forty-nine of 145 (34%) treated children had recurrences as compared to 36 of 136 (26%) controls. The report, which used an intent-to-treat analysis, concluded that any benefit from valproate is likely to be unacceptably small (Newton, 1988).

Valproate has fewer adverse effects on cognition and behavior than does phenobarbital (Vining *et al.*, 1987) and is generally much better tolerated. However, over 100 cases of fatal hepatic failure are on record worldwide (Dreifuss *et al.*, 1987; Scheffner *et al.*, 1988) and the children at highest risk (under 2 years of age and neurologically abnormal) are precisely those most likely to be considered for prophylaxis. Valproate encephalopathy, an easily overlooked condition, is not rare. Other side-effects include weight gain, tremor, gastrointestinal upset, headache, and rare cases of pancreatitis. In summary, valproate is a first line antiepileptic drug (Davis *et al.*, 1994). It seems to be at least as effective as phenobarbital in preventing recurrent febrile seizures. It is generally well tolerated. However, the serious adverse effects of the drug, though rare, disqualify it for routine use in this common, benign condition.

III. INTERMITTENT PROPHYLAXIS

This approach, i.e., anticonvulsant treatment during febrile episodes, is less inconvenient for the child and his family than is chronic prophylaxis with antiepileptic agents. The child is treated for only a few days with each febrile episode, and is exposed to fewer doses of the drug. The acute and chronic side-effects are less than with daily treatment. Being better tolerated by the child, the treatment is more readily accepted by the parents, a necessary prerequisite for optimal compliance. The disadvantage is that for treatment to be effective it must be promptly initiated at the onset of each febrile illness. Although effective strategies for intermittent prophylaxis are available, some widely applied intermittent strategies for febrile seizures are ineffective.

A. INTERMITTENT PHENOBARBITAL

Phenobarbital given orally at times of fever as prophylaxis has been used extensively for decades. It has few side-effects, but is ineffective (Millichap *et al.*, 1960). In an open clinical trial, 355 children were randomized to daily phenobarbital, intermittent phenobarbital at time of fever, and no treatment following a first febrile seizure (Wolf *et al.*, 1977). As previously discussed, daily phenobarbital treatment reduced the recurrence risk. The group treated with intermittent phenobarbital had the same recurrence risk as the no-treatment group. The long half-life of the drug precludes any significant acute seizure control, because adequate serum levels cannot be attained within several days, even on double oral doses (Svensmark and Buchthal, 1963; Jalling, 1974).

Pharmacokinetic data suggest that an initial high, intramuscular dose of phenobarbital (15 mg/kg) followed by 5 mg/kg orally may be effective in preventing new febrile seizures in a hospital setting (Jalling, 1974; Sternowsky and Lagenstein, 1981). In another clinical scenario, intramuscular phenobarbital has also been effective, although with unacceptable morbidity. In children having seizures with fever caused by cerebral malaria, phenobarbital given as a high, single intramuscular dose (20 mg/kg) provided highly effective seizure control. Unfortunately, this high-dose regimen was associated with an increased mortality, and therefore cannot be recommended (Crawley et al., 2000).

In summary, intermittent oral phenobarbital is ineffective and obsolete as a prophylactic agent in the treatment of febrile seizures. Intramuscular phenobarbital at time of fever, although probably effective, is associated with too many adverse effects and is not recommended.

B. INTERMITTENT VALPROATE

The few trials of intermittent valproate therapy have not demonstrated efficacy. In an open, quasirandomized, hospital-based study, 169 children with their first febrile seizure were given either intermittent prophylaxis with rectal diazepam in solution every 12 hours ($n = 89$) or valproic acid as suppositories ($n = 80$), whenever the rectal temperature was 38.5°C or more. The dose of valproate was 15–30 mg/kg every 24 hours at times of fever. On an intention-to-treat basis, the 12-month recurrence rates in the two groups were similar, 27 vs. 20%, a difference that was not significant. The number of complex recurrences was significantly higher in the valproate-treated group. No side effects were seen (Daugbjerg et al., 1990). In summary, the use of intermittent valproate at time of fever to prevent febrile seizures is of doubtful value and is not recommended.

Intravenous valproate is a safe drug for immediate treatment of seizures (Devinsky et al., 1995; Hovinga et al., 1999) and seizure control can be very rapid (Überall et al., 1998). The drug is well tolerated and may be useful in the treatment of seizures in a hospital setting. However, there is very limited experience with the use of intravenous valproate in preventing febrile seizures in the child with a fever or in treating children with febrile seizures.

C. INTERMITTENT CHLORAL HYDRATE

A Japanese, nonrandomized trial used rectal suppositories at the onset of fever in doses of 250–500 mg chloral hydrate in 154 children with febrile seizures. In the treatment group only 6% had recurrences as compared to 31% among untreated controls. Adverse effects were not seen (Tachibana *et al.*, 1985, 1986). Another trial compared the prophylactic efficacy of rectal diazepam (*n* = 72) with chloral hydrate (*n* = 41) in 113 children with febrile seizures and at least one later febrile episode. The 6-month recurrence rates in the two groups were 3.8 vs. 20.4%, showing that diazepam was significantly more effective than chloral hydrate for the prevention of febrile seizures (Shimazaki *et al.*, 1996). In this study the recurrence risk in the chloral hydrate-treated group did not suggest efficacy. Pharmacokinetic data are not available.

In summary, chloral hydrate may be effective as a prophylactic agent, but only few data exist. Unlike the other drugs discussed in this section, it is not a known anticonvulsant so that the mechanism by which it may prevent febrile seizures is unclear. A double-blind, placebo-controlled study as well as pharmacokinetic and safety data are needed before chloral hydrate use in this clinical setting can be recommended.

D. INTERMITTENT BENZODIAZEPINES

This group of anticonvulsant drugs has been widely used for immediate treatment, for intermittent prophylaxis, and for chronic prophylaxis. The most commonly used are diazepam, lorazepam, nitrazepam, and midazolam. Clobazam has been used for childhood epilepsy, but not for febrile seizures (Shorvon, 1998).

1. Intermittent Diazepam

a. Efficacy

Intermittent diazepam prophylaxis, i.e., diazepam during febrile episodes, has been used extensively for decades in many parts of the world, especially in Europe and Japan. The routes of administration for intermittent prophylaxis include oral (Shirai *et al.*, 1987; Autret *et al.*, 1990; Rosman *et al.*, 1993; Rossi *et al.*, 1993; Uhari *et al.*, 1995), sublingual (Nunez-Lopez *et al.*, 1995), and rectal (Knudsen, 1985a,b; Knudsen and Vestermark, 1978; Shirai *et al.*, 1988; Thorn, 1981; Uhari *et al.*, 1995). A variety of formulations of rectal diazepam are available in different countries as discussed below (see Section IV). These include suppositories (Knudsen and Vestermark, 1978; Thorn, 1981; Shirai *et al.*, 1988) rectal in solution (Knudsen, 1985a,b; Uhari *et al.*, 1995), and, more recently, rectal gel (Dreifuss *et al.*, 1998; Cereghino *et al.*, 1998; Kriel *et al.*, 1999). Although there are some differences in their absorption properties and pharmacokinetics, there is no reason to think that their efficacy for intermittent prophylaxis is significantly different. Nasally administered diazepam has not been used for intermittent prophylaxis in febrile seizures.

A total of three randomized, placebo-controlled trials have studied the efficacy of intermittent diazepam prophylaxis in febrile seizures (Autret et al., 1990; Rosman et al., 1993; Uhari et al., 1995). The results are conflicting. Two of the trials showed no significant seizure control (Autret et al., 1990; Uhari et al., 1995), whereas Rosman et al. (1993) found the treatment effective. A meta-analysis, based on these three studies, concluded that intermittent diazepam prophylaxis was ineffective in reducing the recurrence rate significantly (Rantala et al., 1997). However, the validity of combining these trials in a meta-analysis has been questioned (Watanabe, 1997; Knudsen, 2000; Eysenck, 1994). The two trials showing negative results had methodological problems. In the study of Uhari et al. (1995), neither a low dose of acetaminophen nor a low dose of rectal diazepam followed by oral diazepam (0.2 mg/kg three times a day) resulted in effective seizure control. It is quite likely that the low doses of diazepam used were responsible for the lack of efficacy (Rosman, 1996). The study of Autret et al. (1990) is flawed by a severe lack of compliance. In their trial, 185 children with a first febrile seizure were randomized to receive oral diazepam or placebo with fever every 12 hours. The recurrence rate did not differ between the two groups: 16 vs. 19%. However, only one of the 15 children with a recurrence received diazepam as prescribed prior to the seizure. It is likely that the lack of efficacy is caused by poor adherence to the protocol, a possibility not allowed for if data are analyzed on an intention-to-treat basis. Rosman et al. (1993) used oral diazepam (0.3 mg/kg every 8 hours) or placebo with fever in their study. Drug compliance was monitored by means of riboflavin and was good. An intention-to-treat analysis showed a significant (40%) reduction in the recurrence risk for the prophylaxis group, even though the number of febrile episodes occurred 26% more often in this group. The number of new febrile seizures in children actually receiving diazepam was strikingly lower in the treatment group as compared to the placebo group: 7 vs. 38.

In addition, at least 13 clinically controlled, randomized as well as uncontrolled trials (Echenne et al., 1983; Devilat and Masafierro, 1989) have found that diazepam prophylaxis given at time of fever significantly reduces the number of recurrences (Knudsen and Vestermark, 1978; Dianese, 1979; Thorn, 1981; Vanasse et al., 1984; Garcia et al., 1984; Knudsen, 1985a,b; Lee et al., 1986; Ramakrishnan and Thomas, 1986; A. Katalin and J. Borsi, unpublished; Mosquera et al., 1987; Shirai et al., 1988; Rossi et al., 1993; Nunez-Lopez et al., 1995). Seven of these are prospective, randomized trials with concurrent treated or untreated controls (Knudsen and Vestermark, 1978; Garcia et al., 1984; Knudsen, 1985a,b; Ramakrishnan and Thomas, 1986; A. Katalin and J. Borsi, unpublished; Mosquera et al., 1987; Nunez-Lupez et al., 1995). A Danish trial compared intermittent treatment with diazepam suppositories (5 mg three times a day, $n = 83$) at times of fever with chronic phenobarbital prophylaxis ($n = 73$). The 12-month recurrence rates were 15 and 16%, respectively, well below the spontaneous recurrence rate (Knudsen and Vestermark, 1978). A

Spanish trial compared rectal diazepam in solution given at times of fever with long-term phenobarbital treatment. The 18-month rate of recurrences were 8 vs. 10% (Garcia et al., 1984). In a clinically controlled, odd and even dates, randomized trial, 289 children with a first febrile seizure were given either prophylaxis with rectal diazepam in solution (5–7.5 mg every 12 hours) whenever the rectal temperature was >38.5°C ($n = 152$) or no prophylaxis but only rectal diazepam in the event of new seizures ($n = 137$). The 18-month recurrence rate was reduced from 39 to 12% and the number of prolonged recurrences decreased from 5.0 to 0.7%, both highly significant differences (Knudsen, 1985a,b). Another study compared four groups: long-term phenobarbital ($n = 30$), intermittent phenobarbital ($n = 30$), oral intermittent diazepam ($n = 30$), and no treatment ($n = 30$). The recurrence rates in the groups were 30, 17, 0, and 20%, respectively (Ramakrishnan and Thomas, 1986). In an unpublished Hungarian trial, rectal diazepam in solution ($n = 37$) was compared to long-term phenobarbital treatment ($n = 26$). A 20% recurrence rate was found in both groups (A. Katalin and J. Borsi, unpublished). Another Spanish trial compared rectal diazepam in solution ($n = 21$), long-term valproate ($n = 18$), and no treatment ($n = 25$). The 24-month recurrence rates were 29, 0, and 64%, respectively (Mosquera et al., 1987). Nunez-Lopez et al. (1995) compared three treatment groups: chronic phenobarbital (5 mg/kg/day), acetaminophen (10 mg/kg four times a day with fever), and sublingual or rectal diazepam (0.5 mg/kg every 12 hours at times of fever). The recurrence rates were 32, 40, and 7%, respectively.

That intermittent seizure prophylaxis with benzodiazepines is actually feasible and effective is substantiated in recent, double-blind, placebo-controlled studies. Diazepam rectal gel, administered intermittently to children and adults with episodic epilepsy, showed significant superiority over placebo (Dreifuss et al., 1998; Cereghino et al., 1998; Kriel et al., 1999).

There is pharmacological evidence to suggest that two doses of 0.5 mg/kg diazepam at 8-hour intervals result in anticonvulsant plasma concentrations for at least 24 hours (Minagawa et al., 1986). Oral diazepam (0.3 mg/kg given every 8 hours when fever is present) is also effective (Rosman et al., 1993). Despite the fact that many pharmacokinetic data on prophylactic diazepam exist (Agurell et al., 1975; Knudsen, 1977; Dulac et al., 1978; Meberg et al., 1978; Ramsay et al., 1979; Moolenar et al., 1980; Milligan et al., 1981, 1982; Dhillon et al., 1982; Minagawa et al., 1982, 1986; Benchet et al., 1984), the anticonvulsant level is not well established and the recommended doses for prophylaxis are empirical.

b. Side Effects

There is some controversy as to the short- and long-term side effects of intermittent diazepam prophylaxis. The above-mentioned clinical trials included

1253 diazepam-treated patients and not a single serious adverse event occurred (Knudsen, 1991), as compared to 527 untreated controls with one case of sudden unexplained death (Autret *et al.*, 1990). A total of five recent studies of the use of rectal diazepam in the treatment of seizures (Dreifuss *et al.*, 1998; Cereghino *et al.*, 1998; Kriel *et al.*, 1999, 2000; Mitchell *et al.*, 1999) reported no clinically significant episodes of respiratory depression. The treatment has been used extensively for two decades in many parts of Europe and in Japan. In Denmark alone some 30,000 children have been treated with 150,000 doses of diazepam immediately or prophylactically, most often given by the parents at home. Only two cases of diazepam-induced respiratory problems have been reported to the Danish health authorities from January 1975 to July 2000. Outcome was benign, and not a single serious or fatal case is on record. Although reporting systems of side effects to health authorities are not totally reliable, fatal events would hardly have escaped our attention.

There is a striking discrepancy between these safety data from countries with many years of experience from treating a huge number of patients and a prospective study monitoring potential respiratory depression (Norris *et al.*, 1999). Of 91 patient episodes involving rectal diazepam in solution, 8 were reported to have respiratory depression. Three other reports have also emerged, reporting a few cases (Sykes and Okonofua, 1988; Elterman, 1994; Appleton *et al.*, 1995). The reason for the discrepancy is not clear. However, febrile seizures can be accompanied by respiratory arrest or by irregular, slow respiration ictally or postictally. Bedside distinction between seizure-induced and diazepam-induced respiratory problems may be difficult. Furthermore, bedside differentiation between short-lasting, benign apnea and respiratory arrest may be difficult. Apart from the drug dose, respiratory problems appear primarily related to acute seizure control rather than to prophylaxis, to treatment of febrile status rather than to treatment of simple febrile seizures, to polytherapy rather than to monotherapy, and to intravenous rather than to rectal administration. A survey of diazepam and drug-associated deaths in the United States and Canada confirms that diazepam is a very safe drug (Finkle *et al.*, 1979). In our own clinic we have used immediate or preventive, home-based treatment with rectal diazepam in solution routinely for all children with febrile seizures (100–200 per year) for the past 20 years. Because we have never experienced serious adverse effects, we do not use or advocate a test dose of rectal diazepam prior to home treatment or routinely warn the parents about the potential risk of respiratory arrest.

2. Other Benzodiazepines

Other benzodiazepines have been used much less for intermittent prophylaxis of febrile seizures.

a. Nitrazepam

A total of 55 children with febrile seizures, having a high risk of a recurrence, were treated with oral nitrazepam (0.25–0.5 mg/kg/day, divided equally in three doses) during febrile episodes. The recurrence rate among the 31 children actually taking the drug was 19% as compared to 46% in 24 children in whom the parents refused the medication or gave it inadequately, a significant difference (Vanasse et al., 1984). One-third of the patients experienced side effects, including drowsiness, ataxia, and agitation. The drug is only rarely used, and the side effects observed in higher doses seem to make it less acceptable than diazepam for prophylaxis.

b. Lorazepam and Midazolam

These drugs, especially lorazepam, have been used extensively for the treatment of ongoing febrile or afebrile status epilepticus but not for the prevention of febrile seizures. Although they may well be effective, the lack of data on their relative safety and efficacy would make diazepam the preferred treatment for intermittent prophylaxis.

c. Clonazepam

Oral clonazepam (0.1 mg/kg/day in three or four divided doses) reduced the recurrence rate in febrile seizures significantly in one study (Lalande and De Paillerets, 1978). However, drowsiness and ataxia were common, and the regimen can hardly be recommended in the doses prescribed.

3. Practical Approach to Intermittent Diazepam Prophylaxis

Intermittent diazepam prophylaxis given either orally or rectally at time of fever substantially reduces the risk of recurrent febrile seizures if sufficient doses are given, compliance problems are addressed, and children having a very low risk of recurrences are left untreated (Knudsen, 1985a,b). Bedside recurrence risk assessment based on simple, available data (age of the child, family seizure history, height of the fever, type of seizure, and number of febrile illnesses) is important, because the efficacy of the prophylaxis correlates with the recurrence risk. The higher the recurrence risk, the better the seizure reduction during prophylaxis and vice versa (Knudsen, 1985a,b). Thus, the recurrence risk reduction is most impressive in young children with many febrile episodes, with a low-grade fever at the time of seizure, and a positive family seizure history. Efficacy is low in older, healthy children with a high temperature at the time of seizure and no family seizure history. In children with a low risk of a recurrence (see Chapter 3), intermittent prophylaxis appears ineffective (Knudsen, 1985a,b). In addition, the treatment appears to reduce the number of prolonged recurrences significantly. It appears safe, effective, cheap, and can be administered by most parents after a brief instruction. It is to be given only a few times during the child's lifetime, thereby reducing the risks of acute and chronic side effects.

The drawbacks of the treatment include the very idea of giving drugs to small children for a benign condition. The risk of serious adverse events is very small [though the American Academy of Pediatrics (1999) has raised the concern that diazepam at time of fever may mask the symptoms of more serious underlying illness, such as meningitis]. In addition, the parents may be unable to recognize the beginning of a febrile illness and prophylaxis is therefore given too late. We have not seen excessive administration of benzodiazepines to children by anxious parents, abuse of the drug by the parents or caregivers, accidental ingestion, or Munchausen by proxy. One case of nonaccidental poisoning of a small child with rectal diazepam in solution is on record in Denmark.

For prophylactic purposes diazepam may be administered orally or rectally. The efficacy of seizure control is probably more related to the timing and dose of diazepam than to the route of administration. Irrespective of the form and route of administration, the dose of diazepam is 0.5 mg/kg given two or three times a day at times of fever (Knudsen, 1988, 1991). Rectal diazepam in solution or gel may be given every 12 hours, whenever the child has a rectal temperature of >38.5°C. The diazepam dose is 5 mg every 12 hours for children up to 3 years of age, and 7.5 mg every 12 hours for children 3 years of age or older. For infants less than 12 months of age, the dose should be reduced to 2–4 mg/dose. No more than four consecutive doses should be given without further advice, in order to avoid accumulation of diazepam and the main metabolite, N-desmethyldiazepam. Because the seizures often occur at any early stage of fever, the first dose is the most important. The delivery system may be a prepackaged, unit-dose rectal tube with diazepam in solution or in a gel. Diazepam suppositories are used prophylactically in a dose of 5 mg every 8 hours at rectal temperatures >38.5°C (Knudsen and Vestermark, 1978; Thorn, 1981). For the youngest children, doses of 5 mg at 12-hour intervals are recommended.

Following the recognition of the generally benign nature of febrile seizures and the finding that long-term prognosis is similar with prophylaxis and immediate treatment, intermittent prophylaxis with short-acting benzodiazepines as a routine treatment for simple febrile seizures is no longer recommended (American Academy of Pediatrics, 1999). However, there may still be a role for intermittent prophylaxis in a small, selected group of children, which may include those with generalized and focal febrile status epilepticus; prolonged, focal, or a repetitive variety of complex recurrences; or a strong parental pressure for treatment. Some may also include children with multiple simple recurrences or even many risk factors for recurrences (Fukuyama *et al.*, 1996). The administration of benzodiazepines at times of fever or seizures to young children has no detrimental effects on their later intellectual, scholastic, motor, or neurological achievements (Knudsen *et al.*, 1996). However, the data suggest that the long-term prognosis in terms of subsequent epilepsy, neurological, motor, intellectual, cognitive, and scholastic performance is no better with intermittent diazepam prophylaxis as compared to immediate anticonvulsant treatment (Knudsen *et al.*, 1996) (see Chapters 3–5, and 7).

IV. IMMEDIATE ANTICONVULSANT THERAPY

Benzodiazepines, i.e., diazepam, lorazepam, clonazepam, and midazolam, given intravenously are the drugs of choice for the immediate treatment of ongoing febrile and afebrile seizures. In a home setting, intravenous administration of benzodiazepines is not a feasible treatment, and to avoid unnecessary delay in treatment, rectal administration of these drugs is a rational alternative (Knudsen, 1979; Woody and Laney, 1988; Dooley, 1998). In infants and young children, venous access may be difficult or impossible even in a hospital setting and rectal administration is appropriate in that setting as well. Note that in approximately 90% of children the seizures will be short-lasting and do not require treatment. Although many uncontrolled trials and abundant pharmacokinetic evidence suggest that rectal administration of benzodiazepines may effectively treat ongoing seizures, no decisive evidence from double-blind, placebo-controlled trials exists. The two drugs most extensively used in rectal treatment of ongoing seizure activity are diazepam and lorazepam. There is much less experience with clonazepam and nitrazepam. An interesting new option is midazolam.

A. DIAZEPAM

Being the most lipophilic drug among the benzodiazepines, diazepam crosses the rectal mucosa and the blood–brain barrier extremely fast, and enters the brain within few minutes (Agurell *et al.*, 1975; Knudsen, 1977; Ramsay *et al.*, 1979; Franzoni *et al.*, 1983). Single-dose pharmacokinetic data on rectal diazepam in solution show that anticonvulsant plasma concentration levels are achieved within 2–4 minutes (Agurell *et al.*, 1975; Knudsen, 1977; Dulac *et al.*, 1978; Meberg *et al.*, 1978; Dhillon *et al.*, 1982; Mizuno *et al.*, 1987). Blood levels after 5 minutes were 300–800 ng/ml in all studies, i.e., well above the presumed anticonvulsant level, which is, however, poorly defined and probably differs widely among children. The immediate anticonvulsant efficacy of rectal diazepam in solution has been documented in several uncontrolled studies (Knudsen, 1979, 1985a,b; Hoppu and Santavuori, 1981; Ventura *et al.*, 1982; Sykes *et al.*, 1988; Camfield *et al.*, 1989). The efficacy of rectal diazepam gel in terminating seizures has also been demonstrated in several small randomized open studies comparing it with intravenous diazepam in the prehospital treatment of children with status epilepticus of all types (Alldredge *et al.*, 1995; Dieckmann, 1994). Thus, firm pharmacological and clinical evidence suggests that rectal diazepam effectively treats ongoing seizures and is a rational alternative to intravenous treatment. A potential disadvantage of diazepam treatment is its short duration of action as compared to lorazepam, but this is less of an issue with febrile seizures than with other forms of seizures that tend to recur.

For emergency treatment, diazepam should not be given intramuscularly, because of erratic and often slow absorption. A unit-dose rectal tube of plastic or glass and a rectal gel are available. Most, if not all, commercial intravenous diazepam preparations are applicable for rectal use and may be administered with a plastic syringe fitted with a short plastic tip. Diazepam suppository absorption through the rectal mucosa is slow, taking at least 15–20 minutes (Knudsen, 1977) or more (Minagawa *et al.*, 1982) to reach anticonvulsant levels.

The child should be placed in a semiprone position to help maintain the airway (see Chapter 20 regarding first aid). Rectal diazepam may be used as soon as possible after the onset of a seizure. In practice, several minutes will often elapse before it is given. Some prefer waiting 5 minutes, by which time at least 80% of the seizures have stopped spontaneously and the drug can be avoided. Remaining seizures are terminated with rectal diazepam (0.5. mg/kg/dose; i.e., 5 mg to children under the age of 3 years and 7.5 mg to those who are 3 years of age or more). The child's buttocks should be pressed together for 3 minutes after application.

If the seizure continues for more than 5 minutes, the same dose is repeated. In a prehospital setting a maximum of two doses should be given. We have used this policy, i.e., a maximum of two home-based doses, for 20 years in our clinic and have never experienced serious, adverse events. If the seizures continue or recur, the child should be referred to a hospital. In a hospital setting diazepam is given intravenously [0.2–0.5 mg/kg; rate 0.1–0.2 mg/kg/min up to a total (rectal plus intravenous) dose of 2–3 mg/kg over 30 minutes]. A total dose of 20–30 mg diazepam is often required, but higher doses are usually not helpful.

Emergency treatment can be given either at home (Knudsen, 1979, 1985a,b; Hoppu and Santavuori, 1981; Ventura *et al.*, 1982; Camfield *et al.*, 1989; Kriel *et al.*, 1991; De Negri *et al.*, 1991) or in the emergency room (Sykes and Okonofua, 1988; Anthony *et al.*, 1989). The treatment appears safe, simple, cheap, and almost as effective as intravenous diazepam. The parents can easily master the technique after a short instruction. Emergency room visits and hospitalizations can often be avoided because the drug terminates the seizures in about 90% of the cases (Knudsen, 1979, 1985a,b; Rossi *et al.*, 1988; Camfield *et al.*, 1989), with cost-savings for the family (Kriel *et al.*, 1991). The possession of rectal tubes or syringes reduces family stress, improves the family quality of life and parental confidence (Rossi *et al.*, 1993; O'Dell *et al.*, 2000) (see Chapter 20), increases the flexibility of family activities, and enables parents and caretakers to apply immediate emergency treatment and terminate a potentially brain-damaging febrile status epilepticus, even when professional assistance in unavailable. This is especially important in remote areas with a long transit time to medical care. Clinical data suggest that rectal diazepam is most effective if given within the first few minutes after onset of seizures (Knudsen, 1979; Sykes and Okonofua, 1988), and before the cascade of neurochemical dysfunctional advances. Hence, fast treatment may reduce the number of diazepam-resistant seizures. The safety of the treatment is documented in several large series of patients with febrile seizures and from the large-scale use in Scandinavia.

Diazepam-resistant seizures should be treated with standard treatment protocols for convulsive status epilepticus (Dodson *et al.*, 1993; Maytal and Shinnar, 1995). A full discussion of this topic is outside the scope of this chapter. Note, however, that drugs such as phenytoin or fosphenytoin, which are ineffective in preventing recurrent febrile seizures, are effective in the treatment of all forms of convulsive status epilepticus, including febrile status epilepticus (Dodson *et al.*, 1993; Maytal and Shinnar, 1995). They are often preferred to phenobarbital in this setting because they are less likely to cause respiratory depression, particularly if given after a benzodiazepine. Fosphenytoin has clear advantages over phenytoin and will most likely replace it. It is easier to administer and can be given three times more rapidly than phenytoin (Pellock, 1998).

B. OTHER BENZODIAZEPINES

Lorazepam has been widely used in the United States as a benzodiazepine alternative to diazepam in cases of status epilepticus in both adults and children (Walker *et al.*, 1979; Leppik *et al.*, 1983; Levy and Krall, 1984; Lacey *et al.*, 1986). The drug, being less lipophilic, penetrates biological membranes somewhat more slowly compared to diazepam, including the blood–brain barrier and the rectal mucosa (Homan and Walker, 1983), and is absorbed less rapidly. However, the rapidity of its onset of action is quite satisfactory in the clinical setting of prolonged seizures. Furthermore, it has a longer duration of action, as compared to diazepam. The anticonvulsant efficacy of lorazepam and diazepam, given intravenously or rectally, was recently compared in a prospective, open, odd and even dates, randomized trial in 102 children with afebrile seizures. Both drugs had a rapid onset of action, also shown by Giang and

McBride (1988), but lorazepam appeared superior to diazepam (Appleton et al., 1995). After a single dose, convulsions were controlled in 76% of patients treated with lorazepam and in 51% of patients treated with diazepam. Significantly fewer patients treated with lorazepam required additional anticonvulsants to terminate the seizure. The dosages were 0.3–0.4 mg/kg for diazepam and 0.05–0.1 mg/kg for lorazepam. Rectally (Crawford et al., 1987) or intravenously (Lacey et al., 1986) administered lorazepam to control serial seizures or status epilepticus in children was found effective and safe in a hospital setting. The authors recommend a first dose of 0.05–0.1 mg/kg of lorazepam, up to a maximum dose of 4 mg (Crawford et al., 1987).

In children, serial blood levels have documented rapid absorption following rectal administration of liquid lorazepam, with attainment of therapeutic levels within 5 minutes (Dooley et al., 1985), in contrast to the slow rectal absorption in adults (Graves et al., 1987). In all children the seizures were controlled after a dose of 0.05 mg/kg. A concentrated oral solution of lorazepam has a favorable absorption profile and was effective for the immediate and preventive management of hospitalized children with epilepsy (Schroeder et al., 1996). In summary, lorazepam is as effective as diazepam in the acute management of seizures, and has a longer duration of action. Both drugs seem to be safe, and respiratory problems are rare. Data on home-based treatment with lorazepam are not available and no comprehensive data on the efficacy of lorazepam in the treatment of febrile seizures exist. Hence, diazepam is still considered the drug of choice for home-based treatment of febrile seizures with a benzodiazepine.

Midazolam is a water-soluble benzodiazepine that can be given intravenously, orally, rectally, or by the nasal route (Wallace, 1997). At physiologic pH, the ring structure closes; the drug becomes lipid soluble and is rapidly absorbed and quickly passes the blood–brain barrier (O'Regan et al., 1996). It is widely used in children as a preanesthetic agent because of its rapid onset of action, its relatively short duration of action, and because it is less likely than diazepam to accumulate. Midazolam nasal spray has been successfully used to reduce procedural anxiety in children. Adverse effects includes nasal discomfort (Ljungman et al., 2000). Intranasal midazolam has been administered to 19 children under electroencephalogram (EEG) monitoring. At a dose of 0.2 mg/kg the drug was absorbed rapidly though the nasal mucosa and suppressed spike activity effectively within minutes (O'Regan et al., 1996). In a clinically controlled, randomized study buccal midazolam appeared at least as effective as rectal diazepam in the immediate treatment of seizures in children. It may be an effective and convenient anticonvulsant treatment in and outside the hospital (Scott et al., 1999). No data are available on the efficacy of midazolam in the treatment of febrile seizures. Therefore, although midazolam is a useful and promising drug, the emerging experience must be evaluated before it can be recommended for widespread use in treating febrile seizures, especially in an outpatient setting.

Clonazepam reaches mean peak levels within 15 minutes of rectally administering clonazepam solution (Rylance *et al.*, 1986), suggesting that the drug may be used as an alternative to diazepam for the treatment of seizures. Intravenous clonazepam has been effective in the treatment of status epilepticus in children in a small clinical trial (Congdon and Forsythe, 1980). There are no clinical data on the use of the drug in febrile seizures and therefore it is not recommended for use at present.

V. ANTIPYRETIC TREATMENT

Febrile seizures are, by definition, associated with a febrile illness, therefore both parents and physicians assume that giving antipyretics at the time of fever will be an effective means of reducing recurrence risk. Unfortunately this is not the case. Four well-designed placebo-controlled, double-blind studies have all shown that even aggressive antipyretic treatment with fever does not reduce the recurrence rate. Careful verbal and written counseling about antipyretic treatment and close telephone contact with the parents during their children's febrile episodes failed to reduce the recurrence rate among 79 children after an initial febrile seizure, even though the parents were told to give aspirin or acetaminophen every 4 hours in addition to cooling the child with sponge and bath (Camfield *et al.*, 1980). Another trial, comprising 161 children with a first febrile seizure, showed that low doses of acetaminophen (10 mg/kg four times a day) or diazepam or both were ineffective for preventing febrile seizures (Uhari *et al.*, 1995). In a hospital-based study, higher doses of acetaminophen (15–20 mg/kg every 4 hours) failed to prevent another seizure any better than giving the drug on a more sporadic basis (Schnaiderman *et al.*, 1993). In a prospective, nonblinded, randomized study, children with their first febrile seizure were assigned to one of three treatment groups: acetaminophen (10 mg/kg four times a day with fever), sublingual or rectal diazepam (0.5 mg/kg twice a day with fever), or daily prophylaxis with phenobarbital (5 mg/kg). The recurrence rates in the three groups were 40, 7, and 32%, respectively (Nunez-Lopez *et al.*, 1995). Ibuprofen yielded significantly greater reduction of fever than did acetaminophen 4 hours after the first dose (Van Esch *et al.*, 1995), but its value for the prevention of febrile seizures has not been tested. The concomitant rectal administration of an antipyretic suppository may interfere with early absorption of diazepam (Takei *et al.*, 1996). Aspirin may, in very rare cases, precipitate Reye's syndrome and is therefore not recommended for children with febrile seizures (Wilson, 1981). Diazepam and other benzodiazepines have antipyretic properties and produce significant hypothermia in rodents, especially in higher doses (Jackson and Nutt, 1990; Jackson *et al.*, 1992). The potential clinical significance of this finding for the treatment of febrile seizures is unknown. Antipyretic agents may be useful in making the child more comfortable but do not alter the risk of another febrile seizure.

VI. DECIDING WHO AND HOW TO TREAT

The choice of whether to treat, as well as the specific treatment regimen chosen, will depend on several factors:

1. Natural history of the disorder, including short- and long-term prognoses.
2. Efficacy of treatment in altering short- and long-term prognoses.
3. Adverse effects of treatment.

The final decision is based on balancing the risks and benefits of different therapeutic regimens for each patient and assessing whether the potential benefits of treatment exceed the risks. Huge amounts of new data on the issue have emerged and evidence-based treatment can be afforded to most children with simple febrile seizures, but not yet to those with single or serial complex febrile seizures or febrile status epilepticus. Only four sequellae have been associated with febrile seizures:

1. A 30–40% risk of recurrent febrile seizures, which may be higher or lower in individual cases (see Chapter 3).
2. A somewhat increased risk of later epilepsy, particularly in those with complex febrile seizures (see Chapters 5–7).
3. Rare cases of neurological sequellae (see Chapters 4 and 8).
4. Psychological problems for parents concerned about their child (see Chapter 20).

In deciding whether to treat one must be clear as to which of the possible outcomes is being influenced. The recurrence rate may be reduced by means of prophylaxis, but recurrences are benign in most cases and do not influence the child's health. Data document that prevention is no better than termination of recurrent febrile seizures with regard to IQ, cognitive and motor function, academic performance, and development of subsequent epilepsy (Knudsen et al.,1996). There are no data to suggest that prophylaxis reduces the already small risk of later epilepsy and other central nervous system damage (Shinnar and Berg, 1996). Children with focal febrile status epilepticus are at some risk for later hippocampal sclerosis and temporal lobe epilepsy. The risk has probably been exaggerated and the sequence of events is very rare (Camfield et al., 1994). Even if the small high-risk group could be identified in advance, prophylaxis would hardly be more efficacious than prompt home-based immediate treatment. The maximum estimate of the risk of potential preventable epilepsy after a first febrile seizure appears to be about 1.1 per thousand (Addy, 1981). The psychological problems should be solved by means of parental counseling rather than medical intervention.

The potential disadvantages of prophylactic or immediate treatment include short- and long-term side effects, including drug toxicity; the risks of overdose, misuse, and abuse; and the costs for the family and society. The usefulness of the available therapeutic options is summarized in Table 1. The following discussion of recommended treatment options for simple and complex febrile seizures is limited to those options that are of demonstrated efficacy either in reducing recurrence risk or in the immediate abortive home-based therapy of febrile seizures.

A. TREATMENT OF SIMPLE FEBRILE SEIZURES

There is an emerging consensus that in most cases no treatment is needed for simple febrile seizures. The American Academy of Pediatrics (1999) recommends no treatment for children with a simple febrile seizure. The Japanese consensus statement recommends the use of intermittent diazepam with fever in children with at least two risk factors for recurrences plus a history of at least two prior seizures or frequent seizures occurring over a short period of time, i.e., twice in 12 hours, three or more in 6 months, or four or more in a year (Fukuyama et al., 1996). Consensus has emerged that prolonged daily prophylaxis with phenobarbital, valproate, or primidone should be used only in highly selected cases, if at all. This is also true for the management of febrile seizures in the developing countries. In those rare cases in which treatment may be appropriate, intermittent prophylaxis with oral or rectal diazepam at time of fever is preferable to chronic prophylaxis with antiepileptic agents. In the case of simple febrile seizures, however, the American Academy of Pediatrics (1999) finds that the rate of side effects is high and the benefits too low for even intermittent prophylaxis to be recommended as a first-line routine treatment, and even the Japanese consensus statement recommends its use only in selected cases.

Benzodiazepines afford prompt anticonvulsant activity with proved safety and efficacy. Clinical trial data indicate that rectal diazepam and lorazepam are effective in terminating ongoing febrile seizures with almost intravenous efficacy. The treatment has not been subjected to evaluation in randomized double-blind, placebo-controlled studies. It is, however, considered safe, effective, and cheap and is easy for parents and other caregivers to administer. The possession of rectal diazepam reduces family stress, improves its quality of life, and enables the parents to terminate future, potentially brain-damaging, febrile status epilepticus. The drugs have respiratory-depressing properties, but their safety has been documented in several large clinical series and from worldwide use.

They would appear to be the drugs of choice for simple febrile seizures if any treatment is prescribed.

B. TREATMENT OF COMPLEX FEBRILE SEIZURES AND FEBRILE STATUS EPILEPTICUS

In the case of complex febrile seizures there is no consensus on the treatment and there are no evidence-based recommendations. The main objective, and a rational goal, is to prevent the greatest possible number of future episodes of febrile status epilepticus and complex recurrences. Although not associated with a higher risk of subsequent febrile seizures (see Chapter 3), subsequent recurrences are likely to be complex. In particular, children with initial prolonged febrile seizures are particularly prone to prolonged recurrences (Berg and Shinnar, 1996). Complex febrile seizures are associated with a higher risk of subsequent epilepsy (see Chapter 5) and of adverse developmental outcomes (see Chapter 4). However, this does not per se imply a causal relationship. The long-term prognosis even without intervention is much better than hitherto believed (Nelson and Ellenberg, 1978; Ross et al., 1980; Verity and Golding, 1991; Verity et al., 1993; Knudsen et al., 1996; Verity 1998) (see Chapters 4–7). It is probably justified to refrain from chronic daily prophylaxis with antiepileptic drugs for complex febrile seizures and even for cases of febrile status epilepticus in most cases, because the therapeutic gain is insignificant. A rational alternative is intermittent diazepam prophylaxis or immediate treatment of ongoing seizures with rectal diazepam or lorazepam.

Febrile status epilepticus is a serious neurologic emergency requiring prompt and effective treatment. Adverse outcome of febrile status epilepticus is primarily a function of the underlying cause (Maytal et al., 1989; Maytal and Shinnar, 1990; Gross-Tsur and Shinnar, 1993; Verity, 1998). The time interval between onset of seizures and the start of effective therapy, as well as the underlying cause, are important in determining the prognosis. In the case of febrile seizures, the underlying cause is benign, so it is the duration that seems to matter most. The much improved outcome seen currently probably reflects rapid, aggressive treatment and improved intensive care facilities. Several studies have shown a long time interval between seizure onset and treatment in the emergency department (Goldberg, 1998; Jordan, 1994). These studies provide further evidence for the need for effective home-based immediate therapy for prolonged febrile seizures. Rational management of febrile status epilepticus should afford rapid, safe, and effective seizure cessation and should be useful to parents, caretakers, and professionals. Immediate treatment of ongoing seizures with rectal diazepam fulfills these criteria and is therefore considered a first-line treatment in and outside of the hospital.

A small group of children with febrile status epilepticus or complex febrile seizures, having all three complex features (multiple, prolonged, and focal), carry a high risk of epilepsy—about 50% (Annegers *et al.*, 1987) (see Chapters 5–7). The focal variety carries some risk of subsequent hippocampal sclerosis and temporal lobe epilepsy (see Chapters 6–8). Most clinicians will consider intermittent diazepam prophylaxis or even chronic prophylaxis with antiepileptic drugs for these children. Even in these cases, chronic prophylaxis with antiepileptic agents will rarely achieve more than the much better tolerated intermittent prophylaxis with benzodiazepines. Chronic prophylaxis should therefore be applied only if intermittent prophylaxis fails. Other clinicians take the view that epilepsy should not be treated until it occurs and that rapid seizure cessation with benzodiazepines is the main target. In the few cases in which continuous prophylaxis may be justified, the chronic cognitive–behavioral impairment often caused by phenobarbital should be balanced with the extremely rare, lethal hepatic failure caused by valproate. In this situation, the author recommends valproate, but there is no consensus on this matter.

Complex febrile seizures and an abnormal neurological status are both risk factors for subsequent epilepsy. However, a child's neurological status should not influence the choice of treatment, and an abnormal status (mental retardation, cerebral palsy, hydrocephalus, etc.) hardly justifies a more aggressive treatment.

C. Immunization and Febrile Seizures

Vaccination-induced febrile seizures should be treated like all other cases. The immunization program should be given as usual to children with a history of febrile seizures along with advice about the management of fever and seizures. Rectal diazepam may be made available for use should a seizure occur (Research Unit of Royal College of Physicians and British Paediatric Association, London, 1991).

D. Treatment in Developing Countries

In parts of rural Africa common traditional medical practices have included treating convulsing children with a toxic substance, "cow's urine/tobacco mixture," often with fatal outcome (Oyebola and Elegbe, 1975; Voorhoeve, 1980). For emergency treatment in rural child health services, benzodiazepines are the drugs of choice. If benzodiazepines are unavailable, chloral hydrate may be considered as an alternative (Voorhoeve, 1980). There is a simple drug-dose treatment scheme, depending on the child's age: chloral hydrate, administered by a rectal tube—under 3 month of age, 250 mg; 3–6 months of age, 500 mg; and over 6 months of age, 1000 mg. The drug is stored as crystals and dissolved in water before use. The treatment is simple, safe, and cheap. However, as noted earlier, there are insufficient data on efficacy at the present time so the treatment should be reserved for those settings where proved effective therapy, such as benzodiazepine administration, is not available.

VII. SUPPORTIVE FAMILY MANAGEMENT

Efficacious anticonvulsant treatment of febrile status epilepticus and parental counseling are the two most important parts of the treatment. A holistic approach is not always appreciated by the physician and febrile seizures are often mistakenly treated as a psychologically trivial event. However, a febrile seizure is frightening to the parents (Balslev, 1991). They believe that their child is dead or dying, and the parental management is often highly inappropriate (Rutter and Metcalfe, 1978). The catastrophic experience may leave deep traces of anxiety in their minds for years.

The parents should be informed verbally and in writing about the disorder, and be given specific instructions about antipyretic and anticonvulsant treatment (see Chapter 20). Those parents whose children require emergency treatment with rectal diazepam need instruction in the use of the drug and its effects and side effects. Specific instructions as to when and how to seek emergency medical care should be given. Many parents are suffering from "fever phobia" and fear that the child's high fever per se may cause brain damage. There is clearly a need to educate the parents about when and how to help lower the temperature with medication and cooling but also how to avoid unacceptable alternatives. All parents should be given written instructions with all the necessary information (see Chapter 20).

REFERENCES

Addy, D. P. (1981). Prophylaxis and febrile convulsions. *Arch. Dis. Child.* 56, 81–83.

Agurell, S., Berlin, A., Ferngren, H., and Hellström, B. (1975). Plasma levels of diazepam after parenteral and rectal administration in children. *Epilepsia* 16, 277–283.

Aicardi, J. (1994). Febrile convulsions. *In* "Epilepsy in Children" 2nd Ed. (J. Aicardi, ed.), pp. 253–275. Raven Press, New York.

Alldredge, B. K., Wall, D. B., and Ferriero, D. M. (1995). Effect of prehospital treatment on the outcome of status epilepticus in children. *Pediatr. Neurol.* 12, 213–216.

American Academy of Pediatrics (1995). Committee on Drugs. Behavioral and cognitive effects of anticonvulsant therapy. *Pediatrics* 96, 538–540.

American Academy of Pediatrics (1999). Practice parameter: Long-term treatment of the child with simple febrile seizures. *Pediatrics* 103, 1307–1309.

Annegers, J. F., Hauser, W. A., Shirts, S. B., and Kurland, L. T. (1987). Factors prognostic of unprovoked seizures after febrile convulsions. *N. Engl. J. Med.* **316**, 493–498.

Anthony, A., Reisdorff, E. J., and Wiegenstein, J. G. (1989). Rectal diazepam in pediatric status
epilepticus. *Am. J. Emerg. Med.* **70**, 168–172.

Antony, J. H., and Hawke, S. (1983). Phenobarbital compared with carbamazepine in prevention of
recurrent febrile convulsions. *Am. J. Dis. Child.* **137**, 892–895.

Appleton, R., Sweeney, A., Choonara, I., Robson, J., and Molyneux, E. (1995). Lorazepam versus
diazepam in the acute treatment of epileptic seizures and status epilepticus. *Dev. Med. Child Neurol.* **37**, 682–688.

Autret, E., Billard, C., Bertrand, P., Motte, J., Pouplard, F., and Jonville, A. P. (1990). Double-blind,
randomized trial of diazepam versus placebo for prevention of recurrence of febrile seizures.
J. Pediatr. **117**, 490–449.

Bacon, C. J., Hierons, A. M., Mucklow, J. C., Webb, J.K.G., Rawlins, M. D., and Weightman, D.
(1981). Placebo-controlled study of phenobarbitone and phenytoin in the prophylaxis of febrile
convulsions. *Lancet* **2**, 600–604.

Baldy-Moulinier, M., Covanis, A., D'Urso, S., Eskazan, E., Fattore, C., Gatti, G., Herranz, J. L.,
Ibrahim, S., Khalifa, A., Mrabet, A., Neufeld, M. Y., and Perucca, E. (1998). Therapeutic strategies against epilepsy in Mediterranean countries: A report from an international collaborative
survey. *Seizure* **7**, 513–520.

Balslev, T. (1991). Parental reactions to a child's first febrile convulsion. *Acta Paediatr. Scand.* **80**,
466–469.

Benchet, M. L., Tardieu, M., and Landrieu, P. (1984). Prévention des convulsions fébriles et ciné-
tique du diazépam per os. *Arch. Fr. Pediatr.* **41**, 588–589.

Berg, A. T., and Shinnar, S. (1996). Complex febrile seizures. *Epilepsia* **37**, 126–133.

Brent, D. A., Crumrine, P. K., Varma, R. R., Allan, M., and Allman, C. (1987). Phenobarbital treatment and major depressive disorder in children with epilepsy. *Pediatrics* **80**, 909–917.

Byrne, J. M., Camfield, P. R., Clark-Touesnard, M., and Hondas, B. J. (1987). Effects of phenobarbital on early intellectual and behavioral development: A concordant twin case study. *J. Clin.
Exp. Neuropsychol.* **9**, 393–398.

Camfield, C. S., Chaplin, S., Doyle, A. B., Shapiro, S. H., Cunnings, C., and Camfield, P. R. (1979).
Side effects of phenobarbital in toddlers: Behavioral and cognitive aspects. *J. Pediatr.* **95**, 361–
365.

Camfield, P. R., Camfield, C. S., Shapiro, S. H., and Cummings, C. (1980). The first febrile seizure—
Antipyretic instruction plus either phenobarbital or placebo to prevent recurrence. *J. Pediatr.* **97**,
16–21.

Camfield, P. R., Camfield, C. S., and Tibbles, J.A.R. (1982). Carbamazepine does not prevent febrile
seizures in phenobarbital failures. *Neurology* **32**, 288–289.

Camfield, C. S., Camfield, P. R., Smith, E., and Dooley, J. M. (1989). Home use of rectal diazepam
to prevent status epilepticus in children with convulsive disorders. *J. Child Neurol.* **4**, 125–126.

Camfield, P., Camfield, C., Gordon, K., and Dooley, J. (1994). What types of epilepsy are preceded by febrile seizures? A population based study of children. *Dev. Med. Child Neurol.* **36**, 887–
892.

Camfield, P. R., Camfield, C. S., Gordon, K., and Dooley, J. M. (1995). Prevention of recurrent febrile
seizures. *J. Pediatr.* **126**, 929–930.

Campbell, H., Surry, S.A.M., and Royle, E. M. (1998). A review of randomised controlled trials published in Archives of Disease in Childhood from 1982–96. *Arch. Dis. Child.* **79**, 192–197.

Cavazzuti, G. B. (1975). Prevention of febrile convulsions with dipropylacetate (Depakine®).
Epilepsia **16**, 647–648.

Cereghino, J. J., Mitchell, W. G., Murphy, J., Kriel, R. L., Rosenfeld, W. E., Trevathan, E., and the
North American Diastat Study Group (1998). Treating repetitive seizures with a rectal diazepam
formulation. A randomized study. *Neurology* **51**, 1274–1282.

Congdon, P. J., and Forsythe, W. I. (1980). Intravenous clonazepam in the treatment of status epilepticus in children. *Epilepsia* 21, 97–102.

Consensus Development Panel (1980). Febrile seizures: Long-term management of children with fever-associated seizures. *Pediatrics* 66, 1009–1012.

Crawford, T. O., Mitchell, W. G., and Snodgrass, S. R. (1987). Lorazepam in childhood status epilepticus and serial seizures: Effectiveness and tachyphylaxis. *Neurology* 37, 190–195.

Crawley, J., Waruiru, C., Mithwani, S., Mwangi, I., Watkins, W., Ouma, D., Winstanley, P., Peto, T., and Marsh, K. (2000). Effect of phenobarbital on seizure frequency and mortality in childhood cerebral malaria: A randomized, controlled intervention study. *Lancet* 355, 701–706.

Daugbjerg, P., Brems, P., Mai, J., Ankerhus, J., and Knudsen, F. U. (1990). Intermittent prophylaxis in febrile convulsions: Diazepam or valproic acid? *Acta Neurol. Scand.* 82, 17–20.

Davis, R., Peters, D. H., and McTavish, D. (1994). Valproic acid. A reappraisal of its pharmacological properties and clinical efficacy in epilepsy. *Drugs* 47, 332–372.

De Negri, M., Gaggero, R., Veneselli, E., Pessagno, A., Baglietto, M. G., and Pallecchi, A. (1991). Rapid diazepam introduction (venous or rectal) in childhood epilepsy: Taxonomic and therapeutic considerations. *Brain Dev.* 13, 21–26.

Deonna, T. (1982). Traitement des convulsions fébriles. *Helv. Pediatr. Acta* 37, 7–10.

Devilat, M. B., and Masafierro, M.P.G. (1989). Profilaxis selective discontinue en domicilio de recurrencias de convulsiones febriles con diazepam rectal. *Rev. Child. Pediatr.* 60, 195–197.

Devinsky, O., Leppik, I., Willmore, L. J., Pellock, J. M., Dean, C., Gates, J., and Ramsay, R. E. (1995). The intravenous valproate study team. Safety of intravenous valproate. *Ann. Neurol.* 38, 670–674.

Dhillon, S., Ngwane, E., and Richens, A. (1982). Rectal absorption of diazepam in epileptic children. *Arch. Dis. Child.* 57, 264–267.

Dianese, G. (1979). Prophylactic diazepam in febrile convulsions. *Arch. Dis. Child.* 54, 244–245.

Dieckmann, R. A. (1994). Rectal diazepam for prehospital pediatric status epilepticus. *Ann. Emerg. Med.* 23, 216–224.

Dodson, W. E., DeLorenzo, R. J., Pedley, T. A., Shinnar, S., Treiman, D. B., and Wannamaker, B. B. (1993). The treatment of convulsive status epilepticus: Recommendations of the Epilepsy Foundation of America's working group on status epilepticus. *JAMA* 270, 854–859.

Dooley, J. M. (1998). Rectal use of benzodiazepines. *Epilepsia* 39, (Suppl. 1), S24–S27.

Dooley, J. M., Tibbles, J.A.R., Rumney, P. G., and Dooley, K. C. (1985). Rectal lorazepam in the treatment of acute seizures in childhood. *Ann. Neurol.* 18, 412–413.

Dreifuss, F. E., Santilli, N., Langer, D. H., Sweeney, K. P., Moline, K. A., and Menander, K. B. (1987). Valproic acid hepatic fatalities: A retrospective review. *Neurology* 37, 379–385.

Dreifuss, F. E., Rosman, N. P., Cloyd, J. C., Pellock, J. M., Kuzniecky, R. I., Lo, W. D., Matsuo, F., Sharp, G. B., Conry, J. A., Bergen, D. C., and Bell, W. E. (1998). A comparison of rectal diazepam gel and placebo for acute repetitive seizures. *N. Engl. J. Med.* 338, 1869–1875.

Dulac, O., Aicardi, J., Rey, E., and Olive, G. (1978). Blood levels of diazepam after single rectal administration in infants and children. *J. Pediatr.* 93, 1039–1041.

Echenne, B., Cheminal, R., Martin, P., Peskine, F., Rodiere, M., Astruc, J., and Brunel, D. (1983). Utilisation du diazépam dans le traitement préventif à domicile des récidives de convulsions fébriles. *Arch. Fr. Pédiatr.* 40, 499–501.

Elterman, R. D. (1994). Rectal administration of diazepam. *J. Child. Neurol.* 9, 340.

Eysenck, H. J. (1994). Meta-analysis and its problems. *BMJ* 309, 789–792.

Farwell, J. R., Lee, Y. J., Hirtz, D. G., Sulzbacher, S. I., Ellenberg, J. H., and Nelson, K. B. (1990). Phenobarbital for febrile seizures—Effects on intelligence and on seizure recurrence. *N. Engl. J. Med.* 322, 364–369.

Færø, O., Kastrup, K. W., Nielsen, E. L., Melchior, J. C., and Thorn, I. (1972). Successful prophylaxis of febrile convulsions with phenobarbital. *Epilepsia* 13, 279–285.

Finkle, B. S., McCloskey, K. L., and Goodman, L. S. (1979). Diazepam and drug-associated deaths. A survey in the United States and Canada. *JAMA* 242, 429–434.

Frantzen, E., Nygaard, A., and Wulff, H. (1964). Febrile kramper hos børn. *Ugeskr. Læger* 126, 207–211.

Franzoni, E., Carboni, C., and Lambertini, A. (1983). Rectal diazepam: A clinical and EEG study after a single dose in children. *Epilepsia* 24, 35–41.

Freeman, J. M. (1990). Just say no! *Pediatrics* 86, 624.

Freeman, J. M. (1992). The best medicine for febrile seizures. *N. Engl. J. Med.* 327, 1161–1163.

Freeman, J. M., and Vining, E.P.G. (1995). Febrile seizures: A decision-making analysis. *Am. Fam. Physician* 52, 1401–1406.

Fukuyama, Y., Seki, T., Ohtsuka, C., Miura, H., and Hara, M. (1996). Practical guidelines for physicians in the management of febrile seizures. *Brain Dev.* 18, 479–484.

Garcia, F. O., Campos-Castello, J., and Maldonado, J. C. (1984). Fenobarbital oral contiuado o diazepam rectal intermitente para la prevención de la crisis febriles. *An. Esp. Pediatr.* 20, 763–769.

Giang, D. W., and McBride, M. C. (1988). Lorazepam versus diazepam for the treatment of status epilepticus. *Pediatr. Neurol.* 4, 358–361.

Goldberg, A. (1998). Delay in the treatment of patients with acute seizure episodes (ASE). *Epilepsia* 39, (Suppl. 6), 109–110.

Graves, N. M., Kriel, R. L., and Jones-Saete, C. (1987). Bioavailability of rectally administered lorazepam. *Clin. Neuropharmacol.* 10, 555–559.

Gross-Tsur, V., and Shinnar, S. (1993). Convulsive status epilepticus in children. *Epilepsia* 34, (Suppl. 1), S12–S20.

Heckmatt, J. Z., Houston, A. B., Clow, D. J., Stephenson, J.B.P., Dodd, K. L., Lealman, G. T., and Logan, R. W. (1976). Failure of phenobarbitone to prevent febrile convulsions. *BMJ* 1, 559–561.

Homan, R. W., and Walker, J. E. (1983). Clinical studies of lorazepam in status epilepticus. *Adv. Neurol.* 34, 493–498.

Hoppu, K., and Santavuori, P. (1981). Diazepam rectal solution for home treatment of acute seizures in children. *Acta Paediatr. Scand.* 70, 369–372.

Hovinga, C. A., Chicella, M. F., Rose, D. F., Shannan, K. E., Dalton, J. T., and Phelps, S. J. (1999). Use of intravenous valproate in three pediatric patients with nonconvulsive or convulsive status epilepticus. *Ann. Pharmacother.* 33, 579–584.

Jackson, H. C., and Nutt, D. J. (1990). Body temperature discriminates between full and partial benzodiazepine receptor agonists. *Eur. J. Pharmacol.* 185, 243–246.

Jackson, H. C., Ramsay, E., and Nutt, D. J. (1992). Effect of the cyclopyrrolones suriclone and RP59037 on body temperature in mice. *Eur. J. Pharmacol.* 216, 23–27.

Jalling, B. (1974). Plasma and cerebrospinal fluid concentrations of phenobarbital in infants given single doses. *Dev. Med. Child Neurol.* 16, 781–793.

Jordan, K. G. (1994). Status epilepticus. A perspective from the neuroscience intensive care unit. *Neurosurg. Clin. N. Am.* 5, 671–686.

Katalin, A.C.S., and Borsi, J. D. (1990). Intermittent diazepam or continuous pheno-barbitone in the prophylaxis of febrile convulsions: A comparative long term clinical trial. (Unpublished results.)

Knudsen, F. U. (1977). Plasma-diazepam in infants after rectal administration in solution and by suppository. *Acta Paediatr. Scand.* 66, 563–567.

Knudsen, F. U. (1979). Rectal administration of diazepam in solution in the acute treatment of convulsions in infants and children. *Arch. Dis. Child.* 54, 855–857.

Knudsen, F. U. (1985a). Effective short-term diazepam prophylaxis in febrile convulsions. *J. Pediatr.* 106, 487–490.

Knudsen, F. U. (1985b). Recurrence risk after first febrile seizure and effect of short term diazepam prophylaxis. *Arch. Dis. Child.* 60, 1045–1049.

Knudsen, F. U. (1988). Optimum management of febrile seizures in childhood. *Drugs* 36, 111–120.

Knudsen, F. U. (1991). Intermittent diazepam prophylaxis in febrile convulsions: Pros and cons. *Acta Neurol. Scand.* 83, (Suppl. 135), 1–24.

Knudsen, F. U. (1996). Febrile seizures-treatment and outcome. *Brain Dev.* 18, 438–449.

Knudsen, F. U. (2000). Febrile seizures: Treatment and prognosis. *Epilepsia* 41, 2–9.

Knudsen, F. U., and Vestermark, S. (1978). Prophylactic diazepam or phenobarbitone in febrile convulsions: A prospective, controlled study. *Arch. Dis. Child.* 53, 660–663.

Knudsen, F. U., Paerregaard, A., Andersen, R., and Andresen, J. (1996). Long term outcome of prophylaxis for febrile convulsions. *Arch. Dis. Child.* 74, 13–18.

Kriel, R. L., Cloyd, J. C., Hadsall, R. S., Carlson, A. M., Floren, K. L., and Jones-Saete, C. M. (1991). Home use of rectal diazepam for cluster and prolonged seizures: Efficacy, adverse reactions, quality of life, and cost analysis, *Pediatr. Neurol.* 7, 13–17.

Kriel, R. L., Cloyd, J. C., Pellock, J. M., Mitchell, W. G., Cereghino, J. J., and Rosman, N. P. (1999). Rectal diazepam gel for treatment of acute repetitive seizures. *Pediatr. Neurol.* 20, 282–288.

Kriel, R. L., Cloyd, J. C., and Pellock, J. M. (2000). Respiratory depression in children receiving diazepam for acute seizures: a prospective study. *Dev. Med. Child Neurol.* 42, 429.

Lacey, D. J., Singer, W. D., Horwitz, S. J., and Gilmore, H. (1986). Lorazepam therapy of status epilepticus in children in adolescents. *J. Pediatr.* 108, 771–774.

Lalande, J., and De Paillerets, F. (1978). Prevention of hyperthermic convulsions: Utility of discontinuous treatment with clonazepam. *In* "Advances in Epileptology, Psychology, Pharmacotherapy and New Diagnostic Approaches" (H. Meinardi and A. J. Rowen, eds.), pp. 313–317. Swets and Zeitlinger, Amsterdam.

Lee, K., Taudorf, K., and Hvorslev, V. (1986). Prophylactic treatment with valproic acid or diazepam in children with febrile convulsion. *Acta Paediatr. Scand.* 75, 593–597.

Lennox-Buchthal, M. A. (1973). Febrile convulsions. A reappraisal. *Electroencephalogr. Clin. Neurophysiol.* 32 (Suppl.), 1–132.

Leppik, I. E., Derivan, A. T., Homan, R. W., Walker, J., Ramsay, R. E., and Patrick B. (1983). Double-blind study of lorazepam and diazepam in status epilepticus. *JAMA* 249, 1452–1454.

Levy, R. J., and Krall, R. L. (1984). Treatment of status epilepticus with lorazepam. *Arch. Neurol.* 41, 605–611.

Ljungman, G., Kreuger, A., Andreásson, S., Gordh, T., and Sörensen, S. (2000). Midazolam nasal spray reduces procedural anxiety in children. *Pediatrics* 105, 73–78.

Mamelle, N., Mamelle, J. C., Plasse, J. C., Revol, M., and Gilly, R. (1984). Prevention of recurrent febrile convulsions—A randomized therapeutic assay: Sodium valproate, phenobarbital and placebo. *Neuropediatrics* 15, 37–42.

Maytal, J., and Shinnar, S. (1990). Febrile status epilepticus. *Pediatrics* 86, 611–616.

Maytal, J., and Shinnar, S. (1995). Status epilepticus in children. *In* "Childhood Seizures" (S. Shinnar, N. Amir, and D. Branski, eds.), pp. 111–122. S. Karger, Switzerland.

Maytal, J., Shinnar, S., Moshe, S. L., and Alvarez, L. A. (1989). Low morbidity and mortality of status epilepticus in children. *Pediatrics,* 83, 323–331.

Meberg, A., Langslet, A., Bredesen, J. E., and Lunde, P.K.M. (1978). Plasma concentration of diazepam and N-desmethyldiazepam in children after a single rectal or intramuscular dose of diazepam. *Eur. J. Clin. Pharmacol.* 14, 273–276.

Melchior, J. C., Buchthal, F., and Lennox-Buchthal, M. (1971). The ineffectiveness of diphenylhydantoin in preventing febrile convulsions in the age of greatest risk, under three years. *Epilepsia* 12, 55–62.

Millichap, J. G., and Colliver, J. A. (1991). Management of febrile seizures: Survey of current practice and phenobarbital usage. *Pediatr. Neurol.* 7, 243–248.

Millichap, J. G., Aledort, L. M., and Madsen, J. A. (1960). A critical evaluation of therapy of febrile seizures. *J. Pediatr.* 56, 364–368.

Milligan, N., Dhillon, S., Richens, A., and Oxley, J. (1981). Rectal diazepam in the treatment of absence status: A pharmacodynamic study. *J. Neurol. Neurosurg. Psychiatry* 44, 914–917.

Milligan, N., Dhillon, S., Oxley, J., and Richens, A. (1982). Absorption of diazepam from the rectum and its effect on interictal spikes in the EEG. *Epilepsia* 23, 323–331.

Minagawa, K., and Miura, H. (1981). Phenobarbital, primidone and sodium valproate in the prophylaxis of febrile convulsions. *Brain Dev.* 3, 385–393.

Minagawa, K., Miura, H., Kaneko, T., and Sudo, Y. (1982). Plasma concentration of diazepam and N-desmethyldiazepam in infants with febrile convulsions after single rectal administrations of diazepam suppositories or solutions. *Brain Dev.* 14, 11–19.

Minagawa, K., Miura, H., Mizuno, S., and Shirai, H. (1986). Pharmacokinetics of rectal diazepam in the prevention of recurrent febrile convulsions. *Brain Dev.* 8, 53–59.

Mitchell, W. G., Conry, J. A., Crumrine, P. K., Kriel, R. L., Cereghino, J. J., Groves, L., Rosenfeld, W. E., and the North American Diastat Study Group (1999). An open-label study of repeated use of diazepam rectal gel (Diastat) for episodes of acute breakthrough seizures and clusters: Safety, efficacy and tolerance. *Epilepsia* 40, 1610–1617.

Mizuno, S., Miura, H., Minagawa, K., and Shirai, H. (1987). A pharmacokinetic study on the effectiveness of rectal administration of diazepam in solutions: A comparison with intravenous administration (in Japanese). *No To Hattatsu* 19, 1182–1194.

Monaco, F., Secki, G. P., Mutani, R., *et al.* (1980). Lack of efficacy of carbamazepine in preventing the recurrence of febrile convulsions. *In* "Antiepileptic Therapy. Advances in Drug Monitoring" (S. I. Johannessen, P. L. Marselli, C. E. Peppenger, *et al.*, eds.), pp. 75–79. Raven Press, New York.

Moolenaar, F., Bakker, S., Visser, J., and Huizinga, T. (1980). Biopharmaceutics of rectal administration of drugs in man IX. Comparative biopharmaceutics of diazepam after single rectal, oral, intramuscular and intravenous administration in man. *Int. J. Pharm.* 5, 127–137.

Mosquera, C., Rodrigues, J., Cabrero, A., Fidalgo, I., and Fernández, R. M. (1987). Prevención de la recurrencia de crisis febriles: Profilaxis intermitente con diacepam rectal comparada con tratamiento continuo con valproate sódico. *An. Esp. Pediatr.* 27, 379–381.

Nelson, K. B., and Ellenberg, J. H. (1976). Predictors of epilepsy in children who have experienced febrile seizures. *N. Engl. J. Med.* 295, 1029–1033.

Nelson, K. B., and Ellenberg, J. H. (1978). Prognosis in children with febrile seizures. *Pediatrics* 61, 720–727.

Nelson, K. B., and Ellenberg, J. H. (1981). *In* "Febrile Seizures" (K. B. Nelson and J. H. Ellenberg, eds.), p. 1–360, Raven Press, New York.

Newton, R. W. (1988). Randomized controlled trials of phenobarbitone and valproate in febrile convulsions. *Arch. Dis. Child.* 63, 1189–1191.

Newton, R. W., and McKinlay, I. (1988). Subsequent management of children with febrile convulsions. *Dev. Med. Child Neurol.* 30, 402–406.

Ngwane, E., and Bower, B. (1980). Continuous sodium valproate or phenobarbitone in the prevention of "simple" febrile convulsions. *Arch. Dis. Child.* 55, 171–4.

Norris, E., Marzouk, O., Nunn, A., McIntyre, J., and Choonara, I. (1999). Respiratory depression in children receiving diazepam for acute seizures: A prospective study. *Dev. Med. Child Neurol.* 41, 340–343.

Nunez-Lopez, L. C., Espinosa-Garcia, E., Hernandez-Arbelaez, E., *et al.* (1995). Efficacy of diazepam to prevent recurrences in children with a first febrile convulsion. *Acta Neuropediatr.* 1, 187–195.

O'Dell, C., Shinnar, S., Ballaban-Gil, K., Kang, H., and Moshe, S. L. (2000). Home use of rectal diazepam gel (Diastat). *Epilepsia* 41 (Suppl. 7), 246.

O'Regan, M. E., Brown, J. K., and Clarke, M. (1996). Nasal rather than rectal benzodiazepines in the management of acute childhood seizures. *Dev. Med. Child Neurol.* 38, 1037–1045.

Oyebola, D.D.O., and Elegbe, R. A. (1975). Cow's urine poisoning in Nigeria. *Trop. Georgr. Med.* **27**, 194–202.

Pellock, J. M. (1998). Management of acute seizure episodes. *Epilepsia* **39** (Suppl. 1.), S28–S35.

Ramakrishnan, K., and Thomas, K. (1986). Long term prophylaxis of febrile seizures. *Ind. J. Pediatr.* **53**, 397–400.

Ramsay, R. E., Hammond, E. J., Perchalski, R. J., Wilder, B. J. (1979). Brain uptake of phenytoin, phenobarbital and diazepam. *Arch. Neurol.* **36**, 535–539.

Rantala, H., Tarkka, R., and Uhari, M. (1997). A meta-analytic review of the preventive treatment of recurrences of febrile seizures. *J. Pediatr.* **131**, 922–925.

Research Unit of Royal College of Physicians and British Paediatric Association, London (1991). Guidelines for the management of convulsions with fever. *BMJ* **303**, 634–636.

Rosman, N. P. (1996). Diazepam to reduce the recurrence of febrile seizures. *J. Pediatr.* **128**, 303–304.

Rosman, N. P., Colton, T., Labazzo, J., Gilbert, P., L., Gardella, N. B., Kaye, E. M., Van Bennekom, C., and Winter, M. R. (1993). A controlled trial of diazepam administered during febrile illnesses to prevent recurrence of febrile seizures. *N. Engl. J. Med.* **329**, 79–84.

Ross, E. M., Peckham, C. S., West, P. B., and Butler, N. R. (1980). Epilepsy in childhood: Findings from the national child development study. *BMJ* **280**, 207–210.

Rossi, L. N., Rossi, G., Bossi, A., Cortinovis, I., and Brunelli, G. (1988). Behaviour and confidence of parents instructed in home management of febrile seizures by rectal diazepam. *Helv. Paediatr. Acta* **43**, 273–281.

Rossi, L. N., Chiodi, A., Bossi, A., Cortinovis, I., and Alberti, S. (1993). Short-term prophylaxis of febrile convulsions by oral diazepam. *Acta Paediatr.* **82**, 99.

Rutter, N., and Metcalfe, D. (1978). Febrile convulsions—What do parents do? *BMJ* **2**, 1345–1346.

Rylance, G. W., Poulton, J., Cherry, R. C., and Cullen, R. E. (1986). Plasma concentrations of clonazepam after single rectal administration. *Arch. Dis. Child.* **61**, 186–188.

Scheffner, D., König, S., Rauterberg-Ruland, I., Kochen, W., Hofmann, W. J., and Unkelbach, S. (1988). Fatal liver failure in 16 children with valproate therapy. *Epilepsia* **29**, 530–542.

Schnaiderman, D., Lahat, E., Sheefer, T., and Aladjem, M. (1993). Antipyretic effectiveness of acetaminophen in febrile seizures: Ongoing prophylaxis versus sporadic usage. *Eur. J. Pediatr.* **152**, 747–749.

Schroeder, M. C., Wolff, D. L., Maister, B. H., Norstrom, S., Leppik, E. I., and Graves, N. M. (1996). Lorazepam intensol for the management of hospitalized pediatric patients with epilepsy. *Epilepsia* **37**, (Suppl. 5), S154.

Scott, R. C., Besag, F.M.C., and Neville, B.G.R. (1999). Buccal midazolam and rectal diazepam for treatment of prolonged seizures in childhood and adolescence: a randomized trial. *Lancet* **353**, 623–626.

Shimazaki, S., Kuremoto, K., Sato, H., Onishi, M., Motohashi, T., Oyama, S., and Takahashi, K. (1996). The efficacy of rectal diazepam in comparison with rectal chloral hydrate for febrile convulsion prophylaxis. *Brain Dev.* **18**, 477–478.

Shinnar, S., and Berg, A. T. (1996). Does antiepileptic drug therapy prevent the development of "chronic" epilepsy. *Epilepsia* **37**, 701–708.

Shirai, H., Miura, H., Minagawa, K., and Mizuno, S. (1987). Pharmacokinetic study on the effectiveness of intermittent oral diazepam in the prevention of recurrent febrile convulsions. *Adv. Epileptol.* **16**, 453–455.

Shirai, H., Miura, H., and Sunaoshi, W. (1988). A clinical study on the effectiveness of intermittent therapy with rectal diazepam suppositories for the prevention of recurrent febrile convulsions: a further study (in Japanese). *Tenkan Kankyu (Tokyo)* **6**, 1–10.

Shorvon, S. D. (1998). The use of clobazam, midazolam and nitrazepam in epilepsy. *Epilepsia* **39** (Suppl. 1), S15–S23.

Smith, M. C. (1994). Febrile seizures. Recognition and management. *Drugs* 47, 933–944.

Sternowsky, H. J., and Lagenstein, I. (1981). Phenobarbital bei Fieberkrämpfen im Kindesalter. *DWM* 106, 49–51.

Svensmark, O., and Buchthal, F. (1963). Accumulation of phenobarbital in man. *Epilepsia* 4, 199–206.

Sykes, R. M., and Okonofua, J. A. (1988). Rectal diazepam solution in the treatment of convulsions in the children's emergency room. *Ann. Trop. Pediatr.* 8, 259–61.

Tachibana, Y., Yamada, T., Seki, T., *et al.* (1985). Effect of intermittent administration of chloral hydrate suppositories in the prevention of recurrences of febrile convulsions. *Brain Dev.* 7, 258.

Tachibana, Y., Seki, T., Hidenori, Y., *et al.* (1986). Effect of intermittent administration of chloral hydrate suppositories for the prevention of recurrent febrile convulsions. *Brain Dev.* 8, 560.

Takei, K., Miura, H., Takanashi, S., *et al.* (1996). The effects of concurrent rectal administration of an antipyretic on the rectal absorption of diazepam suppositories: A pharmacokinetic study in children with febrile convulsions [in Japanese]. *Shonika Rinsho (Tokyo)* 49, 245–252.

Thilothammal, N. K., Krishnamurthy, P. V., Kamala, K. G., Ahamed, S., and Banu, K. (1993). Role of phenobarbitone in preventing recurrence of febrile convulsions. *Ind. Pediatr.* 30, 637–642.

Thorn, I. (1975). A controlled study of prophylactic long-term treatment of febrile convulsions with phenobarbital. *Acta Neurol. Scand.* 60 (Suppl.), 67–73.

Thorn, I. (1981). Prevention of recurrent febrile seizures: Intermittent prophylaxis with diazepam compared with continuous treatment with phenobarbital. *In* "Febrile Seizures" (K. B. Nelson and J. H. Ellenberg, eds.), pp. 119–26. Raven Press, New York.

Überall, M. A., Lauffer, H., and Wenzel, D. (1998). Parenterale intervallbehandlung mit natrium-valproat-injektionslösung bei kindern und jugendlichen mit zerebralen anfällen. *Nervenheilkunde* 17, 278–282.

Uhari, M., Rantala, H., Vainionpää, L., and Kurttila, R. (1995). Effect of acetaminophen and of low intermittent doses of diazepam on prevention of recurrences of febrile seizures. *J. Pediatr.* 126, 991–995.

Vanasse, M., Masson, P., Geoffroy, G., Larbrisseau, A., and David, P. C. (1984). Intermittent treatment of febrile convulsions with nitrazepam. *Can. J. Neurol. Sci.* 11, 377–379.

Van Esch, A., Van Steensel-Moll, H. A., Steyerberg, E. W., Offringa, M., Habbema, J.D.F., and Derksen-Lubsen, G. (1995). Antipyretic efficacy of ibuprofen and acetaminophen in children with febrile seizures. *Arch. Pediatr. Adolesc. Med.* 149, 632–637.

Ventura, A., Basso, T., Bortolan, G., *et al.* (1982). Home treatment of seizures as a strategy for the long term management of febrile convulsions in children. *Helv. Paediatr. Acta* 37, 581–587.

Verity, C. M. (1998). Do seizures damage the brain? The epidemiological evidence. *Arch. Dis. Child.* 78, 78–84.

Verity, C. M., and Golding, J. (1991). Risk of epilepsy after febrile convulsions: A national cohort study. *BMJ* 303, 1373–1376.

Verity, C. M., Ross, E. M., and Golding, J. (1993). Outcome of childhood status epilepticus and lengthy febrile convulsions: Findings of a national cohort study. *BMJ* 307, 225–228.

Vining, E.P.G., Mellits, E. D., Dorsen, M. M., *et al.* (1987). Psychologic and behavioral effects of antiepileptic drugs in children: A double-blind comparison between phenobarbital and valproic acid. *Pediatrics* 80, 165–174.

Voorhoeve, H.M.A. (1980). Childhood convulsions in the tropics. *Trop. Doct.* 10, 122–123.

Walker, J. E., Homan, R. W., Vasko, M. R., Crawford, I. L., Bell, R. D., and Tasker, W. G. (1979). Lorazepam in status epilepticus. *Ann. Neurol.* 6, 207–213.

Wallace, S. J. (1975). Continuous prophylactic anticonvulsions in selected children with febrile convulsions. *Acta Neurol. Scand.* (Suppl.) 75, 62–66.

Wallace, S. J. (1988). "The Child with Febrile Seizures." Butterworth, London.

Wallace, S. J. (1997). Nasal benzodiazepines for management of acute childhood seizures? *Lancet* 349, 222.

Wallace, S. J., and Smith, J. A. (1980). Successful prophylaxis against febrile convulsions with valproic acid or phenobarbitone. *BMJ* **280**, 353–354.

Watanabe, T. (1997). Pros and cons of treatments and studies of recurrent febrile seizures. *J. Pediatr.* **133**, 715.

Wilson, J. T. (1981). Antipyretic management of febrile seizures. *In* "Febrile Seizures" (K. B. Nelson and J. H. Ellenberg, eds.), pp. 231–239. Raven Press, New York.

Wolf, S. M. (1979). Controversies in the treatment of febrile convulsions. *Neurology* **29**, 287–290.

Wolf, S. M., and Forsythe, A. (1978). Behavior disturbance, phenobarbital, and febrile seizures. *Pediatrics* **61** (5), 728–731.

Wolf, S. M., Carr, A., Davis, D. C., Davidson, S., Dale, E. P., Forsythe, A., Goldenberg, E. D., Hanson, R., Lulejian, G. A., Nelson, M. A., Treitman, P., and Weinstein, A. (1977). The value of phenobarbital in the child who has had a single febrile seizure: A controlled prospective study. *Pediatrics* **59**, 378–385.

Woody, R. C., and Laney, S. M. (1988). Rectal anticonvulsants in pediatric practice. *Pediatr. Emerg. Care* **4** (2), 112–116.

Wright, S. W. (1987). The child with febrile seizures. *Am. Fam. Phys.* **36**, 163–167.

CHAPTER 20

What Do We Tell Parents of a Child with Simple or Complex Febrile Seizures?

CHRISTINE O'DELL

Comprehensive Epilepsy Management Center, Montefiore Medical Center, Bronx, New York 10467

Febrile seizures are a common pediatric problem. Although generally benign, they are very frightening events. Parents of children who experience a febrile seizure have many questions for the clinician regarding causation, the chance of another event, and prognosis. The content of information conveyed to the parents must not only answer their questions, but also instruct them in how to manage another febrile seizure, because many children will have another event. In particular, parents must be instructed regarding first aid for a seizure and on the "dos and don'ts" of seizure management. The manner in which the education is done will influence whether there is understanding of the information, and will form a basis for the parents' conceptualization of the event and for their view of the long-term outcome. With suitable communication and education, the family will adapt to the diagnosis of a febrile seizure without undue disruption of their quality of life. © 2002 Academic Press.

I. INTRODUCTION

Parents of a child who has had a febrile seizure have many questions for the physicians and nurses. Although the clinician is aware that a febrile seizure is a generally benign event, it is a very frightening experience for the parents. Many parents are convinced that their child was dying during a febrile seizure (Baumer *et al.*, 1981). Some of the diagnostic procedures, especially a lumbar puncture, that are necessary to exclude more serious illnesses such as meningitis (see Chapter 18) may also cause great concern to parents. The clinician must convey to the parents that febrile seizures are usually benign, and must inform them about prognosis, treatment, and steps to take should a seizure happen again.

The questions parents will have will depend on their level of medical knowledge, whether they are seeing the clinician in the emergency department or at a later time, whether there is a family history of febrile seizures, and other less well-defined variables. What the physicians and nurses tell the parents depends on several factors, including the practitioners' level of expertise, how certain they are of the diagnosis and etiology, the setting of the visit, and the individual clinician's biases regarding patient education. This chapter discusses an approach to conveying our current knowledge of febrile seizures to parents in a manner that addresses their concerns and takes into account how parents learn. The goal is to help the parents of a child with a febrile seizure better understand the diagnosis and cope with its implications in such a way as to minimize the impact of the event on the family and to maximize their ability to cope with a recurrence.

II. INFORMATION

A. QUESTIONS—WHAT DO PARENTS WANT TO KNOW?

What parents want to know will depend on when they see the clinician. The closer it is to the seizure the more alarmed the parents will be. The type of seizure may make a difference in the way the parents react to the episode. Febrile illness in combination with a seizure may be confusing and frightening, and parents who witnessed the seizure may have thought that their child was about to die (Baumer *et al.*, 1981). Parents will ask the doctor a number of basic, generic questions:

- What was it?
- What caused it?
- Is it related to the illness that caused the fever?
- How is it related . . . ?
- Has it caused harm to the child?
- Will it cause harm to the child in the future?
- Is it a sign that something worse will happen?
- Will it happen again?
- Is there a way of preventing it from happening again?
- What do I do if it does happen again?
- Do we need to do any more tests?
- Is it something that they as parents have done wrong, or not done right?

It is important for the clinician to realize that almost all parents have these basic questions, whether or not they successfully articulate them. In the emergency department they may be too stressed to think through anything more than "Is my child going to be all right?"—but later all these questions do arise.

B. CONTENT—WHAT PARENTS SHOULD BE TOLD

In order to provide needed information to parents, their questions must be answered in a manner understandable to them. One starts with a definition of a febrile seizure, including its association with fever and age dependence, the difference between febrile seizures and epilepsy, and the fact that although febrile seizures are very frightening, they are generally benign and that they occur in 2–4% of the overall population (see Chapters 1–3). Parents will want to know that they are not alone in having a child who has had a febrile seizure, but they will also want to know specifics about their child. In the emergency department, it is important to provide an explanation of the tests being done and, in particular, the need for a lumbar puncture or the clinical certainty that this is not meningitis. Referring to the practice parameter of the American Academy of Pediatrics (1996) about the necessity of doing or not doing specific tests will reassure the parents that the clinician is not being too aggressive or is failing to be aggressive enough in the evaluation (see Chapter 18).

Afterward, parents will want to know the long-term prognosis and the chances that brain injury has occurred. Again, an explanation of the generally benign nature of febrile seizures is appropriate. There should be an explanation of whether their child's seizure was simple or complex (see Chapter 1) and what that implies. The risk of subsequent febrile seizures (Chapter 3) in their particular case as well as the risk of subsequent epilepsy (Chapters 5–7) should be discussed. Parents will want to know about risk of brain injury. In the case of simple and most complex febrile seizures one can be very reassuring (Chapter 7). In the case of very prolonged febrile seizures one should discuss the available data (Chapters 6–8) that in rare cases damage may occur, while emphasizing that most children do well even after prolonged febrile seizures (Ellenberg and Nelson, 1978; Maytal and Shinnar, 1990; Shinnar and Babb, 1997; Verity et al., 1993, 1998). The favorable cognitive outcomes following febrile seizures (Chapter 4) should be emphasized and, in the author's experience, are a very important reassuring factor for parents.

Much of the above discussion is theoretical. However, many parents focus on the more practical aspects of the risk of another febrile seizure, how to avoid it, and what to do if and when it occurs. If parents are told that 30–40% of children who have a first febrile seizure will have a second seizure (Chapter 3), they can prepare emotionally. Telling the parents about the ages of onset and when febrile seizures are outgrown (Chapter 1) provides information that febrile seizures are a time-limited phenomenon. This information will give them hope that their child will outgrow the episodes and a sense of relief that they will not continue throughout the child's life. This information will decrease the parents' level of anxiety and make them ready to process more information. For those children with an initial brief febrile seizure, one can also reassure them that if another one does occur, it too will most likely be brief (Berg and Shinnar, 1996) (see Chapter 3).

Predictors of recurrence will be of some interest to most parents, but this topic must be individualized to their child for it to be meaningful. Because risk of a first febrile seizure is associated with a parent, sibling, aunt, uncle, or grandparent having had a febrile seizure (Berg *et al.*, 1995; Bethune *et al.*, 1993) (Chapter 2), this information can be used by the physician as an explanation and as reassurance if the child fits into this category. Family history is also associated with recurrence risk (see Chapter 3). Although a family history of febrile seizures is associated with a higher recurrence risk, it is also associated with a lower level of stress because these families are often familiar with the entity and have first-hand evidence of its generally benign nature.

C. What Do Parents Need to Know?

Parents need to know the answers to any of the questions that they have asked, regardless of how peripheral the practitioner thinks that they may be. After each of the parents' questions are answered they will need some basic information about febrile seizures as stated above. Finally, parents will need to know what to do if the child has another febrile episode or another febrile seizure, including some first aid training (Table 1).

What is the risk in having another febrile seizure? There are both direct consequences for the child as well as psychosocial or emotional consequences for the parents. For the child, there is no convincing evidence that a brief febrile seizure causes brain damage. Furthermore, by definition febrile seizures are isolated events associated with a febrile illness without an acute neurological insult. These children, because of their age, are likely to be in a supervised environment at the time of a febrile seizure. Injury related to seizures in general is rare, especially in the younger age groups because they are less likely to be independently active or participating in sports. The seizure in these children may be the first sign of febrile illness (Al-Eissa *et al.*, 1992; Berg *et al.*, 1992). The clinician should underscore the information that outcome is generally favorable for cognitive, behavioral, and academic function (Verity *et al.*, 1998) (see Chapter 4).

Febrile seizures are different from unprovoked seizures in the need for medical evaluation. The child with a brief, unprovoked seizure does not usually need acute medical care unless it is the first event. However, in the case of febrile seizures, medical evaluation will be needed not so much for the seizure but to

TABLE 1   Guidelines for Parents during and after a Seizure

What to do	What not to do

Protect
  Move the child away from danger
  Do not try to restrain the child except if
    he/she is in danger of injuring self
  Keep airway open—turn the child on his/her
    side to allow secretions to drain from mouth
Observe
  Stay with the child and watch what
    is happening
Comfort
  The child may be agitated or dazed after the
    seizure; stay calm and be reassuring
Medical evaluation
  Call your doctor or follow instructions the
    doctor has given you
Call Emergency Medical Services
  If the seizure lasts more than 5 minutes or
    there is more than one seizure (unless
    your doctor tells you otherwise)
  If the child does not recover or is injured
	Do not panic
	Do not put anything in the child's
	  mouth
	Do not hold the child's tongue
	Do not throw water on the child
	Do not put the child in the bathtub
	  while he/she is having a seizure
	Do not restrain any part of the child
	  (unless he/she is in danger)

determine the cause of the fever and to provide treatment if indicated. Tell parents when it is necessary to call the doctor. Discuss with the parents what information should be given to other adults having contact with the child, such as siblings, grandparents, and babysitters. Once the child has had a febrile seizure, persons having contact with the child can be told about the child's seizures, including what they look like and what to do if another seizure occurs. This gives a baseline from which the observer can administer first aid and can curtail the confusion and panic typically seen in the public arena during a seizure. Parents can also ask for assistance of these persons to describe the characteristics of these events, should they happen, so that accurate information can be given to the medical provider in follow-up. This information is of importance to the physician in diagnosis and treatment decisions (see Chapters 18 and 19).

1. Prevention and Treatment

Parents will want to know about treatments available to prevent the next episode. A discussion needs to emphasize that although treatments are available to reduce the risk of another febrile seizure, they are associated with side effects and do not alter the long-term outcome (Knudsen *et al.*, 1996; Shinnar and Berg, 1996; Shinnar, 1999) (see Chapters 3 and 19). A study has shown that although most parents would want medications prescribed to prevent another febrile seizure, their enthusiasm for medications markedly diminishes when they are told about potential side effects (Gordon *et al.*, 2000). For children with a simple febrile seizure, one can reassure the parents using the published practice parameter of the American Academy of Pediatrics (1999), which recommends no treatment for these children. As daily prophylactic medication is only rarely indicated for either simple or complex febrile seizures (see Chapter 19); we will focus the discussion on other treatment modalities.

a. Antipyretics

Antipyretics are almost universally prescribed for children who have had a febrile seizure. This remains the case despite the fact that controlled trials (Camfield *et al.*, 1980) (see Chapter 19) have shown that they are no more effective than placebo. The reasons for this are unclear, though they may have to do with the fact that a febrile seizure is often the first clinical manifestation of the fever. If antipyretics are prescribed, it is important to instruct to the parents about rational use so that they are not given too often—such as every time the child feels warm. It is also important to emphasize to the parents that even if they give the medications conscientiously as prescribed, another febrile seizure may still occur and it is not their fault (Camfield and Camfield, 1995). Feelings of guilt and blame are common in this setting and need to be addressed both after the first seizure and again after subsequent seizures, should they occur.

b. Intermittent Diazepam

One widely used therapy is intermittent diazepam at the time of illness (see Chapter 19). This is usually given orally in the United States (Rosman *et al.*, 1993), though in Europe rectal administration has also been used (Knudsen, 1985). If this mode of treatment is chosen, clear instruction as to when to initiate it must be given. Giving diazepam at every perceived sniffle will result in overmedicating the child with a potent sedative. However, delaying the treatment until the child is clearly sick may reduce its efficacy. This treatment does reduce the risk of another febrile seizure, but it certainly does not eliminate it. Therefore, the same caveats discussed above about dealing with feelings of guilt and blame are even more relevant.

c. Rectal Diazepam at Time of Seizure

In some cases, the physician may prescribe rectal diazepam to be given when the child has a seizure (Camfield and Camfield, 1995; Knudsen, 1979; Shinnar 1999) (see Chapter 19). The assumption underlying this treatment is that it is not so important to prevent a febrile seizure as to make sure that we are preventing prolonged ones. This approach minimizes how often diazepam is used because it limits it to when the child is actually convulsing, which necessitates the rectal route. The precise instructions to be given are described below. The importance of clear instructions in this setting is even greater, because parents will be under considerable stress.

2. First Aid for Febrile Seizures

A febrile seizure is a dramatic and frightening event for a parent. The emotional consequences can be striking, and the physician will need to counsel the parents to overcome this. A portion of this guidance should include information about what to do should the child have another febrile seizure. First aid information will be important for the parents, because 30–40% of children will experience at least one additional seizure. Typically the parents should be told to follow the ABCs of first aid (O'Dell, 2000): Assess level of consciousness. Is the child fully conscious? If so, observe until there is a return to baseline status. If consciousness is impaired the observer must assess for breathing. If breathing is intact the observer should stay with the child and take note of the features of the seizure, such as which side of the body is involved and how long the event lasts. If breathing is impaired or absent the airway must be opened. This may involve tipping the head back to open the throat. Sometimes breathing stops during the tonic (or "tightening") phase of a generalized seizure; breathing will resume once this phase is over and other measures, such as mouth-to-mouth resuscitation, are not needed. After the seizure is over the child should be assessed for injury. Additional support can be given at that time if needed.

In the case of the child who has had prolonged or repetitive febrile seizures, rectal diazepam can be used as an abortive measure independent of whether the child is also on prophylactic medications (see Chapter 19). Diazepam is also useful when the parents are far away from medical care or are unusually anxious about a recurrence. It can be administered at home, at daycare, or in school. In the United States, the available preparation is rectal diazepam gel (Diastat). In other countries, other forms of rectal diazepam, including solutions and rectal capsules, are used. All forms of rectal diazepam are effective (see Chapter 19). Our research (O'Dell *et al.*, 2000) has shown that even in families where parents do not need to use the rectal diazepam gel for prolonged or repetitive seizures, quality of life is improved by having medication available, in that this reduces worry and stress. Parents and other caregivers will need instruction as to when and how to administer this medication. With education, lay persons can administer rectal diazepam gel quite easily to abort seizure activity and potentially avoid prolonged febrile seizures, which are the main concern in terms of potential adverse consequences. As the caregivers will have to administer the medications in a time of great stress, to a convulsing child, thorough instruction is necessary. The practitioner should use a visual tool for demonstrating the administration technique and give written information to the parents regarding when to administer the rectal diazepam.

In some instances emergency assistance will be needed during or after a febrile seizure. If a there is an injury, emergency medical assistance should be called. Sometimes the seizure will stop and then restart without the child regaining consciousness. Emergency medical assistance should be called in this instance also. If a generalized tonic–clonic seizure lasts longer than 5–10 minutes, medical intervention is usually needed, either by administering rectal diazepam or via emergency medical services. If a child has not responded to rectal diazepam within a reasonable period of time, emergency medical services should also be called. The clinician has to be very clear in giving instructions on this issue, regardless of whether rectal diazepam is also being prescribed. On the one hand, one wants to reassure the family and not have them panic. On the other hand, it is important to provide clear guidelines for when it is appropriate to call emergency medical services, taking into account the individual circumstances, including how far away from medical care the family is and how long the first febrile seizure lasted.

D. MANNER—WHY, WHERE, HOW, WHEN, AND BY WHOM IS IT TOLD?

Information is given to the parents of a child who had a febrile seizure in order to help them manage the situation should it happen again and to allay their fears about the initial event. The setting in which information is given will make a difference in how and by whom the education is done. If the information is first given in the emergency department, it is likely that the parents will not "absorb" most of it. If the child is admitted to the hospital, follow-up information and reenforcement of previous information can be given in a more relaxed atmosphere the following day by the physician or nurse. If the child is seen in the office for follow-up, an educational session can take place there. In the office setting, the child has usually recovered both from the febrile seizure and the precipitating illness, and the information can be conveyed without the distractions and uncertainties inherent in the emergency department setting.

Follow-up questions are usually based on information that the doctor has given the parents during the course of the initial explanations—issues that the parents did not initially understand. Unless they have written down explicit questions prior to the doctor's visit, parents seldom have independent questions. Discussion of possible outcomes that are not relevant to the immediate situation, such as the possibility of subsequent epilepsy (Chapter 5) or the possibility of developing mesial temporal sclerosis (Shinnar, 1998; VanLandingham *et al.*, 1998) (Chapters 6–8), should be delayed until the acute episode is over and the parents begin asking questions about prognosis.

Education and counseling are best supplemented by written information. This is one of the most useful tools that can be used when educating parents because they can refer to written material after they leave the doctor's office. If the parents are able to visit the physician more than once they will be able to learn more— in part because they will be more relaxed by this time and also because retention of information is greater when issues are reinforced. For simple febrile seizures a single visit is usually sufficient to address the family's concerns, but a return visit to address subsequent issues is sometimes also useful in selected cases. Availability of the staff to answer future questions is also important. A list of resources available to families and clinicians is provided at the end of this chapter.

III. LEARNING THEORIES

Adult learning theories can help the practitioner decide how to style the patient education information given to parents (Knowles, 1984). Adults have life experiences from which analogies can be drawn to explain complicated material. Building on the adult's previous learning recognizes his acquired knowledge and promotes his understanding of related data. If someone else in the family has a history of having had febrile seizures the parents can then identify with the experience more readily. Parents will be able to retain information if they are given it at a point of low anxiety. Explaining about febrile seizures in the emergency department is not conducive to retention of information. Parents must believe that the facts being discussed will be of some help to them or their situation. The material must be meaningful and the parent must be ready to learn or "hear it"; practical advice is usually the most beneficial. With this in mind the clinician can convey information that parents will need in order to understand their child's condition, to act appropriately should the child have another seizure, and to help them cope with this new situation.

IV. CONCLUSIONS

Knowledge of febrile seizure disorder empowers parents and helps them cope. Physicians and nurses can improve the quality of life of the families that they care for by providing data that will help parents understand and manage their child's febrile seizures. Various resources available for patient education can be used by the clinician (see Section V). By using principles of adult learning, valid information can be transmitted in a way that is meaningful for the parents and can help them to adapt to a new situation. Knowledge is a resource that parents can utilize to foster coping so that the child who has a febrile seizure receives not only appropriate care, but the seizure causes only minimal disruption in the child's and family's life activities.

V. AVAILABLE RESOURCES

The following selected organizations and web sites contain generally reliable information about febrile seizures that will be of interest to both parents and professionals. Note the specific caveats in the comments on some sites. The printed publications listed are those directly related to febrile seizures, or are catalogs, and are not a complete listing of the publications available from the organizations.

American Academy of Pediatrics (AAP), 141 NorthWest Point Boulevard, Elk Grove Village, IL 60007-1098. Tel: 847/434-4000; fax: 847/434-8000; home page: www.aap.org.
  In addition to information for AAP members, the web site has a large amount of information available to consumers and nonmembers. This includes an information fact sheet about febrile seizures (also available directly from AAP), practice guidelines relating to the diagnostic evaluation of febrile seizures, and on the treatment of febrile seizures as well as a variety of other information that is updated on a regular basis. Printed publications: *Fact Sheet About Febrile Seizures.*

American Association of Neuroscience Nurses (AANN), 4700 W. Lake Avenue, Glenview, IL 60025. Tel: 888/557-2266 or 847/375-4733; fax: 847/375-6333; e-mail: info@aann.org; home page: www.aann.org.
  The web site has a variety of materials that will be of interest to both parents and professionals. In particular, the publication, *Seizure Assessment Guidelines* (also available directly from AANN), contains instructions on how to assess a seizure. Printed publications: *Seizure Assessment Guidelines* (1998).

American Epilepsy Society (AES), 342 North Main Street, West Hartford, CT 06117-2507. Tel: 860/586-7505; fax: 860/586-7550; e-mail: info@aesnet.org; home page: www.aesnet.org.
  Research, treatment, and management data as well as a reference guide for nurses, families, and patients. Much of the material on the web site is about epilepsy rather than febrile seizures, but there is also information on febrile seizures. The web site is regularly updated. Printed publications: *Epilepsy Reference Guide for Nurses and Epilepsy Reference Guide for Persons with Epilepsy* (2001). Listing of journals, books, videos, networking groups, and web sites.

Epilepsy Foundation, 4351 Garden City Drive, Landover, MD 20785-2267. Tel: 301/459-3700; home page: www.epilepsyfoundation.org.

This is an excellent resource for all consumers and clinicians who want to find out more about seizures of all kinds, including febrile seizures. Printed publications: Catalog listing available books, videos, and pamphlets that can be purchased from the Epilepsy Foundation.

National Institute of Neurological Disorders and Stroke (NINDS), National Institutes of Health (NIH), Bethesda, MD 20892-2540. Home page: www.ninds .nih.gov.
Clinicians and researchers will find a variety of useful information. Patient section contains information related to management, studies, publications, and health organizations on a variety of neurological disorders and also on febrile seizures. Printed publications: *National Institute of Health Publication No. 95-3930 (1995)*. Fact sheet: *Febrile Seizures*. Office of Scientific and Health Reports, National Institute of Neurological Disorders and Stroke, National Institutes of Health, Bethesda, MD 20892-2540.

Nervous System Diseases: National Guideline Clearinghouse: Home page: www.guideline.gov.
Clinical practice guidelines about many disorders, including seizures. This web site is an excellent one, but not all the guidelines listed are equally valuable and some may be out of date. Readers should look not just at the guideline but also at the date of the guideline and who originated the guideline (i.e., a national organization such the American Academy of Pediatrics or Epilepsy Foundation versus a local hospital).

Exceptional Parent Magazine (2000). Publication of PSY-ED Corporation, 555 Kinderkamack Road, Oradell, NJ 07649. *Contemporary Issues in Epilepsy: What families need to know about childhood seizures.*
This publication, although not focused on febrile seizures per se, contains many articles (particularly the article on first aid) that are applicable to all seizures, including febrile seizures.

REFERENCES

Al Eissa, Y. A., Al Omair, A. O., Al Herbish, A. S., *et al.* (1992). Antecedents and outcome of simple and partial complex febrile convulsions among Saudi children. *Dev. Med. Child Neurol.* **34**, 1085–1090.
American Academy of Pediatrics, Provisional Committee on Quality Improvement, (1996). Practice Parameter: The neurodiagnostic evaluation of the child with a simple febrile seizure. *Pediatrics* **97**, 769–775.
American Academy of Pediatrics, Committee on Quality Improvement, Subcommittee on Febrile Seizures (1999). Practice Parameter: Long-term treatment of the child with simple febrile seizures. *Pediatrics* **103**, 1307–1309.

Baumer, J. H., David, T. J., Valentine, S. J., *et al.* (1981). Many parents think their child is dying when having a first febrile convulsion. *Dev. Med. Child Neurol.* 23, 462–464.

Berg, A. T., and Shinnar, S. (1996). Complex febrile seizures. *Epilepsia* 37, 126–133.

Berg, A. T., Shinnar, S., Hauser, W. A., *et al.* (1992). A prospective study of recurrent febrile seizures. *N. Engl. J. Med.* 327, 1122–1127.

Berg, A. T., Shinnar, S., Shapiro, E. D., Salomon, M. E., Crain, E. F., and Hauser, W. A. (1995). Risk factors for a first febrile seizure: A matched case-control study. *Epilepsia* 36, 334–341.

Bethune, P., Gordon, K., Dooley, J., Camfield, C., and Camfield, P. (1993). Which child will have a febrile seizure? *Am. J. Dis. Child.* 147, 35–39.

Camfield, P., and Camfield, C. (1995). Febrile Seizures. *In* "Childhood Seizures" (S. Shinnar, N. Amir, and D. Branski, eds.), pp. 32–38. Karger, Switzerland.

Camfield, P. R., Camfield, C. S., Shapiro, S., *et al.* (1980). The first febrile seizure—Antipyretic instruction plus either phenobarbital or placebo to prevent a recurrence. *J. Pediatr.* 97, 16–21.

Ellenberg, J. H., and Nelson, K. B. (1978). Febrile seizures and later intellectual performance. *Arch. Neurol.* 35, 17–21.

Gordon, K. E., Dooley, J. M., Camfield, P. R., Camfield, C. S., Wood, E., and MacSween, J. (2000). Treatment of febrile seizures: The influence of treatment efficacy and side effect profile on value to parents. *Epilepsia* 41 (Suppl. 7), 177.

Knowles, M. (1984). "The Modern Practice of Adult Education: From Pedagogy to Andragogy." Follett Publ. Co., Chicago, IL.

Knudsen, F. U. (1979). Rectal administration of diazepam in solution in the acute treatment of convulsions in infants and children. *Arch. Dis. Child.* 54, 855–857.

Knudsen, F. U. (1985). Effective short-term diazepam prophylaxis in febrile convulsions. *J. Pediatr.* 106, 487–490.

Knudsen, F. U., Paerregaard, A., Andersen, R., and Andresen, J. (1996). Long-term outcome of prophylaxis for febrile convulsions. *Arch. Dis. Child.* 74, 13–18.

Maytal, J., and Shinnar, S. (1990). Febrile status epilepticus. *Pediatrics* 86, 611–616.

O'Dell, C. (2000). First aid for seizures. *Contemporary Issues in Epilepsy: What Families Need to Know about Seizures. Exceptional Parent Magazine, Special Report on Epilepsy,* pp. 14–18.

O'Dell, C., Shinnar, S., Ballaban-Gil, K., Kang, H., and Moshe, S. L. (2000). Home use of rectal diazepam gel (Diastat). *Epilepsia* 41 (Suppl. 7), 246.

Rosman, N. P., Colton, T., Labazzo, J., *et al.* (1993). A controlled trial of diazepam administered during febrile illnesses to prevent recurrence of febrile seizures. *N. Engl. J. Med.* 329, 79–84.

Shinnar, S. (1998). Prolonged febrile seizures and mesial temporal sclerosis. *Ann. Neurol.* 43, 411–412.

Shinnar, S. (1999). Febrile seizures. *In* "Pediatric Neurology; Principles and Practice," 3rd ed. (K. E. Swaiman and S. Ashwal, eds.), pp. 676–682. Mosby, St. Louis, MO.

Shinnar, S., and Babb, T. L. (1997). Long-term sequelae of status epilepticus. *In* "Epilepsy: A Comprehensive Textbook" (J. Engel, Jr. and T. A. Pedley, eds.), pp 755–763. Lippincott-Raven, Philadelphia, PA.

Shinnar, S., and Berg, A. T. (1996). Does antiepileptic drug therapy prevent the development of "chronic" epilepsy? *Epilepsia* 37, 701–708.

VanLandingham, K. E., Heinz, E. R., Cavazos, J. E., and Lewis, D. V. (1998). Magnetic resonance imaging evidence of hippocampal injury after prolonged focal febrile convulsions. *Ann. Neurol.* 43, 413–426.

Verity, C. M., Ross, E. M., and Golding, J. (1993). Outcome of childhood status epilepticus and lengthy febrile convulsions: Findings of national cohort study. *Br. Med. J.* 307, 225–228.

Verity, C. M., Greenwood, R., and Golding, J. (1998). Long-term intellectual and behavioral outcomes of children with febrile convulsions. *N. Engl. J. Med.* 338, 1723–1728.

CHAPTER 21

Human Data: What Do We Know about Febrile Seizures and What Further Information Is Needed

SHLOMO SHINNAR

Departments of Neurology and Pediatrics, and Comprehensive Epilepsy Management Center,
Montefiore Medical Center, Albert Einstein College of Medicine, Bronx, New York 10467

Much progress has been made in the past 25 years in clinical and basic research on febrile seizures. The results of this work are summarized in this volume. However, although much knowledge has been gained, many questions remain unanswered. This final analysis will attempt to give a brief overview of what the author sees as the important areas of clinical investigations that will be the focus of clinical research in the next decade.

I. GENETICS

As reviewed in Chapter 17, there is substantial evidence that susceptibility to febrile seizures has a genetic component. A history of febrile seizures in a first- or second-degree relative is a major risk factor both for the occurrence of febrile seizures (Chapter 2) and for recurrent febrile seizures (Chapter 3). There is also evidence for an underlying predisposition to prolonged febrile seizures or status epilepticus from both epidemiological and twin studies (Berg and Shinnar, 1996; Corey *et al.*, 1998; Shinnar *et al.*, 2001a). The recent finding of a strong association between a polymorphism at the interleukin-1β (IL-1β) locus and mesial temporal sclerosis (MTS) in patients with temporal lobe epilepsy suggests that genetic factors may also predispose to the development of MTS following a prolonged febrile seizure (Kanemoto *et al.*, 2000; Berkovic and Jackson, 2000). Although there is strong evidence that genetic susceptibility is an important contributor to risk for the occurrence, duration, recurrence, and sequelae of febrile seizures, little is known about the precise genes involved or the mechanism by which their influence might be exerted. Although several loci that are associated with an increased risk of febrile seizures have been identified thus far, it is clear that these account for only a small fraction of cases (Chapter 17). Studies such as that by Briellmann *et al.* (2001), who utilized monozygotic twin pairs discordant for the presence of epilepsy to study environmental influences after controlling for genetic influences, also offer another approach of using genetic techniques to study the association between febrile seizures and temporal lobe epilepsy. Thus, further studies on the genetic mechanisms involved in both the susceptibility to febrile seizures in general and prolonged febrile seizures in particular, as well as in predisposing to seizure-induced injury, are an exciting avenue of future research.

II. ROLE OF MAGNETIC RESONANCE IMAGING AND FUNCTIONAL IMAGING IN DEFINING SEIZURE-INDUCED HIPPOCAMPAL INJURY

Hippocampal magnetic resonance imaging (MRI) abnormalities following status epilepticus have been demonstrated in both children and adults (Chapter 8). MRI also shows signal changes secondary to status epilepticus in animal models. These changes may be transient and therefore not detected unless MRI is performed shortly after the prolonged seizure. MRI is essential to detect chronic hippocampal injury, i.e., MTS. Although hippocampal MRI abnormalities can be seen following prolonged seizures in general and prolonged febrile seizures in particular, it is not clear how to predict whether a hippocampal abnormality seen on an acute MRI will be permanent. Other functional imaging modalities have not yet been well studied. Timing of the studies appears to be even more critical in functional imaging studies such as spectroscopy, compared to MRIs. The demonstration that we can detect acute imaging abnormalities will lead to new studies in both animals and humans that will help define who is at risk for developing sequelae and what are the anatomical and physiological substrates for these acute changes.

III. ROLE OF PREEXISTING ABNORMALITIES
IN SEIZURE-INDUCED INJURY

It is clear that seizure-induced injury can occur in humans (Chapters 6–8). It remains unclear what are the necessary substrates for it to occur. In the study of vanLandingham *et al.* (1998), two of three children who demonstrated acute hippocampal changes that progressed to MTS had evidence of preexisting pathology. Many patients with temporal lobe epilepsy have dual pathology consisting of both MTS and other lesions, most commonly cortical dysgenesis. Rat pups with induced cortical dysgenesis are more susceptible to hyperthermia-induced seizures and hyperthermia-induced hippocampal neuronal death than are controls (Chapter 10). Thus, both clinical and experimental data suggest that focal cortical dysplasia or other preexisting pathology could have a role in producing febrile seizures that are both focal and prolonged and possibly enhance seizure-induced neuronal injury. Further studies are needed to clarify whether preexisting MRI abnormalities are an independent risk factor for hippocampal injury in humans or if they simply predispose to prolonged and lateralized seizure activity.

IV. FEVER VERSUS HYPERTHERMIA

Animal models of febrile seizures have used hyperthermia to induce seizures. Hyperthermia clearly does produce seizures in the appropriate developmental window, as elegantly described in Chapters 9–16. However, the clinical phenomenon is somewhat more complex. Whether a febrile seizure occurs is a function of the age of the child, the peak temperature, the family history of febrile seizures, and the nature of the febrile illness (Chapter 2). In addition, febrile seizures do not always occur at the same time as the peak temperature nor necessarily at the onset of fever. Although hyperthermia is clearly a key component, fever is the body's response to a variety of stimuli and involves the release of cytokines and particularly interleukins. The finding of a strong association between a polymorphism at the IL-1β locus and MTS in patients with temporal lobe epilepsy (Kanemoto *et al.*, 2000) is particularly intriguing due to evidence that IL-1β is associated with febrile response to external pathogens and to new data that it is proconvulsant and exerts its effect via the N-methyl-D-aspartate receptor. The data reviewed in Chapter 12 are very exciting and suggest how one may proceed to the next step in studying the effects of fever beyond those of hyperthermia, which, although a key component of the febrile response, may not be the entire story.

V. ROLE OF SPECIFIC PATHOGENS

The cause of the febrile illness may influence not only whether a febrile seizure occurs (Chapter 2), but also its duration and whether it results in hippocampal injury. Some of these differences may be due to the differential response of the human immune system to different pathogens and the resultant differences in the febrile response, as elegantly reviewed in Chapter 12. The potential role of human herpesvirus-6 (HHV-6) and HHV-7 in causing very prolonged febrile seizures and hippocampal damage is of particular interest. HHV-6 infection appears to be universally acquired by age 3 years (Hall et al., 1994). In a study by Caserta et al. (1998) HHV-6 and HHV-7 combined accounted for 53% of first febrile seizures presenting to the emergency department in children below age 3 years. Suga et al. (2000) reported that children with primary HHV-6 infection were more likely to have prolonged, focal febrile seizures and to have postictal paralysis than those with febrile seizures not occurring with HHV-6 infection. It remains unclear whether these viruses are associated with prolonged febrile seizures due to the high fevers associated with them or whether they are also involved with the pathogenesis of seizure-induced damage (Chapter 2). Further investigations are needed on the precise role of HHV6 and HHV7 as well as other potential pathogens in febrile seizures, and particularly in prolonged febrile seizures in childhood.

VI. EPILEPSY SYNDROMES

Older studies focused on the risk of epilepsy following febrile seizures and did not specifically analyze by epilepsy syndrome. Because a history of febrile seizures is more common in many forms of epilepsy than in the general population (Chapters 5 and 7), it is important to try and tease out the specific association with temporal lobe epilepsy. Modern epidemiological studies of childhood-onset seizures have demonstrated that it is possible to classify epilepsy syndromes with good interrater reliability in prospective epidemiological studies (Berg et al., 1999). Future studies of the risk of epilepsy following febrile seizures need to be analyzed with specific attention to epilepsy syndromes to see if the increased risk of epilepsy is specific to temporal lobe epilepsy. Long-term outcome studies on children with febrile status epilepticus are particularly needed and are currently being planned (Shinnar et al., 2001b).

VII. THE CONTROVERSIAL RELATIONSHIP BETWEEN PROLONGED FEBRILE SEIZURES, MESIAL TEMPORAL SCLEROSIS, AND TEMPORAL LOBE EPILEPSY

Clarifying this issue is the most critical area in clinical research in febrile seizures today. Retrospective studies reviewed in Chapter 6 report that many adults with intractable temporal lobe epilepsy have a history of prolonged febrile seizures in childhood (Chapters 5–7). In contrast, recent cohort studies of prolonged febrile seizures in children (reviewed in Chapter 7) have minimized the potential role of prolonged seizure activity in causing MTS and, later, temporal lobe epilepsy. Instead, these investigators have attributed both the febrile seizures and ensuing epilepsy to preexisting pathology (Chapters 5–7). In these epidemiological studies, MRIs were not performed. Because hippocampal injury may have no clinical correlate for many years, it is unclear whether some of these children may have suffered permanent hippocampal injury due to prolonged febrile seizures. Recent imaging studies reviewed in Chapter 8 suggest that the negative findings from epidemiological studies may simply reflect the rarity of febrile status epilepticus even in large studies. Further studies are needed to clarify the risk of developing MTS, epilepsy in general, and temporal lobe epilepsy in particular, following prolonged febrile seizures in childhood. Ultimately, one needs to combine epidemiological and imaging techniques and possibly genetic analysis as well to answer the question.

VIII. COGNITIVE AND BEHAVIORAL OUTCOMES AND MEMORY

The data reviewed in Chapter 4 indicate that children with febrile seizures, even prolonged ones, seem to do well in terms of global measures of cognition and behavior. A study that appeared as this book was going to press reported that children with febrile seizures also performed well on memory tasks (Chang *et al.*, 2001). The exception were children whose febrile seizures occurred under 1 year of age, a group also implicated with worse cognitive outcomes in other studies. However, as noted in the commentary (Baram and Shinnar, 2001), this population-based study included only a small number of children with prolonged febrile seizures. Why be concerned about memory and hippocampal function in children with febrile seizures? It is well-known that memory performance is highly dependent on intact hippocampal function. Patients with temporal lobe epilepsy and MTS have memory deficits, but it is unclear whether these deficits are secondary to the MTS alone, the effects of the subsequent seizures, the antiepileptic drugs used to treat them, or a combination of these factors. Both human (Chapter 8) and animal (Chapters 9, 10, and 13–15) data indicate that at least transient injury to hippocampus and related limbic structures can occur in individuals with prolonged febrile seizures. Neuroimaging studies have demonstrated acute swelling of hippocampus after very prolonged febrile seizures. In a rat model of prolonged febrile seizures, cytoskeletal changes in neurons were evident within 24 hours and persisted for several weeks without leading to cell loss (Chapter 9). However, altered functional properties of these neuronal populations were evident (Chapters 14 and 15). Thus, it is conceivable that exposure of hippocampal neurons to febrile seizures early in life may lead to transient injury and more sustained dysfunction of these neurons. This may in turn result in impairment of memory, which is a specific hippocampal function even if global measures of cognition are preserved. Future research will focus on the relationship between prolonged febrile seizures and impairment of hippocampal functions such as memory.

IX. TREATMENT AND NEUROPROTECTION

There is now a broad consensus that simple febrile seizures are benign and rarely require treatment (Chapter 19). There is less consensus on complex febrile seizures, though many authorities feel that the optimal treatment is abortive therapy, which will prevent the occurrence of status epilepticus. This analysis is based on a risk–benefit basis, including the facts that outcome is benign in most cases and that antiepileptic drug therapy does not alter long-term prognosis and is associated with significant potential adverse effects (Chapter 19). However, there is a small group of children in whom seizure-induced injury does occur. Furthermore, although the human data indicate that seizures must be very prolonged to cause demonstrable injury (Chapters 6–8), the animal data suggest that a seizure lasting 20 minutes can produce long-lasting physiological changes (Chapters 14 and 15). If we had treatments that did not simply suppress seizures but prevented epilepsy, then the risk–benefit analysis may be quite different. This would be particularly true if the treatment could be given for only a short period of time following the prolonged seizure, because most of the adverse effects of antiepileptic drugs are associated with long-term therapy. Before such trials can be undertaken, one would have to identify the population at risk and define a suitable surrogate for epileptogenesis. The development of clinical epilepsy following prolonged febrile seizures is variable and may not occur for many years (Chapters 5–7). MTS may be a suitable surrogate early marker but this has not been clearly demonstrated (Chapter 8). A search for drugs that not only suppress seizures but are also truly antiepileptogenic, in the sense that they alter the natural history and prevent epilepsy, is needed. To date no such effect has been proved with any of the standard antiepileptic drugs (Shinnar and Berg, 1996). Once we identify the target population and the suitable surrogate markers, prevention of epileptogenesis will be the ultimate goal of therapy.

X. SUMMARY

Although much information has been gained, much remains to be learned. With the advent of new techniques in imaging, genetics, and neuropsychology, and the availability of animal models, the tools to further increase our understanding of febrile seizures are now available. The new studies will require large cohorts and sophisticated techniques and will therefore be expensive. They will also have to take into account that we are studying children so that risks and discomforts associated with the research have to be minimized and acceptable. With these caveats, the recent findings in clinical and basic science offer the opportunity for elucidating the epidemiology, genetics, and prognosis of the most common form of childhood seizures. This will also allow us to identify the large majority who have a benign disorder, so that we can reassure the families (Chapters 19 and 20), as well as the smaller number of children in whom the febrile seizure is a more serious event and who may be candidates for therapeutic interventions.

REFERENCES

Baram, T. Z., and Shinnar, S. (2001). Do febrile seizures improve memory? *Neurology* 57, 7–8.

Berg, A. T., and Shinnar, S. (1996). Complex febrile seizures. *Epilepsia* 37, 126–133.

Berg, A. T., Levy, S. R., Testa, F. M., and Shinnar, S. (1999). Classification of childhood epilepsy syndromes in newly diagnosed epilepsy: Interrater agreement and reasons for disagreement. *Epilepsia* 40, 439–444.

Berkovic, S. F., and Jackson, G. D. (2000). The hippocampal sclerosis whodunit: Enter the genes. *Ann. Neurol.* 47, 571–574.

Briellmann, R. S., Jackson, G. D., Torn-Broers, B. A., and Berkovic, S. F. (2001). Causes of epilepsies: Insights from discordant twin pairs. *Ann. Neurol.* 49, 45–52.

Caserta, M. T., Hall, C. B., Schnabel, K., Long, C. E., and D'Heron, N. (1998). Primary human herpesvirus 7 infection: A comparison of human herpesvirus 7 and human herpesvirus 6 infections in children. *J. Pediatr.* 133, 386–389.

Chang, Y. C., Guo, N. W., Wang, S. T., Huang, C. C., and Tsai, J. J. (2001). Working memory of school-aged children with a history of febrile convulsions: A population study. *Neurology* 57, 37–42.

Corey, L. A., Pellock, J. M., Boggs, J. G., Miller, L. L., and DeLorenzo, R. J. (1998). Evidence for a genetic predisposition for status epilepticus. *Neurology* 50, 558–560.

Hall, C. B., Long, C. E., Schnabel, K. C. *et al.* (1994). Human herpesvirus-6 infection in children: A prospective study of complications and reactivation. *N. Engl. J. Med.* 331, 432–438.

Kanemoto, K., Kawasaki, J., Miyamoto, T., Obayashi, H., and Nishimura, M. (2000). Interleukin (IL)-1β, IL-1β, and IL-1 receptor antagonist gene polymorphisms in patients with temporal lobe epilepsy. *Ann. Neurol.* **47**, 571–574.

Shinnar, S., and Berg, A. T. (1996). Does antiepileptic drug therapy prevent the development of "chronic" epilepsy? *Epilepsia* **37**, 701–708.

Shinnar, S., Berg, A. T., Moshe, S. L., and Shinnar, R. (2001a). How long do new-onset seizures in children last? *Ann. Neurol.* **49**, 659–664.

Shinnar, S., Pellock, J. M., Berg, A. T., O'Dell, C., Driscoll, S. M., Maytal, J., Moshe, S. L., and DeLorenzo, R. J. (2001b). Short-term outcomes of children with febrile status epilepticus. *Epilepsia* **42**, 47–53.

Suga, S., Suzuki, K., Ihira, M. *et al.* (2000). Clinical characteristics of febrile convulsions during primary HHV-6 infection. *Arch. Dis. Child.* **82**, 62–68.

VanLandingham, K. E., Heinz, E. R., Cavazos, J. E., and Lewis, D. V. (1998). MRI evidence of hippocampal injury after prolonged, focal febrile convulsions. *Ann. Neurol.* **43**, 413–426.

CHAPTER 22

Mechanisms and Outcome of Febrile Seizures: What Have We Learned from Basic Science Approaches, and What Needs Studying?

Tallie Z. Baram

Departments of Pediatrics, Anatomy/Neurobiology, and Neurology, University of California at Irvine, Irvine, California 92697

I. WHAT ARE THE KEY QUESTIONS?

The epidemiological, genetic, and imaging chapters of this book clarify several important issues: febrile seizures are the most common of all seizures in the developing child. They affect individuals and families throughout the world, causing fear and anxiety. The mechanisms by which fever leads to seizures (Chapter 12), the neuronal matrix of the seizures (Chapters 8, 9, and 14–16), and the outcome of these seizures are currently undergoing reevaluation, using newer, more sophisticated methods as they become available. Despite the growing understanding of these seizures, several topics have not been fully resolved:

A. WHAT IS THE MECHANISM BY WHICH FEVER CAUSES SEIZURES, AND WHY ARE THESE LIMITED TO A SPECIFIC DEVELOPMENTAL AGE?

New evidence for the involvement of cytokines in the process by which fever leads to seizures is presented in Chapter 12. These data are particularly fascinating in view of recent data on genetic variability in the interleukin 1 gene, which may enhance the production of this cytokine in individuals manifesting febrile seizures (Kanemoto *et al.*, 2000). Concurrently, better understanding of neurotransmission and neuromodulation mechanisms (Chapter 11; Baram and Hatalski, 1998), which may facilitate the triggering of febrile seizures during specific developmental states, is being uncovered. These two lines of study would ideally culminate in specific, targeted drugs that will prevent fever-induced seizures without untoward effects.

B. What Is the Relationship of Childhood Febrile Seizures to Adult Temporal Lobe Epilepsy?

Here, human data strongly support the notion that simple febrile seizures bear no relationship to temporal lobe epilepsy (Chapters 5–7). However, the more intricate interaction of complex (particularly prolonged) febrile seizures to this limbic epilepsy is not fully clarified. As indicated in Chapters 5 and 7, prospective epidemiological studies have not shown a progression of febrile seizures to temporal lobe epilepsy, whereas retrospective analyses of adults with this seizure type have demonstrated a high prevalence of a history of prolonged (longer than 10–15 minutes) febrile seizures during early childhood, suggesting an etiological role for these seizures in the development of epilepsy (Chapter 6). However, this high correlation should not be taken to indicate a causal relationship, and alternative mechanisms may exist for the correlation of prolonged febrile seizures and temporal lobe epilepsy. These involve preexisting—genetic or acquired—functional or structural neuronal changes that underlie both the prolonged febrile seizures and the subsequent epilepsy (see Chapters 7, 10, and 17). A simplified depiction of these alternatives is shown here:

Alternative I:
Normal hippocampus → prolonged febrile seizures → neuronal damage → TLE

Alternative II:
Preexisting injury/lesion → fever-triggered seizure = first sign of TLE

Because human studies are limited by the inability to induce febrile seizures of controlled length and analyze potential molecular and functional changes resulting from them, animal models have been used (Chapters 9, 10, and 13–15). These allow induction of febrile seizures of controlled duration, and prospective studies focused on dissecting out the nature of these seizures and of their consequences.

C. What Is the Role
of Genetic Predisposition?

Models based on individual animals of a rather homogeneous genetic makeup are valid only if the occurrence and consequences of febrile seizures do not depend exclusively on specific genetic predisposition. Whereas a large number of genes may predispose individuals to having fever-triggered seizures, it is quite clear that genetic makeup is but one of several determinants required for the seizures, and other determinants include primarily age and hyperthermia. Indeed, studies using monozygotic twins with identical genetic makeup have shown that these twins may be discordant for febrile seizures, as well as for seizure-induced structural and functional changes (Jackson *et al.*, 1998). Clearly, a major issue for future research involves the nature and extent of genetic predisposition for the occurrence of febrile seizures and of their sequelae.

II. WHAT HAVE WE LEARNED SO FAR?

- Animal models of febrile seizures have been devised for both "normal" and "injured" brain, and for both simple and complex seizures. Studies using these models have shown that a preinjured or abnormal brain sustains worse seizures and more neuronal injury compared to a normal brain (Chapter 10).
- Studies of neuronal survival and integrity found that a single prolonged experimental febrile seizure can alter neuronal structure, but does not result in cell death (Chapter 9).
- Importantly, experiments described in Chapters 9, 14, and 15 demonstrate that neuronal death is not required for induction of persistent and profound changes in the function of neurons in hippocampus and related brain regions. These changes appear unique to experimental febrile seizures and lead to a predisposition to having further seizures later in life.

III. WHAT ARE THE GOALS
FOR EXPERIMENTAL APPROACHES
TO FEBRILE SEIZURES?

The focus of research should be on prolonged or complex febrile seizures. The mechanisms by which fever or hyperthermia cause seizures should be studied, using genetically engineered animals, selective agonists and antagonists of candidate molecules, and, hopefully, novel recording methods of neuronal activity.

The precise molecular changes that result from experimental prolonged febrile seizures should be delineated. The sequence of changes and the genes, molecules, and pathways involved should be clarified. The time frame involved is critical if intervention and prevention are to be attempted. In addition, a vigorous search for selective and unique mechanisms (Chapters 14 and 15) that may trigger and underlie seizure-induced changes in excitability and in vulnerability to further seizures should be sought. These would then provide molecular targets for prevention and intervention. It is quite clear that compounds (medications) with broad-spectrum activities may be less suitable as agents for prevention of febrile seizures or of the consequences of prolonged febrile seizures. This is because such agents (e.g., glutamate receptor antagonists, barbiturates) have actions on large numbers of neurons involved in critical functional and maturational processes, leading to unacceptable side effects.

The ultimate goal of experimental approaches to febrile seizures should then involve delineating targets for specific and selective therapies that will either prevent these seizures or interfere with early and specific mechanisms resulting from them and leading to a more excitable, epilepsy-prone brain. These agents will then be available to the appropriate at-risk candidates, determined by ongoing and future human studies (see Chapter 21), for intervention strategies aimed at preventing any potential adverse outcome of complex fever-induced seizures in infants and young children.

Let us head back to the clinic and the laboratory. There is a great deal of work to be done. . . .

REFERENCES

Baram, T. Z., and Hatalski, C. G. (1998). Neuropeptide-mediated excitability: A key triggering mechanism for seizure generation in the developing brain. *Trends Neurosci.* **21**(11), 471–476.

Jackson, G. D., McIntosh, A. M., Briellmann, R. S., and Berkovic, S. F. (1998). Hippocampal sclerosis studied in identical twins. *Neurology* **51**, 78–84.

Kanemoto, K., Kawasaki, J., Miyamoto, T., Obayashi, H., and Nishimura, M. (2000). Interleukin (IL)-1β, IL-1α, and IL-1 receptor antagonist gene polymorphisms in patients with temporal lobe epilepsy. *Ann. Neurol.* **47**, 571–574.

INDEX